A Stranger Among Us

Understanding Sexual Addiction

D. E. WILKIE

First Edition – 2015

ISBN
978-1-4602-4177-6 (Hardcover)
978-1-4602-4178-3 (Paperback)
978-1-4602-4179-0 (eBook)

Produced by:

FriesenPress
Suite 300 – 990 Fort Street
Victoria, BC, Canada V8V 3K2

www.friesenpress.com

Distributed to the trade by The Ingram Book Company

Table of Contents

Dedication

To my wife:

When we got married in July of 1988, we memorized and quoted Corinthians 13:4-8 in our vows.

"Love is patient, love is kind. It does not envy, it does boast. It is not rude, it is not self-seeking, it is not easily angered; it keeps no record of wrongs. Love does not delight in evil but rejoices with the truth. It always protects, always trusts, always hopes, always perseveres. Love never fails..."

Although I have fallen short of this standard of love in our marriage at times, I want to publically declare that my wife's commitment to me and our marriage, to protect, to trust, to hope and persevere has not failed despite all I have put her through in these years. Thank you; I know others have not seen the depth of your love, but I have and for that I am very thankful and love you.

To my three children:

Like my wife, they have been directly impacted by my actions and to this day continue to live with the hurt and shame of their fathers actions. Children are a gift from God and I have been so blessed with the three beautiful children. Since concluding this book I have also been given a very beautiful grand-daughter with another one on the way. I have written this book in part, with the hope that they and my wife would better understand who I am and see God in the midst of all the heartache and pain.

Friends, Doug and Jack and others:

From the moment that my world fell apart 6 years ago they came beside me and have loved and supported me as a brother in the Lord. Unlike Job's friends they have comforted me when I have cried or screamed in anger and felt betrayed by God and the church. They have never judged me or condemned me but have believed in me when I could not believe in myself. Thank you for being God's love with skin on it. I have been blessed with others who have followed suit and have walked with me in the journey, wept and prayed with me, and encouraged me, when all seemed black with despair.

Brother, sister and brother-in-law:

My brother has been a wonderful sounding board and emotional and spiritual support for me, as one who has journeyed down the road of heartache, pain and disillusionment. I thank my sister and brother-in-law for their moral and financial support, for without their aid I could not get this book published.

Joann, Cara, Albert and my wife:

For their editing support and constructive feedback.

Last but not least, God:

Who continues to reveal to me that He is able to make all things work together for good, to those who love Him and are called according to His purpose. Truly His grace is sufficient to meet all our needs according to His riches. I continue to acknowledge that apart from Him I can do nothing, but with Him all things are possible. For that I can say thank you, that your grace abounds and despite me you still love me. You truly are a very patient God.

Preface

This book simply began as a paper in which I was attempting to integrate my understanding of psychology and theology as it relates to my own story in the narrative of sexual addiction. I was hoping that it would have some therapeutic benefit to me as I tried to work through the pain and suffering caused by my addiction. In hindsight it has become a book that explores the Trinitarian nature of man and reflects my Theology of God and the implications and personal impact on recovery from Sexual Addiction. Secondly, it was also my hope that by writing my story it would assist my wife and children to put into some context all that has happened in the past few years. Thirdly, that it would be a benefit to others who are wrestling with like minded questions and issues.

I can take some comfort in knowing that I am not alone in my struggle, as the old cliché says, "misery loves company" and yet I am disturbed with how common a problem it has become and perhaps even more disturbing that these numbers are growing by the day. Recent statistics tell us seventy-two million people view adult websites monthly. Seventy percent of men from 18-34 years of age visit pornographic sites in a typical month. One in three porn viewers are women and twenty-eight percent admit sexual addiction (defined as spending eleven hours or more per week online looking at porn). Sex is the number one topic for internet searches and seventy percent of the internet traffic occurs between the hours of 9-5 workdays. Every second thirty thousand people are viewing porn. Wendy and Larry Maltz in their book *The Porn Trap* point out that a whopping twenty-five percent of all daily Internet search engine requests and thirty-five percent of all downloads are for pornography.

How has this affected the family? Perhaps the most disturbing statistic is that the age of onset is becoming younger and younger. Research shows that nine out of ten children between the ages of eight and sixteen have viewed pornography on the internet and the average age is eleven. The depth of the problem on the partners of porn users was driven home when two-thirds of the members of the American Academy of Matrimonial Lawyers reported that compulsive Internet use had played a significant role in divorces and that well over fifty percent of those cases involved pornography. Fifty-eight percent suffer considerable financial loss and one-third lost their jobs.

Dr. Mark R. Laaser, author of *Healing the Wounds of Sexual Addiction* and recovering sex addict himself states,

> "Christians are not exempt from this disease. A 1996 Promise Keepers survey at one of their stadium events revealed that over fifty percent of the men in attendance were involved with pornography within one week of attending the event. With fifty-seven percent of pastors say that addiction to pornography is the most sexually damaging issue to their congregation *(Christians and Sex Leadership Journal Survey, March 2005).*

Luke Gilkerson who is the author of *Covenant Eyes* website published on February 19, 2013 the following research.

> Regular church attenders are 26% less likely to use porn then non-church attenders but those self-identified "fundamentalists" are 91% more likely to look at porn.

By 2015 mobile adult content and services are expected to reach 2.8 billion and adult video's on tablet will triple world wide.

Of course we cannot be naive in thinking that it is simply those in the congregation that are battling with this issue. Fifty-one percent of pastors say cyber-porn is a possible temptation and thirty-seven percent say it is a current struggle (Christianity Today, Leadership

Survey, 12/2001). Over half of evangelical pastors admit viewing pornography last year. Roger Charman of *Focus on the Family's Pastoral Ministries Reports,*

> "That approximately twenty percent of the calls received on their Pastoral Care Line are for help with issues such as pornography and compulsive sexual behavior. In a *2000 Christianity Today* survey, thirty-three percent of clergy admitted to having visited a sexually explicit Web site. Of those who had visited a porn site, fifty-three percent had visited such sites "a few times" in the past year, and eighteen percent visit sexually explicit sites between a couple of times a month and more than once a week."

Although the primary focus of this book is overcoming sexual addiction in which internet pornography is only one small part of that (see Appendix 1 for definition of Sexual Addiction). I believe the biological-psychological-social and spiritual principles that I outline are universal in their application to all humanity. It is eighty percent that is behind the addiction that is most common to us all. The false self that we come to hide behind and dramatically shape our personalities and attitudes. Only twenty percent of the issue is related to our drug of choice (whatever that may be in your life) to medicate the ill-at-ease which only seems to perpetuate more dis-ease.

I have done my best to describe and explain how despite my very good intentions growing up, I ended up aligning myself with a very unholy trinity - the sense of worthlessness, the striving for niceness, and pretending all is well-which inevitably stole all vestiges of freedom to be a real person in a relationship. At best to pretend and wear masks that would keep the world from knowing the real me.

Consider these words that I came across several years ago.

> The Masks We Wear (Please hear what I'm not saying)
>
> Don't be fooled by me. Don't be fooled by the face I wear.
>
> For I wear a mask, I wear a thousand masks, masks that I'm afraid to take off, and none of them are me.

Pretending is an art that's second nature with me, but don't be fooled, for God's sake don't be fooled.

I give you the impression that I'm secure, that all is sunny and unruffled with me, within as well as without, that confidence is my name and coolness my game, that the water's calm and I'm in command, and that I need no one.

But don't believe me, please!

My surface may seem smooth, but my surface is my mask, my ever - varying and ever - concealing mask.

Beneath lays no smugness, no complacency.

But I hide this.

I don't want anybody to know it.

I panic at the thought of my weakness and fear of being exposed.

That's why I frantically create a mask to hide behind, a nonchalant, sophisticated façade, to help me pretend, to shield me from the glance that knows.

But such a glance is precisely my salvation, my only salvation. And I know it.

It's the only thing that can liberate me, from myself, from my own self-built prison walls, from the barriers that I so painstakingly erect.

It's the only thing that will assure me of what I can't assure myself: that I'm really worth something.

But I don't tell you this, I don't dare. I'm afraid to. I'm afraid your glance will not be followed by acceptance and love. I'm afraid you'll think less, that you'll laugh, and your laugh would kill me.

I'm afraid that deep down I'm nothing, that I'm just no good, and that you'll see this and reject me.

So I play my game, my desperate pretending game, with a façade assurance without, and a trembling child within.

And so begins the parade of masks, the glittering but empty parade of masks. And my life becomes a front.

I idly chatter to you in the suave tones of surface talk. I tell you everything that's really nothing, and nothing of what's everything, of what's crying within me. So when I'm going through my routine do not be fooled by what I'm saying.

Please listen carefully and try to hear what I'm not saying, what I'd like to be able to say, what for survival I need to but what I can't say. I dislike hiding. Honestly. I dislike the superficial game I'm playing, the superficial, phony game. I'd really like to be genuine and spontaneous, and me, but you've got to help me.

You've got to hold out your hand even though that's the last thing I seem to want, or need. Only you can wipe away from my eyes the blank stare of the breathing dead. Only you can call me into aliveness. Each time you're kind, and gentle, and encouraging, each time you try to understand because you are really caring, my heart begins to grow wings, very small wings, very feeble wings, but wings.

With your sensitivity and sympathy, and your power of understanding you can breathe life into me. I want you to know that. I want you to know how important you are to me, how you can be the creator of the person that is me if you choose to.

> You alone can break down the wall behind which I tremble, you alone can remove my mask, and you alone can release me from my shadow-world of panic and uncertainty, from my lonely prison.
>
> So do not pass me by. Please do not pass me by. It will not be easy for you. A long conviction of worthlessness builds strong walls. The nearer you approach to me, the blinder I may strike back. It's irrational, but despite what the books say about man, I am irrational. I fight against the very thing I cry out for. But I am told that love is stronger than strong walls. And in this lies my hope
>
> Please try to beat down these walls with firm hands, but with gentle hands – for a child is very sensitive. Who am I? you may wonder. I am someone you know very well. For I am every man you meet and I am every woman you meet.

C. Baxter Kruger in *Across All Worlds* speaks to this very conflict with self by stating,

> Inside our beings, behind the layers of our defense mechanisms, pain arises from deep parts of us like smoke from the fires of our hidden brokenness. In these areas we believe we are not acceptable in one form or another. We are trapped in our own vision of God and cannot see the acceptance of the Father.

Yet the irony of God the Father, Son and Holy Spirit is that it is not in fearing ourselves, but rather in being honest about what we have done and not done, in staring our shame in the face and feeling the sheer sadness of it all, that we encounter the Father's unflinching heart and find the courage to remove our masks. How can I do this? I am hoping this book will answer that question, as one who has believed I am not worthy, not good enough and too bad for His love.

Part I

My Journey

Chapter 1
Addict or Saint?

The Early Years

Let me begin this book with a brief theological sketch of my spiritual history and how I came to believe. Theologically, I didn't grow up in an Evangelical Christian home and as dysfunctional as it was at times, I knew I was loved. Both my parents were very active in our lives and encouraged us kids to get involved in extracurricular activities. This had its advantages and disadvantages as I will describe later in the book. As a middle class family growing up in a middle class neighborhood, both my parents worked hard, careers by day apartment building owners and landlords by night. For the most part I was your classic "latch key kid." At the time I thought nothing of it and don't necessarily regret it to this day.

As I reflect on my parent's marriage, I can see that they had a volatile relationship with a degree of emotional isolation. I saw my mother's role to be a good co-dependent, keeping the peace by trying to please and appease my father. I saw my father as a tyrant at times and at 6' 4 and well over 200 pounds with a very volatile temper, someone to fear and appease. This bred insecurity and secrets in the family as loyalties became divided. My father equated love with obedience and fulfilling his expectations. As a result I grew up experiencing a lot of fear, guilt, shame, inferiority, inadequacy and fearing any authority figure. I also felt this way towards my brother who was four years my senior and at the time appeared to be more intelligent and far more athletic than me.

These experiences were filtered through a personality that some might call phlegmatic and melancholic. My personality, like my mothers, is a peace keeper and a people pleaser. To describe my personality using a few different profiles, Myers Briggs Personality Profile would peg me as an ISFJ (Introvert, Sensory, Feeling, Judging). My talents lay in supporting others and supplying them in what they need. Other characteristics include warm, considerate, thoughtful, friendly, respectful, agreeable, loyal, conscientious, committed, dedicated, sympathetic, kind and dependable. I thrive on helping others and bringing people together. I make sure everything is taken care of so others can succeed and accomplish their goals. I most recently did a DISC Personality Inventory and discovered that my primary characteristic is a covert perfectionist. This has manifested itself in my life as a person who is very driven to be the best he can be and yet lives under the constant threat and fear of failure.

My earliest theological influence as a child was with a neighbor across the street who taught a Good News Club which was basically a Sunday School Class Curriculum taught out of a residential home. As a young child I would come home and go over with my sister who was my senior by two and a half years. These same neighbors also drove us to church and other church activities. I began to learn that there was a God in heaven that loved me and died for me and if I believed this I would go to heaven. So one day the teacher asked me if I believed that Jesus died on the cross for my sins and I said yes, we prayed together and I told God in a child like prayer that I believed and wanted to go to heaven one day. As the years past and teen years approached, church activities gave way to hockey and other sporting activities. However, the Christian foundation that was laid as a child would not be wasted but would be temporarily forgotten.

Teen Years

All through my preteen and teen years I struggled with low self-esteem. I felt very inadequate academically and socially inferior to my peers. In grade six it was clear to the educators that I had some academic deficiencies in which the school board wanted to hold me back. In my own minds eye this meant that I was stupid and less intelligent than everyone else in my class. Over the next years of junior high and high school I felt inferior to others and believed the teachers were just there to push me through. At thirteen years of age I began to isolate myself in the world of weight lifting and running. In both these activities I found great satisfaction and fulfillment. I was able to set personal goals and not fear being compared to or failing others. By age seventeen I had run my first marathon and competed in a power lifting competition all in the same week.

At the age of sixteen, I started going back to church via my brother-in-law, who was a Christian and ten years my senior. He encouraged me to play church league hockey (under the condition that I would have to attend church every Sunday) I agreed. Through the Plymouth Brethren Denomination I was reintroduced to the Bible and what God had done for me on the cross. At the age of seventeen on January 18, 1981 I accepted the Lord as my personal Savior, forgetting that I had made this decision when I was much younger. This was truly a life-changing event because it brought great hope to an emotionally scared and insecure teenager.

Within a few months of accepting the Lord as my Savior, I was eager to learn as much as I could about the Lord. To that point in my life I rarely ever read simply because I was told that I was a very poor reader. This new found hunger for understanding would catapult me into reading and would bring me to Briercrest Bible College. After several opportunities to give my testimony and trying to decide what I wanted to do as a career, I felt encouraged to consider ministry. Over those years I discovered that although I was very fearful of public speaking, when I trusted God to do so, I felt a real strength and presence of the Lord. As a result of these ministry opportunities and some very clear directives I changed my program from the two year General

College program to the four year Bachelor of Religious Education with a Pastoral Major and Minors in Administration and Counseling. This was truly the grace of God for I did not even believe that I would ever be intelligent enough to go to College, let alone do any type of public speaking of which I was generally petrified.

Adult Years

Immediately upon changing programs I was mandated to be preaching on a weekly basis at an extend-a-care in Moose Jaw Saskatchewan and The Salvation Army Core in Regina. Again individuals were reconfirming that God was calling me to the Pastoral Ministry. Perhaps one of the most confirming experiences that I had to my calling was my pastoral internship in an Evangelical Free Church in Nebraska. Over the next twenty plus years the Lord would open up the door to Pastoral Ministry opportunities but with a primary focus being in the field of Counseling and Therapy, both in the Christian and secular setting.

I made it my goal to be the best that I could be and I made it my primary responsibility to know as much as I could know. I pursued higher education, achieving Masters Degree in counseling and theology and diplomas in administration, counseling, fitness and nutrition amongst other things, bringing lifelong learning to a whole new level. I brought this same drive and discipline to every area of life including fitness and nutrition and training for marathons. Hoping that one day when I crossed over the finish line God would say to me, "well done my good and faithful servant, you ran the race of life in such a way as to receive the prize."

This brings me to the here and now and a reflection on some of my spiritual challenges throughout these years. These past sixteen years have been met with a lot of highs and lows. Our middle child has a seizure disorder along with a number of other delays and has not been very stable medically. With more questions than answers and her condition worsening she was subjected to a Lobectomy (removing her left temporal lobe and part of the frontal lobe of her brain) in May of 2003.

The results did not yield a cure, but rather, the pathologists' report indicating something far worse: a rare neurological disease called Cortical Displacia. These years were traumatic for the whole family as we lived with so much uncertainty from medical crisis to medical crisis.

These kinds of experiences will do one of two things: drive you away from God or draw you to God. They will either make you bitter or better as a person. My wife and I drew unto God; however, we appeared to have more questions than answers and the long term prognosis for our daughter is not fully determined. God has taught us through the difficult circumstances of these past years but I have also begun to see God's word in a new light. I believe Dr. Larry Crabb in his book *Shattered Dreams* would best describe what I have been learning as I seek to align my reality with my theology. I am discovering how truly paradoxical God's kingdom is compared to my own. That making my own plans, setting my own goals, promoting my own agenda, nurturing my own ambition (in short, living out my own dreams) are sure ways to get less than God wants to give me. Even though all along I believed that I was doing exactly what God wanted me to do, and making what I thought were Godly sacrifices to reach that end.

Present Years: Reflection of my Addiction

What I have discovered over the past five years is that I still didn't get it. Woven through all these years has been the fact that I struggled with sexual compulsive behaviors, a sexual addiction from about age twelve or thirteen which often left me feeling confused, guilty, ashamed and yet at the same time, comforted and relieved. Was it a friend or a foe? I would oscillate between feeling that I am normal with a healthy sex drive to feeling abnormal and wondering what was wrong with me. Fear of rejection and ridicule left me in silence and emotional isolation with my secret. On the other hand it also made me feverish with religious pursuit to make it up to God and appease Him. What I didn't realize was that I was on a one way track to self-destruction.

People don't initially make decisions about life with the intention of destroying themselves. People become addicted through a series of choices they make in the process of growing up. Today I am a child of God who is recovering from a sexual addiction and although I felt I understood God's love and acceptance despite my actions, it didn't take care of my low self-esteem and life-controlling problem. Underneath the veneer, I was the same old person who couldn't quite get it, despite my over achieving ways. In the journey of the past couple of years I have only began to realize that I have been the biggest barrier to my freedom, because of my pride, my strength, my plans, my goals and my agenda. Many of the things I have tried have been good but have all failed, I believe for four reasons:

1. I tried to change my behavior instead of the underlying belief that determined my behavior.

2. I focused on me and what I should do instead of focusing on God and what He had already done.

3. I relied on my own efforts instead of trusting God and living by the power of the Holy Spirit.

4. I accepted a failure identity instead of appropriating my true identity in Christ.

I lived under the law through my own efforts instead of under grace by faith in the power and wisdom of God. The results of living under the law are clear in Romans 7:5, "For when we were controlled by the sinful nature, the sinful passions aroused by the law were at work in our bodies, so that we bore fruit for death."

I believed the saying that is not biblical and yet was my mantra, that "God helps those who help themselves." Instead, God doesn't help those who help themselves, but leaves them to their misery and to their own devices until they come to the end of their resources and trust in Him.

In the past few years God has been breaking me, to quote Chapter 1 in the *Sex Addicts Anonymous Big Book,* using the first person narrative to describe myself. I was addicted to sexual behaviors that I returned to over and over, despite the consequences. The compulsive desires were irresistible, persistent, and insatiable. They went off like alarms in my head that made it difficult to focus on anything else. They intruded into my thoughts, especially when I was under pressure. I used sexual fantasy to deal with emotions and situations that I didn't want to face.

I would try to establish boundaries around my behavior, but eventually I'd violate these boundaries. I decided that I would engage in certain behaviors that were not dangerous, cause harm to others, or were illegal. I would act out in so-called "safe" ways, and only fantasize about acting out. Then one day, I crossed those boundaries. I bought a pornographic magazine and masturbated in the car. Before long, I did it repeatedly hoping I could stop, while praying that I wouldn't get caught. I recall thinking to myself "please someone notice me" as I felt invisible and alone yet at the same time wanting someone to tell me how disgusting and bad I was as a person. I tried to stop my behaviors, knowing that at times I was seen and feeling embarrassed and ashamed. I would swear to never act out again, and then I would be right back into my addiction within days, hours, or even minutes. I would promise myself, and sometimes my wife, that I wouldn't repeat my behavior. Sometimes I could keep my promises for weeks, months, or years. But eventually I would act out again. I believed that, given time or changed circumstances, I could stop acting out. I lived a double life. To hide my acting out, I lied to my family, friends, and co-workers. I also tried to hide my addiction from myself—by working hard, being a covert perfectionist, and being very religious. Still, with all the self-discipline I could muster, it wasn't very long before I felt compelled to act out again.

Sexual addiction impaired my judgment. In my obsession, I acted as if I were invisible, immortal, and invincible. Being a sex addict felt like being trapped in endless contradictions. At times I avoided sex with my wife, preferring the unknown, and the solitary. I sought comfort and security through dangerous and risky behaviors that left me more wounded, abused, and traumatized than when I started. My sexuality, which should have been a source of happiness and pleasure, became destructive and dangerous to myself and others.

These consequences were many and varied. Some came as a direct result of my acting out; I was arrested and charged with Indecent Act. Although it was not my intent to be seen, it was irrelevant, I was and was charged accordingly. It resulted in a night in jail, a criminal record, loss of job, career, income and now nearing bankruptcy due to my sexually inappropriate behavior. My reputation and livelihood have been damaged by publicity, by both radio and printed press about my charge and have placed an unbearable amount of stress upon my wife and children. I have lost friendships, family and community. I have suffered tremendous emotional grief and loss and at times find myself contemplating suicide. I often feel dissatisfied with my life.

The high usually wasn't as "good" as I hoped it would be. It rarely matched my fantasies, and didn't recapture the excitement that it once did. When I realized that I had been seduced by my fantasies again, I often felt despair. The strange thing was that my despair, rather than deterring me, led me right back to acting out. My feelings of pain and shame were often more than I could take. Without having any reason to hope I could stop, I looked for ways to dull the pain.

Shame was also a common feeling and expression. It was the lingering feeling that I am never good enough, that there is something wrong with me and that I am a bad person. Shame played a part in my addictive cycle, undermining my resistance to acting out. To the extent that I felt that I was unworthy, it didn't matter if I acted out or not. Acting out helped me to escape or hide from my shame. Sometimes shame itself became part of my addictive high, so that I'd actually get a sexual thrill from being "bad." Shame also caused me to hide and isolate from others so that I didn't seek the help I needed.

Even when I tried to quit, the distress of withdrawal impelled me to act out again despite myself. Abstaining from my addictive sexual behaviors prompted a reaction in my mind and body that could only be deemed as very similar to a drug addict going through withdrawal. I could not tolerate the physical and emotional discomfort I felt when I stopped my behaviors. So I acted out again.

One of the most dangerous aspects of my addiction is my inability to see it for what it is; this difficulty recognizing what I am doing, and how serious and risky it is, and how much harm it causes. It is called denial and conceals the awful truth of my addiction by convincing me that what I am doing is not that bad or dangerous, or that other people or external circumstances are responsible for my behavior. Denial is very subtle. I remember acting out, but at times would deny the pain of acting out, the consequences, the risks, or my inability to stop.

My sexual addiction has led me to a place of hitting bottom. It is a very low point mentally, physically, emotionally, and spiritually. I am discovering that my sex addiction is not just a bad habit. Nor is it the result of poor self-control, a lack of morals, or a series of mistakes. If it was something I could stop on my own, the negative consequences would have been enough to make me stop. As I started out by saying, I tried to cure myself with religion and spiritual practices, moral discipline, and self-improvement. Despite my sincerity and my best efforts, I continued to act out. My behavior eluded all rational attempts at explanation or correction. I have had to swallow my pride and face the fact that I could not and cannot stop the addictive behavior by myself.

In correlation of what I have stated earlier, "God doesn't help those who help themselves" but on the contrary, "He helps those who can't help themselves."

Chapter 2
Freedom

Through my struggle for freedom from the bondage of sexual addiction, I never questioned my beliefs or my theology. I tried many different things, but throughout I stubbornly held to some established beliefs that prevented my freedom. Why did I hold onto these beliefs? Simply because from my perspective, I had been taught the "truth." I was convinced my problem wasn't my beliefs, but my inability to put my beliefs into action.

The piece I have never really understood is *Romans 6:6* "Our old self was crucified with Christ." I could grasp that Christ died for our sins, but I did not understand that I also died with Christ. Because of this death, "I am a new creation because the old self, the person I used to be is no more, and I am in Christ." Romans 6:6,7 says, "For we know that our self was crucified with Him so that the body of sin might be done away with, that we should no longer be slaves to sin because anyone who has died has been freed from sin." It isn't something you do, it's something that has been done; our death with Christ is past tense, the old person that we were "was crucified," and "anyone who has died has been freed from sin." The implication, I am dead to sin (Romans 6:11). Even if I don't feel dead to sin, act dead to sin or even look dead to sin; it doesn't change the positional truth that I am dead to sin. "Anyone who had died has been freed from sin" (verse 7). Jesus said, "Then you will know the truth and the truth will set you free" (John 8:32).

If I don't believe I am free then I won't live like I am free. We act according to our beliefs. The central issue is always identity. If you don't know the truth about your identity" in Christ," then as I discovered it doesn't make any difference what programs you are involved in or what spiritual exercises you are doing.

A great example of this is the Declaration of Emancipation on December 18th, 1865. Because of this Thirteenth Amendment, on December 19, 1865 there were no more slaves in the United States. In reality, none, but many still lived like slaves. Many did, because they never learned the truth. Others knew and even believed that they were free, but chose to live as they had been taught.

I like the way Neil Anderson describes it in his book, *Freedom from Addictions.*

> Several plantation owners were devastated by the Emancipation Proclamation. "We're ruined! Slavery has been abolished. We've lost the battle to keep our slaves." But their chief spokesman slyly responded, "Not necessarily, as long as these people think they're still slaves, the Emancipation will have no practical effect. We don't have a legal right over them anymore, but many of them don't know it. Keep your slaves from learning the truth, and your control over them will not even be challenged."
>
> One cotton farmer asked, "But, what if the news spreads?" "Don't panic. We have another bullet in our gun. We may not be able to keep them from hearing the news, but we can still keep them from understanding it. They don't call me the 'father of lies' for nothing. We still have the potential to deceive the whole world. Just tell them that they misunderstood the Thirteenth Amendment. Tell them that they are going to be free, not that they are free already. The truth they heard is

just positional truth, not actual truth. Someday they may receive the benefits, but not now."

"But they'll expect me to say that. They won't believe me." "Then pick out a few persuasive ones who are convinced they are still slaves and let them do the talking for you. Remember, most of these free people were born as slaves and have been their whole lives. All we have to do is to deceive them so they still think like slaves. As long as they continue to do what slaves do, it will not be hard to convince them that they must still be slaves. They will maintain their slave identities because of the things they do. The moment they try to profess that they are no longer slaves, just whisper in their ear, "How can you even think you are no longer a slave when you are still doing things that slaves do?" After all, we have the capacity to accuse the brethren day and night."

Years later, many have still not heard the wonderful news that they have been freed. Quite naturally they continue to live the way they have always lived. Some have heard the good news, but evaluated it by what they are presently doing and feeling. They reason, "I'm still living in bondage, doing the same things I have always done. My experience tells me that I must not be free. I'm feeling the same way I was before the proclamation, so it must not be true. After all, your feelings always tell the truth," So they continue to live according to how they feel, not wanting to be hypocrites!

One former slave hears the good news, and receives it with great joy. He checks out the validity of the proclamation, and discovers that the highest of all authorities has originated the decree. Not only that, but it personally cost the authority a tremendous price which He willingly paid so the former slave could be free. His life is transformed. He correctly reasons that it would be

> hypocritical to believe his feelings, and not believe the truth. Determined to live by what he knows to be true, his experiences begin to change rather dramatically. He realizes that his old master has no authority over him and does not need to be obeyed. He gladly serves the one who set him free.

People living in sexual sin and addiction are caught in a web of faulty thinking. Those of us who struggle with addiction constantly entertain thoughts such as: I'm different from others. Christianity works for others, but it doesn't work for me. Maybe I'm not a Christian. When I was younger I can't count the number of times that I asked the Lord to be my Savior, just in case. I have often thought that God doesn't love me. How could He? I'm such a failure. I'm just a miserable sinner with no hope of ever breaking the chains of sexual addiction.

Why, despite my great and valiant effort, did I live a defeated life? Like me most Christians are trying to become what God says they've already achieved or have already accomplished. I had been encouraged to "die to self," and struggled to make it happen. Yet Scripture couldn't be clearer. It says, "For we know that our old self was crucified with Him" (Romans 6:6). Not only have we been crucified, died and buried with Christ, but we have also been "raised up with Him and are now seated with Him in heavenly places" (Ephesians 2:6). "It was for freedom that Christ set us free" (Galatians 5:1). If we believe that we have to work, sweat and strain, God will allow us to work, sweat and strain, until we collapse in frustration and failure.

Watchman Nee writes:

> Oh, it is a great thing to see that we are in Christ! Think of the bewilderment of trying to get into a room in which you already are! Think of the absurdity of asking to be put in! If we recognize the fact that we are in, we make no effort to enter.

As I wrestle with the fact that I died with Christ on the Cross and all that implies, it has been equally challenging for me to understand my identity "in Christ." If I am a new creation "in Christ" (2 Corinthians 5:17), then I am no longer a sinner and I don't have to sin. For many years I had been taught, believed and also preached that everyone, including Christians, had a sin nature.

The *Bible* says, "Therefore if any man is in Christ, he is a new creature; the old things passed away; behold, new things have come." (2 Corinthians 5:17). "I am a child of God" (1 John 3:1) and a "partaker of the divine nature" (2 Peter 1:4). A new "me" was raised up with Christ (Romans 6:5) and "by the grace of God I have become the righteousness of God in Christ" (2 Corinthians 5:21).

The most practical, immediate benefit of being a child of God then, is freedom. We are free from our pasts. "Because you are sons, God sent the Spirit of His Son into our hearts, the Spirit who calls out, 'Abba Father'. So you are no longer a slave, but a son; and since you are a son, God has made you also an heir. Formerly, when you did not know God, you were slaves to those who by nature are not gods" (Galatians 4:6-8). As children of God, we are no longer products of our pasts; we are primarily products of Christ's work on the cross. We have a new heritage; we are heirs of God.

Over the past couple of years this truth is becoming clearer to me. I had bought the lie that I can't ever overcome sin and lust in my life. My theology and beliefs had been formulated on my experience instead of God's Word. Experience convinces us that we're sinners because we have sinned. I need to throw out my presuppositions and turn to God's Word for a fresh perspective. Who was I "in Christ" and according to God's Word? As I learn this my experience could change. I need to embrace the Word that says, "Christ's grace is sufficient for you, for your power is made perfect in weakness. Therefore we can boast all the more gladly about our weaknesses, so that Christ's power may rest on us" (2 Corinthians 12:9).

Some have called these positional truths, as I stated earlier and claim that our nature doesn't really change until we get to heaven, so all these passages are irrelevant for us today. God's Word says that the believer is in Christ and He ascribes certain characteristics to any man in Christ. If God says that is the way it is, then that's the way it is right now. Christian faith is simply looking at things through God's eyes and agreeing with Him. I believe that this will then begin to control my performance and I can experience a victorious walk!"

The key to knowing Christ is understanding that I died with Him. Paul says, "For you have died and your life is hidden with Christ in God" (Colossians 3:3).

Without this understanding we try to become somebody we already are. We try to do for ourselves what Christ has already done for us. This is an exercise in futility as I have clearly demonstrated in my own story. God has no interest in improving our old natural life. He desires that we exchange our life in Adam for a new life in Christ.

Henry Warkentin, a counselor I had seen on several occasions helped me to better understand these truths, by stating in his book, *Answers and Hope for the Struggling Christian* that:

> "He died as our representative. Paul says in, 1 Corinthians 15:45, 47, "And so it is written, the first man Adam was made a living soul; the last Adam was made a quickening spirit... the first man was of the dust of the earth the second man from heaven."
>
> Notice it does not say the first Adam and the second Adam; it says the first Adam and the last Adam. Through the first man Adam, we received all that was in Him. When Jesus came as the last Adam, everything that was in Adam was nailed to the cross. Jesus was the last, and there can be nothing beyond that which is last. The Enemy will always try to get us to focus on what we have to try to do to get out of Adam, thereby getting us to focus on "self." Nevertheless, the first Adam is finished because the last Adam, Jesus Christ, finished everything that we ever inherited through Adam. Jesus ended all that was started with Adam, thereby starting a new race. The first man started a sinful race; the second man started the redeemed race." On the cross Jesus cried out, "it is finished," complete nothing to be added.

I take comfort in knowing that I have not been alone in this theological struggle, Watchman Nee also struggled with this truth. He wrote the following in *The Normal Christian Life*:

> "For years after my conversion I had been taught to reckon. The more I reckoned that I was dead to sin, the more alive I clearly was. I simply could not believe myself dead and I could not produce that death. Whenever I sought help from others I was told to read Romans 6:11, and tried to reckon, the further away death was: I could not get at it. One morning I prayed and said, "Lord open my eyes!" And then in a flash I saw it. I saw my oneness with Christ. I saw that I was in Him and that when He died I died. I saw that the question of my death was a matter of the past and not of the future, and that I was just as truly dead as He was because I was in Him when He died. I was overcome with such joy that I cried out, "Praise the Lord, I am dead!"

I have come to realize that feelings will not always match the truth, but I choose to believe what God says is true: "For we know that our old self was crucified with him so that the body of sin might be done away with, that we should no longer be slaves to sin—because anyone who has died has been freed from sin" (Romans 6:6, 7).

The truth set me free. My freedom is coming as I understand who I am "in Christ." I had always believed that Christians are "sinners saved by grace," God says that our identity has changed. "For you are all sons of God through faith in Christ Jesus...there is neither slave nor free man, there is neither male nor female; for you are all one in Christ Jesus" (Galatians 3:26, 28). It is not what we do that determines who we are; it is who we are that determines what we do.

Upon this discovery JohnWommack in his book *Spirit, Soul & Body* shared that;

> "I've recognized that the Christian life isn't a process of "getting from God." Instead, it's a process of renewing my mind and learning to release what I've already received. It's much easier to release something I've already got than to go get something I don't yet have.

Neil Anderson says;

> "You are not primarily a product of your past; you are primarily a product of the work of Christ on the cross and His resurrection. Your beliefs determine how you live. He goes on to say that the proper response to scriptural truth is to believe it. The only proper response to a biblical promise is to claim it and the only response to a command is to obey it."

The concept is simple but, as I have shared it can get twisted.

"If the Son, then, sets you free, you are really free!" (John 8:36). Freedom is the assurance that your need for security, significance, love, acceptance and worth are always met in Christ. They can't be taken away by changing circumstances or personal bondages. Because I am free, "I can count myself dead to sin and alive to God" (Romans 6:11). "When I choose to not let sin rule in my body and not obey its evil desires" (verse 12), "I offer myself and my body to God" (verse 13). Once we understand this truth, we will experience victory in our situation. We are no longer hopeless and helpless. This is not positive thinking, but positive believing. We experience freedom when we choose to believe God, and then act on the basis of the truth regardless of our feelings. I don't feel the world is round; I believe it is because I know it for a fact.

Let me give you an example of what I mean. Many of us live our lives trying to avoid failure. God's purpose, however, is to show us what a failure we are in our own resources. We can then give up on our lives in the flesh and find our life in Christ. One thing we know for sure: we are going to fail and no one's life is perfect. It is very difficult to give up the right to succeed, so that you can be free to fail. And you aren't really free to succeed until you are free to fail. As a covert perfectionist this is a very difficult concept for me - that with this kind of perspective you can enter life without worrying about the results. Colossians 3:23 says, "Whatever you do, work at it with all your heart, as working for the Lord, not for men."

I had believed I was a failure in ministry. As I learn more about freedom in Christ, I am beginning to understand my problem in ministry. I was trying to meet my needs for self-worth and self-acceptance through success in my ministry. My ministry was hooked to my identity. When things didn't go the way I thought they should, I felt like a failure.

I assumed the responsibility and ownership of the ministry belonged to me. As I stated earlier, I just wanted God to say to me one day, "well done good and faithful servant." As it would turn out, I always felt like a failure and that whatever I did was not good enough. I lived in a constant state of failure and/or the fear of failure.

Despite the fact that I am progressively learning what it means to "be in Christ" and "know the truth that sets me free" I still find the law of sin and the pathology of sexual addiction to be operative, powerful and constantly making its appeal. You may find all this very theology deep, confusing and difficult to digest. Please bare with me as I will unpack all these theological principles later on in the book. I think it is at this point that we need to explore what is the pathology of sexual addiction?

This leads us to Dr. Patrick Carnes who I believe is the leading psychologist and researcher on the pathology of Sexual Addiction. I believe he was also a significant influence in the recently released 2013 movie, *Thanks for Sharing* that stars Gwyneth Paltrow, Pink and Tim Robbins that depicts the life of several sex addicts and their road to recovery. To give due respect to his model I am going to summarize some of his research and evaluate it through a more Theological perspective.

Part II

Pathology of Sexual Addiction

Chapter 3
The Larger Addictive System

Belief System

The first component of this system is the belief system, which in turn is followed by impaired thinking and unmanageability. The driving force of the addictive system is the belief system, the addict's filtering lens through which he or she views the world. This includes all the messages, conclusions about self, family rules, myths, meanings, information, "self-evident truths," prejudices, and guesses regarded as fact gathered from life experience and combined to form an interlocking mosaic of beliefs. Through this belief system all decisions are filtered and the foundation of a false sense of self is formulated.

The addict possesses faulty beliefs which give the addiction its momentum. During the early stages of the addiction, the most important indication of faulty beliefs is when the addiction increases the addict's negative feelings about him or herself. Being out of control comes to mean, "I am a bad, unworthy person." This reinforces what Jesus tells us: that we can believe in the lie or the truth. But it also reaffirms what was stated earlier "When you know and believe the truth, the truth will set you free" (1 John 8:32).

For those of us in caught in addiction, it is our incorrect beliefs rather than our behaviors that hold us there. Neil Anderson has said that if Satan can get you to believe a lie, he can control your life. This is the plight of many Christians. Psalm 4:2 "How long, O men, will you turn my glory into shame? How long will you love delusions and seek false gods?"

Anderson teaches that a true knowledge of God and our identity in Christ are the greatest determinants of our mental health. Two of Satan's primary strategies are to present a false concept of God and a distorted understanding of our identity in Christ. If Satan can encourage us to believe either one of these lies, our lives will be miserable and in bondage.

Every person grows up with a false concept of God. When we become Christians, we don't automatically believe the truth about our identity in Christ. Our minds have been programmed to believe certain things about ourselves. God doesn't push the CLEAR button when we become Christians. Through the years, I have counseled hundreds of people who have believed the lie. It took us years to develop a false self and a distorted perception of reality and God.

Most of us try to create the impression of strength instead of inadequacy or insecurity. I certainly didn't introduce myself in the past by saying, "Hi, my name is Wilkie. I'm insecure, inadequate and worthless." Yet deep down, I felt that way and believed it. Satan wants you to believe these lies about your identity. His plan is not to get us to drink alcohol, do drugs or be sexually immoral. He knows that if we believe a lie about who we are, the steps into a life-controlling addiction are easy. If you believe the truth about your true identity in Christ, rather than the lies associated with one's false sense of self you'll be free from life-controlling addiction and will no longer engage in addictive, self-destructive behavior.

Mike Quarles the Co-author with Neil Anderson in the book *Freedom from Addiction* states that many who have addictive behaviors exhibit at least one of the following four incorrect beliefs or feelings in their lives. Patrick Carnes in his book, *Out of the Shadows Understanding Sexual Addiction* also talks about four Core Beliefs of every sex addict and how the 12 Steps to Sex Addicts Anonymous enable the addict to change those incorrect or false beliefs. Let me begin with what

Anderson and Quarles calls incorrect beliefs of any addict. The first incorrect belief that they state is, "I have no hope."

I have no hope. Every person in addiction feels hopeless and those who have these feelings believe they have no hope. I lost hope when I struggled with my addiction and failed time after time. I was stuck in a vicious cycle of "using" followed by inevitable remorse and guilt. As I wallowed in self pity and remorse, I thought, "it's hopeless and I'm a hopeless incurable sex addict who is never going to change. I had bought the lie. The second incorrect belief is that I am a victim and in turn feel helpless.

I'm a victim. It doesn't matter what behavior or addiction enslaves you, if you feel helpless, and your situation is hopeless, you will never change. Individuals who feel hopeless will become depressed and will often experience high volumes of anxiety. Inherent in hopelessness is the incorrect belief that "I'm a victim." Defeated Christians believe they are victims of circumstances, the past or their own bad characters. A great misunderstanding occurs because Christians don't understand their identity in Christ and do not experience victory over the world, the flesh and the Devil.

Our victory in Christ is explained in Ephesians 2:6 "If we know where the heavenly realms are we'll never consider ourselves victims and be defeated again." Ephesians 1:20, 22 tell us the exact location of the heavenly realms. Verse 20 says, "He raised him [Christ] from the dead and seated him at his right hand in the heavenly realms." The next verse describes exactly where they are; "Far above all rules and authority, power and dominion, and every title that can be given, not only in the present age but also in the one to come. And God placed all things under his feet and appointed him to be head over everything for the church" The heavenly realms are a place of spiritual authority and because we are "in Christ," we are appointed over everything." One preacher stated that, "Nothing under Christ's feet can be over your head, because you are in Christ and everything is under Christ's feet."

Christ was seated in the heavenly realms and we were seated with Him to live in victory. "How much more will those who receive God's abundant provision of grace and of the gift of righteousness reign in life through the one man, Jesus Christ?" (Romans 5:17). The key is understanding that we aren't fighting for victory, but coming from victory. "Thanks be to God, who gives us the victory through our Lord Jesus Christ" (1 Corinthians 15:57). Christians aren't victims: "We are more than conquerors through him who loved us" (Romans. 8:37). Our beliefs determine the difference between victory and defeat—the lying schemes of Satan or the truth of God. The third false belief stated by Quarles and Anderson is the belief that I'm somehow different than everyone else.

"I'm different" Another incorrect belief of hopelessness. People believe that they are different and their problems are different and that they need a different answer. Throughout my growing up years, I believed I was different from most people. All through public and secondary school I felt very different. As I shared earlier, in grade six it was recommended that I stay back that year because of my lack of scholastic ability. I didn't read a book, not even a comic book until I was in grade ll. It took me three years to get through grade ten English and five years to get through a four year general program. My friends all spoke of going to College and University and I wondered if I could ever get through High School. I felt inferior to all those around me.

I perceived myself as being different from those I played sports with. Often I was compared to a much more athletically gifted brother. My parents were always very involved, when it came to sports, which I appreciated. Unfortunately, my dad would spend more time telling me what I did wrong than what I did right. I became very self-conscious and considered myself the weakest player on any team. I believed I was deficient in character and deep inside something was wrong. Many times I wished I could be like that other person and do the right thing or be smarter, more muscular and more athletic, 'just more like everyone else.' As an adult, I find myself struggling with the same thoughts. With a special needs daughter, I often feel different than others around me - not able to dream the same dreams, excluded or uninvited to social events - When we are, we find ourselves so preoccupied with attending to our daughters needs that we don't enjoy the event. I still find myself struggling with the fact that no one has quite gone through what I've gone through or are living the nightmare that I'm living, which would suggest that my problems are different, a thought that I have to fight against and take captive.

God's truth applies to everyone regardless of differences such as the past, education, age, sex, color, appearance, character or IQ. At the cross of Christ, the ground was level. Over the past twenty plus years since high school I have gone on to study Psychology and Counseling. What you are taught is a bill of goods that would suggest that the problems of the alcoholic, addict, anorexic, bulimic or sex addict are so different from each other that each needs some specialist to understand the problem. Granted, each of these addictions involve many different factors, but because the behavior is different, we erroneously believe each problem is unique and requires a different answer. Each of these behaviors is a manifestation of the flesh, the soul and not the real root problem. Neil Anderson says, "We suffer from the paralysis of analysis." We have become convinced that their problems are unique and require a unique answer.

The fact is Christians are not different because they are without hope, but rather we have "hope in Christ" (1 Corinthians 15:19). We don't receive hope as the world does, hoping things will work out. We receive hope by believing God's truth, then putting our trust in Him: "May the God of hope fill you with all joy and peace as you trust in Him, so that you may overflow with hope by the power of the Holy Spirit" (Romans. 15:13).

A Christian shouldn't ever be without hope. "We are in Christ and He is in us" (John 14:20). "We are more than conquerors" (Romans 8:37), "have been given the victory" (1 Corinthians15:57) and are "always led in triumph in Christ" (2 Corinthians 2:14).

One of the predominant feelings of the addict is guilt, which often feeds into their false belief regarding self.

Guilty. Without exception, alcoholics and addicts are mired and consumed with guilt. In my struggle with sexual addiction, I was laden with guilt. As my constant companion, guilt accused me, threatened me and reminded me of my failing life as a Christian. My seminary degrees and experience as a Christian counselor and an ordained minister only made things worse, when I stood before the mirror of self-evaluation.

The false guilt that I carried from childhood as the result of feeling blamed became so generalized that I could not cross the border into the United States without experiencing anxiety for fear of being questioned. I became so self-conscious of looking guilty that I looked guilty to the border patrol; this often precipitated more questions. My wife was often amused by this whole process and I was left feeling like I had just gone through some kind of trauma. This generalized guilt has plagued me my whole life.

What exactly is guilt, anyway? Sigmund Freud said that "guilt is a result of social restraint." To Freud, guilt was born in the mind of a child whose parents scolded him or her; it was rooted in the child's fear of losing the love of someone significant to him or her. Therefore, according to Freud, we experience guilt when we fear a loss of social esteem, when instinctive drives cause us to act in ways other than the accepted social norm. Alfred Adler wrote that "guilt arises from a refusal to accept one's inferiority. Therefore, he concluded, guilt feelings are those pangs of self-incrimination we feel anytime we think or behave inadequately." Both Freud and Adler tried to explain the pain of guilt from a perspective that denies the righteous judgment of God and our personal responsibility for sin. To them, guilt could only be explained on a human, existential basis.

Christian authors Bruce Narramore and Bill Counts represent a more biblical perspective when they differentiate between true guilt and false guilt. True guilt, they explain, "is an objective fact, but false guilt is a subjective feeling of pain and rejection. They emphasize that while the Bible discusses the fact of legal or theological guilt, it never tells the Christian to feel psychological guilt." These distinctions are helpful, but they may not clarify the issue for those who equate any guilt with condemnation. For this reason, it is important to distinguish between guilt and conviction and between the condemnation our sin deserves and the loving motivation prompted by God to live in a way that brings honor to Him. Though many people confuse these two concepts, they are actually worlds apart.

I like what Robert S. McGee in his book *The Search for Significance* states on this topic,

> "Perhaps no emotion is more destructive than guilt. It causes a loss of self-respect. It causes the human spirit to wither, and it eats away at our personal significance. Guilt is a strong motivation, but it plays on our fears of failure and rejection; therefore, it can never ultimately build, encourage, or inspire us in our desire to live for Christ."

No one can experience peace, freedom or joy when consumed with guilt. Satan uses this scheme to rob Christians of their freedom. Those who permit guilty feelings to rob them of their freedom let the past control them. They believe they are products of their pasts as Freud would suggest, rather than products of the Cross. Addicts are prone to this cycle of using followed by remorse and guilt. It is repeated endlessly.

The stronghold of guilt involves a strange paradox. To be guilt free, we must be honest, admit our problem and confess our sin or may I say lust. One of the first major barriers for the addict is the admission of a problem. Most of us fear exposure. We'll go to great length to create the impression that we are OK; but we won't ask for help until the great wall of denial is broken.

How do we face the awful truth about ourselves and our past? Only through the Cross. First we have to admit the problem. For guilt to be removed, the wrongdoing must be admitted. We admit God accepts us because of Christ's death on the cross, which paid for our sins. Roman 8:1 says, "There is therefore now no condemnation for those who are in Christ Jesus." Sin—past, present and future—has been eliminated. Romans 4:8, "Blessed is the man whose sin the Lord will never count against him." Only those who are honest admit their wrongs and confess their sins and lust will ever be free.

When we learn it's unnecessary to justify ourselves, we can begin to walk in freedom. Because of the Cross, we can find the courage to face the truth and experience God's liberating grace. The J.B.Phillips translation, *The New Testament in Modern English* of Colossians 2:13-15 summarizes this truth.

> "He has forgiven you all your sins: He has utterly wiped out the written evidence of broken commandments which always hung over our heads, and has completely annulled it by nailing it to the cross. And then, having drawn the sting of all the powers and authorities ranged against us, He exposed them, shattered, empty and defeated, in His own triumphant victory!"

So it is not only unnecessary to justify ourselves, but its paramount that we recognize that we can't simply change ourselves by willpower. Addicts have the incorrect belief that they can change themselves through self-help.

Self-Help: I Can Change Myself. By nature I am a self-starter and self driven. Since High School I have done several degrees, both undergraduate and graduate, competed in body building, ran marathons, and sought to balance pastoring a church full time and directing a Christian Counseling Centre. All this while simultaneously caring for a special needs daughter with a rare neurological disease who was medically unstable throughout this time. I carried this into my relationship with God believing that I could change myself. Of course what is inherent in the stronghold of self-help is the incorrect belief that I can change myself.

This of course is nothing more than bootstrap religion and positive legalism. It's just another form of my old mantra that said, "God helps those who help themselves." For some strange reason, most people believe that if they can change their behaviors, they will be able to change as a person. This is simply untrue as I have clearly proven in my own life.

Only God can change a person. I am coming to believe that when Christians understand their identities in Christ, their behaviors will change. Most Christians are trying to be someone they already are and get something they already have. The truth is we are in Christ, dead to sin, freed from it, alive to God, victorious and righteous in Him. When we believe these truths, our behavior will change.

One of the greatest deceptions is the belief that if we do something spiritual, our lives will automatically change. Nothing can be further from the truth. Martin Luther pointed out that nothing we do helps us spiritually. Only faith helps—only what we believe. I believed for many years that if I could spend enough time in prayer, and say the right prayer, read my Bible enough, memorize enough Scripture, it would change me; it didn't.

When we give up on ourselves, then we're ready to look to God and get some help. Trust me when I say it is most difficult to let go of our beliefs and devices. The last five years have been showing this to me. I never considered myself a self reliant and prideful person and yet I am discovering how true that has actually been. God only responds to faith, not our empty promises and futile strivings. Isaiah 50:11 tells us what happens to those of us who try to work it out by ourselves: "But now, all you who light fires and provide yourselves with flaming torches, go, walk in the light of your fires and of the torches you have set ablaze. This is what you will receive from my hand: You will lie down in torment."

The major reason for the anemic condition of today's Church is our lapse into positive legalism. If we do enough of the right things, we believe all will be well. Paul addressed this in his letter to the Galatians. Eugene Peterson's *The Message Bible* captures it vividly:

> "You crazy Galatians! Did someone put a hex on you? Have you taken leave of your senses? Something crazy has happened, for it's obvious that you no longer have the crucified Jesus in clear focus in your lives. His sacrifice on the Cross was certainly set before you clearly enough.

> Let me put this question to you: How did your new life begin? Was it by working your heads off to please God? Or was it by responding to God's Message to you? Are you going to continue this craziness? For only crazy people would think they could complete by their own efforts what was begun by God. If you weren't smart enough or strong enough to begin it how do you suppose you could perfect it? Did you go through this whole painful learning process for nothing? It is not yet a total loss, but it certainly will be if you keep this up!
>
> Answer this question. Does the God who lavishly provides you with His own presence, His Holy Spirit, working things in your lives you could never do for yourselves, does He do these things because of your strenuous moral striving or because you trust Him to do them in you?" (Galatians 3:1-5).

Those who are ready for God's help know they can do nothing. When it comes to self-help strongholds, I was the world's worst offender. I have completed multiple self help work books including *12 steps to a Spiritual Journey, Celebrate Recovery* by John Baker, *Facing the Shadow* from Dr. Patrick Carnes, *Ministering Steps to Freedom in Christ* and *Freedom From Addiction* by Neil Anderson only to name a few. Read many books on sexual addictions, attended group therapy and several types of support groups including, OA, AA, CODA, SA, SAA and support groups within the Church. I have seen a multitude of Christian and secular counselors, therapists, Psychologists and Psychiatrists. I have buffeted my body, tried spiritual disciplines including journaling, meditation, memorization, praying, fasting, baptism of the Holy Spirit, deliverance on several occasions, and very deep exegetical personal studies of the Word of God. I have made promises to God and to my wife and kids with determined willpower. I have had several personal accountability partners, sponsors and of course spent years going to school and have graduate degrees in theology and counseling and a two year specialty in addictions.

I came from the school that said, "Just tell me what to do and I will do it." The most difficult people to help are those who think they can do it, are willing to do it and are going to do it. I gave it my best shot. We need to come to an end in ourselves and our own resources. That is a very difficult process as I have discovered. I want to make one thing clear, I am not saying that any of the things that I have tried are bad things and not relevant to recovery. I continue to see a psychologist, attend a Sex Aholics Anonymous group and have a sponsor. On the contrary they are all very positive if put into proper context. If we believe they will fix us then they are wrong; they can't do this. However when we understand who we are in Christ then any and all of these tools can help us in the process of recovery. They are simply a means to the end not an end in themselves. The Cross is that.

You and I don't have to shape up the old person in ourselves in an all-out spiritual boot camp. That isn't Christianity. The stronghold of self-help is nothing but self-improvement. God doesn't want us to improve the flesh and soul, as "it is hostile to God." (Romans 8:7), and "the mind-set on it is death" (verse 6). "Those who belong to Christ Jesus have crucified the flesh with its passions and desires." (Galatians 5:24). Today's secular programs are designed to improve the flesh and to modify behavior. Unfortunately, many "Christian" programs, that I've been a part of, do the same but have a spiritual slant. Neil Anderson has said, "It is nothing but Christian behaviorism, which is legalism."

When we admit failure, God doesn't do a retread job on our old person. Galatians 2:20 can't be improved. "I have been crucified with Christ and I no longer live, but Christ lives in me. The life I live in the body, I live by faith in the Son of God, who loved me and gave himself for me."

I stated a few moments ago that guilt is a predominant emotion amongst addicts, so too is the feeling of insecurity.

Insecurity. I have never counseled an alcoholic or addict who did not struggle with insecurity. That inability to accept oneself or feel accepted and loved by others is always predominant. Larry Crabb in his book, *Effective Biblical Counseling* states,

> "People have one basic personal need which requires two kinds of input for its satisfaction. The most basic need is a sense of personal worth, an acceptance of oneself as a whole, real person. The two required inputs are significance (purpose, importance, adequacy for a job, meaningfulness, impact) and security (love—unconditional and consistently expressed; permanent acceptance)."

> He goes on to say that he, "believes that before the Fall Adam and Eve were both significant and secure. From the moment of their creation their needs were fully met in a relationship with God unmarred by sin. Significance and security were attributes or qualities already resident within their personalities, so they never gave them a second thought. When sin ended their innocence and broke their relationship with God, what formerly were attributes now became needs. After the Fall Adam hid from God, fearing His rejection. They both blamed another for their sin, afraid of what God might do. They were now insecure. The earth was cursed and Adam was instructed to work by the sweat of his brow. There was now a struggle between man and nature. Would Adam have the strength to handle the job? He now was wrestling with threatened insignificance." Crabb concludes by stating, "Significance depends upon understanding who I am in Christ. I will come to feel significant as I have an eternal impact on people. My need for security demands that I be unconditionally loved, accepted and cared for, now and forever. When God has seen you at your worst and still loves you to the point of giving his life for you."

You and I are completely acceptable to Him regardless of our behavior. My acceptability to God depends only on the fact that Jesus' death was counted as full payment for my sins.

What is our greatest need? It is to be loved and accepted. God made us that way; and God's design is for us to meet that need through a relationship with Him. As the old song says, many people are "looking for love in all the wrong places."

As a young child growing up I always remember feeling insecure. I would listen to my mom and dad fight, and at times my father would rage. As stated earlier my father was 6' 4" and well over 200 pounds. There was always something that went wrong and it was never his fault. I recall most of the time it was my mother who was blamed and she would work hard to appease my father and keep the peace. She was valiant in her attempt to protect us children, but it wouldn't stop the insults, criticism, blaming, or showing physical aggression. It was like walking on egg shells, you were never quite sure what was going to set my father off. It seemed every good occasion was overshadowed by another eruption in which everyone recoiled into silence.

I learned as a child that it was not safe to express negative emotions, never disagree, and do whatever you can to keep the peace and please dad. As I grew up I became out of touch with my emotions and learned that it was better to stuff them. In my early years I don't ever remember telling anyone at anytime how I felt about anything and no one ever asked. As a teenager I began to look for love in all the wrong places. I often fantasized what a perfect or ideal relationship would be. At times it might even become sexual in my fantasy life. When I first saw pornography in my twenties, it opened up a whole new reality to my fantasy life and provided an escape from my imperfect self.

The greater the insecurity, the more you develop insecure patterns. No one could get too close to me. At all costs, I avoided intimacy. Anyone who got too close might discover the real me and I could not let that happen. I learned to not disagree and do whatever it takes to avoid any conflict. To keep the peace and try not to draw any negative attention to myself that would initiate any kind of interrogation, in which I would instantly feel guilty. My insecurity demanded that it was far safer to isolate than to initiate. I developed the fine art of avoidance.

For years I have struggled with the fact that my wife could love me. I was convinced it would only be a matter of time before she would reject me. To my amazement and despite all that I have put her through, as a testament to her character and love, she has not rejected me.

Thankfully God has spoken clearly and acted decisively. He said that we are so worthy that He sent His one and only Son to die for our sins. Then we could have relationship with Him. In Hebrews 13:5, God tells us of His commitment to us: "For He [God] Himself has said, I will not in any way fail you nor give you up nor leave you without support. [I will] not in any degree leave you helpless nor forsake nor let [you] down [relax my hold on you]!"

How much does God love us? Hundreds of verses in the Bible tell us of God's love. I want to point out one: Jesus said, "As the Father has loved me, so have I loved you. Now remain in my love" (John 15:9). I think what most of us struggle with, and I know I do is the commandment to, "remain in His love." We may say, but I just don't feel his love. That is irrelevant; addiction is nothing but lies that comprise of strongholds in our mind. Freedom believes the truth that sets us free.

This brings me to the four core incorrect beliefs that Carnes identifies and I believe are in conjunction with what I have just stated. The first false belief that he shares is, I am basically a bad, unworthy person.

I am basically a bad, unworthy person. The root of this belief is shame. Joseph Chilton Pearce, who quotes Schores in his book *The Biology of Transcendence*, states,

> "That the introduction of shame is a blatant form of the accusation of sin, and because most of us have heard this and been the recipients of such accusations from the beginning of life, we unconsciously and impulsively inflict the same on our children. He goes on to say that this shame perfectly articulates the tone of the accusation: "You are no good. You are bad." Shamed in this sense, we forget who we are. We actually become the protective mask we adopt to shield us from the

> accusing fingers pointed toward us. Cut off from our spirit, we spend the rest of our lives trying to prove our innocence.

According to Gershen Kaufman in his book, *SHAME,*

> "Shame is..."a sickness of the soul. It is the most poignant experience of the self by the self, whether felt in humiliation or cowardice, or in a sense of failure to cope successfully with challenge. Shame is a wound felt from the inside, dividing us both from ourselves and from one another."
>
> According to Kaufman, shame is the source of most of the disturbing inner states which deny full human life. Depression, alienation, self-doubt, isolating loneliness, paranoid and schizoid phenomena, compulsive disorders, splitting of the self, perfectionism, a deep sense of inferiority inadequacy or failure, the so-called borderline conditions and disorders of narcissism, all result from shame. Shame is a kind of soul murder. Once shame is internalized, it is characterized by a kind of psychic numbness, which becomes the foundation for a kind of death in life. Shame conditions every relationship in our lives. It is a total non-self acceptance.

Shame differs greatly from the feeling of guilt. Guilt says I've done something wrong; shame says there is something wrong with me. Guilt says I've made a mistake; shame says I am a mistake. Guilt says what I did was not good; shame says I am no good.

It is from our state of shame that this inner speech arises, full of accusation and fault-finding. Many of us are driven to try to prove our worth (our innocence) to our accusing world by earning success with it and at any cost. Each accused soul scrabbles for gain at any price because wealth alone is deemed proof of authenticity and freedom from censure.

This belief expresses the self-concept of addicts. A positive sense of self precedes any possibility of closeness or intimacy. Without that fundamental acceptance of self, nurturing and intimacy can be closed out. Addicts who have experienced intense shame in their early development regard themselves as "unworthy." They survive in a secret world in which obsession blocks pain and loneliness and in which they are accountable to no one. Only the addicts know the whole truth. Each effort to quit but fails, adds to an addict's sense of hopelessness, shame and belief that "I am bad." By keeping it a secret and wearing the mask, the addict maintains an illusionary sense of control and responsibility. One way to break out is Step 1 in the 12 step program. An admission removes the veil of secrecy and allows others to help. It is the path to reclaiming reality. Steps 2 and 3 help them discover they are not alone, abandoned, or bad and unworthy. They learn to trust a higher power and begin to internalize a new belief: "I am a worthwhile person." My biggest concern with the 12 Step program is that it is to general with the use of a generic higher power rather than having faith in the words and declarations of a very personal God who actually determines and declares one's personal worth. God states in Ephesians, "I am God's workmanship" (2:10), "I am a saint" (1:1), "I am adopted (chosen) as God's child." (1:5). A second false belief that Carnes observes that addicts have about themselves, is no one loves me as I am.

No one would love me as I am. "Addicts conclude that they are basically bad people and thus do not love themselves. They add the parallel belief that the only path for them is to project an unreal image that protects the secrets of the addiction. They live in constant tension, fearing the truth will be discovered and made public. Rejection and abandonment would follow. Step 4 is a moral inventory of the addict's strengths and weaknesses. This helps to dismantle the basic convictions about being unworthy and unlovable. Step 5 challenges their belief that if someone really knew them they would reject them. This also enables the addict to experience reconciliation and forgiveness. They learn that if they make a mistake they don't need to retreat into the secret world. Steps 4, 5, 8 and 9 reveal to them that they are loved and accepted by people who know who they are. However, that being said, we know that people can still reject you because of their own fears and insecurities but "God will never leave you nor forsake you and we are free from condemning charges against us" (Romans 8:33-39). The third false belief states, my needs are never going to be met if I have to depend upon others.

My needs are never going to be met if I have to depend upon others. "While the first two core beliefs dealt with self-acceptance and intimacy, the third core belief deals with dependency. Addicts distrust other people, believing themselves to be unworthy and unlovable. Therefore they conclude they cannot depend on others. This leaves addicts feeling resentful, manipulative, and secretive. Addicts have to be taught, or have to relearn, how to let others know about their needs. As they learn to ask, they discover a new belief: "My needs can be met by others if I let them know what I need." Steps 6 and 7 demand a complete surrender to their dependency needs." This in essence is living in true community. I believe this includes God in the equation. Let me explain what I mean. Dr. Larry Crabb in his book *Connecting a Radical New Vision* states,

> "I have come to believe that the root of all our personal and emotional difficulties is a lack of togetherness, a failure to connect that keeps us from receiving life and prevents the life in us from spilling over onto others." He goes on to say, "Communities that heal are communities that probe and expose, that help people to see what's going on inside and encourage them to handle their struggles more effectively.
>
> We were designed to connect with others. Connecting is life. Loneliness is the ultimate horror. In connecting with God, we gain life. In connecting with others, we nourish and experience that life as we freely share it. Rugged individualism, proud independence, and chosen isolation violate the nature of our existence as much as trying to breathe under water. The capacities that distinguish us as human beings from all other creations (including angels and animals) were given to us

> so we could connect with each other the way the three divine persons connect. We have the capacity to enjoy the wonder of a relationship built on grace that no angel has ever personally experienced."

Let me illustrate what Crabb is saying by considering the person who struggles with pornography. His personal problem is sex addiction. Committed to managing life without God and afraid to face his emptiness and guilt, the highest goal is that he "make it," that he experience some level of internal satisfaction. Over the course of thousands of learning experiences, he settles into a basic life strategy, continuing to do whatever creates personal pleasure and working hard to avoid whatever brings pain. His life becomes thoroughly and strategically self-centered. Whatever kindness he extends or responsibility he takes on is prompted by the hope of personal advantage. No one is taking care of him as he wants to be taken care of, so he looks after himself. He therefore never connects. Nothing comes out of him that is aimed at arousing the good in another. Every choice is in the service of self. He is a slave to lust.

His disconnection is complete. He finds himself separated from God, himself, and others. He is foolishly independent and unaware of his destiny and purpose. He is committed to a justice that revolves around himself and scared that he's inadequate, desperately insecure and angry when things don't go his way. He is incapable of loving anybody and not terribly bothered that he doesn't, finally alone with himself, either settling for lesser satisfactions and "doing fine" or troubled by any one of dozens of symptoms of his terrified, angry, selfish internal life. Communion with God means nothing. It isn't felt, tasted, or experienced. At best, it is a transitory Sunday morning happening that lasts until the closing hymn. That man senses a void that yearns to be filled but lacks the sense to realize that he longs for love, not pleasure. He has lost touch with his humanity, with his longing for love, and with his moral design.

Experience with life teaches him that no one is especially interested in his well-being. Perhaps he discovers few talents within himself or opportunities that reliably provide him with a taste of the satisfaction he craves. While keeping up appearance as a responsible, good man, he inwardly gives up on relationships or achievement as a means of finding what he wants. His capacity for sexual pleasure, intended to provide a physical excitement that more deeply bonds him to his wife, becomes, in the absence of connection with her, the means of experiencing nothing more than a moment of predictable pleasure. Because sexual excitement from pornography becomes the closest thing in his experience to soul satisfaction, because it seems justified and reliable, and because it provides pleasure without risk, it becomes the centre of his life. Lust controls him. He is a sex addict.

The cause of his addiction is released badness, wrong desires that are honored, urges that result from disconnecting, first from God then from self and others. The cure, is found in a reconnecting with God, believing that "God can meet all your needs according to His riches in Christ" (Philippians 4:19) and as Dr. Carnes states "in connecting with others."

In our natural state, before we accept what Christ did for us on the cross in our place, we all walked in the lusts of our flesh. That was our only option. Our entire approach to life was built on the conviction that God wasn't good enough to fully trust. The root of all our choices therefore was self-dependence, self-interest, self-preoccupation, the exact opposite of the choices that govern relationships with the Trinity. We were filled with bad urges. "Every inclination of the thoughts of his heart was only evil all the time" (Genesis 6:5).

However, those who believe in the finished work of Christ on the cross are no longer in their natural state. They have been given a new nature and their spirit has been reborn. "Therefore if any man be in Christ, he is a new creation, old things have passed away and behold all things have become new" (2 Corinthians 5:17). We were created and designed to be connected with God, ourselves and then others. *Sexaholics Anonymous Big Book* states, "without this essential core of our being plugged in somewhere, life is unbearable. We can't survive alone, cut off, disconnected." This brings me to the last false belief that Cairns espouses.

Sex is my most important need. The idea that old obsessions, rituals and behaviors will bring peace dies hard, especially under stress. Only by living the program daily and experiencing other people's care continuously does that belief diminish. Step 10 and 11 are ongoing disciplines. Urging them to take an inventory and when wrong promptly admit it. Step 11 asks the addicts to improve their conscious contact with God through prayer and meditation. In time the addicts discover that sex is but one expression of their need and care for others." What the 12 Steps state and Dr. Carnes advocates and what I would suggest is that we need a daily time with God for self-examination, Bible reading, and prayer in order to know God and His will for our life.

One of the greatest ways to prevent relapse is to maintain an "attitude of gratitude." God's Word states that we "need not be anxious (worry) about anything, but in everything with prayer and petition with thanksgiving let your requests be made known to God and the peace that surpasses all comprehension will guard your heart and mind in Christ Jesus." (Philippians 4:4). Rejoice and celebrate the small successes along your road to recovery! Always remember you're on a journey, a journey of several steps. Maintaining an "attitude of gratitude" is like taking spiritual vitamins. Share your victories-no matter how small-with others. "Be joyful always, pray at all times, and be thankful in all circumstances. This is what God wants from you in your life in union with Christ Jesus" (1 Thessalonians 5:16).

Today, one of the greatest truths I am learning is that one of my biggest sins is unbelief—not believing how much God loved me and how much He accepts me. This affected my identity and security and as a result I have suffered from these last two components of the larger addictive system.

Impaired Thinking

The second component of the larger addictive system is impaired thinking. Impaired thinking usually involves a distortion of reality. Other types of impaired thinking include denial, rationalization, self-delusion, self-righteousness, or blame of others. But the addict's problem is that despite all the denial and distortion, reality does creep in. No amount of self-justification can account for all the complications in the addict's life. Anxiety and alienation occur in the family. Relationships are neglected. The addict violates personal values such as honesty or fidelity. Procrastination and low productivity at work may compound the difficulties.

> *Sexaholics Anonymous Big Book* shares that "it is an attitudinal force that shapes the person and their character. It is a process at work in the development of addiction. Many a sexaholic is seething with resentment, hostility, anger, envy, rebellion and rage. We may not be consciously aware of it or of the powerful life-altering significance of such a disposition, but the more we discover about this aspect of our condition, the more we realize that our behavior was the manifestation of inner attitudes and impaired thinking. Our attitudes enabled the addiction. We are what we think. We nourish, defend, and deny it.
>
> We become increasingly closed off and defensive, unteachable and willful, and a kind of hardening sets in. The greater the self-obsession, the greater the con to disguise it. From our very first attitude change, we isolate ourselves. We start building a wall around us, especially between us and those we are close to.
>
> We can be outgoing, warm, personable, charming, lovable, and kind as long as it serves the self. We are separating ourselves from God and self. The duplicity of holding resentments on the inside while being something else on the outside creates a split that not

> only isolates us from others but from our true selves-separation at the very core of our being.
>
> As soon as we set into motion the process of covering our wrongs, there is an increasing inability to see ourselves as we really are and others as they really are. The alcoholics call this "pride-blindness." The blindness starts as we deny the truth about our wrongs and hold on to the lie of our own rationalizations.
>
> We choose the course that sets us against ourselves and others so we can persist in wrong. Our diseased attitude is an irresistible force driving us away from others, ourselves and God and into our addiction. To stop means we must face the truth about ourselves, and that is like the very threat of death. But unless we do stop and face the truth about ourselves, we remain in death." The addict's life becomes progressively more unmanageable.

Unmanageability

This brings us to the third component of the larger addictive system: unmanageability.

Reality, i.e. the consequences which the addict cannot rationalize completely away, keeps the addict's life unmanageable. The split between delusion and reality eats away at the addict's sense of self. An eroding self-concept adds to the addict's pain and contributes negative emotional energy to core beliefs about his or her unworthiness.

When the addictive cycle has become fully established, the addictive system becomes an autonomous, closed system, feeding upon itself, maintaining regularity and priority. Signs that an addictive system has formed are: Preoccupation becomes a routine way to avoid problems. Rituals emerge which usually precede sexual behavior. A baseline of regular behavior can be established...behavior becomes a priority over other meaningful aspects of life. Periods of depression are sometimes followed by efforts to curb beliefs about self. Thought process distorts reality, creating unrealistic confidence and negating potential problems. Reversal of life priorities causes complications in family, work, relationship, and values, and the addict starts to live a double life. When the addiction moves beyond the early stages, greater degrees of intensity are experienced, as well as greater suffering. *Sexaholic Anonymous Big Book* calls this the addictive Process and summarizes by stating:

- It begins with an overpowering desire for a high, relief, pleasure, or escape.
- It provides satisfaction
- It is sought repeatedly and compulsively.
- It then takes on a life of its own.
- It becomes excessive.
- Satisfaction diminishes.
- Distress is produced.
- Emotional control decreases.
- Ability to relate deteriorates.
- Ability for daily living is disturbed.
- Denial becomes necessary.
- It takes priority over everything else.
- It becomes the main coping mechanism.
- The coping mechanism stops working.
- The party is over.

This brings me to the growth of the addictive system in which *Sexaholic Anonymous Big Book* states that there are three aspects of our condition that commonly identify addiction: tolerance, abstinence, and withdrawal. If someone experiences these three phenomena in some area of his or her life, that person is generally regarded as being addicted.

> It states that the term "tolerance refers to the tendency to tolerate more of the drug or activity and get less

> from its use, hence need for increasing dosage to maintain or recapture the desired effect. It can also include the need for increasing amounts of obsessive thinking, interaction, or activity, with less and less effect.
>
> The term abstinence refers to the phenomenon where the typical addict tries to quit using the addictive agent or activity. They swear off again and again. Perhaps we should call it "attempting abstinence."
>
> The last term is withdrawal and is applied to the symptoms the addict may experience when deprived of the drug or activity. Such symptoms can be physical, emotional, or both. This gives rise to the deception and demand that they got to have sex."

I have spent several pages describing the larger addictive system which included a faulty belief system, impaired thinking, unmanageability, tolerance, abstinence and withdrawl. I will now take some time to describe the addictive cycle and the addictive growth that operates within the larger addictive system. Let's look first at the addictive cycle.

Each person travels a private path to addiction, but the downward spiraling cycles are all remarkably similar. Dr. Patrick Carnes, in his book "Contrary to Love" states the following about the addictive cycle and how it develops and maintains itself in the addict's life.

Chapter 4
The Addictive Cycle

The first clue that an addiction is established and is an issue is regularity. As I examine my own case history, I can see that my sexual life became predictable as opposed to spontaneous. As an integral part of established, addictive behavior, a cycle emerges with four distinct and sequential components: preoccupation; ritualization; sexual compulsivity; and shame.

Preoccupation

The addictive cycle begins at the point where the addict's thoughts become focused on the behavior. It was not uncommon for me to be spending time obsessing in anticipation of acting out and euphorically recalling the event before. My mental state was a kaleidoscope of feelings, fantasies, memories, hopes, and expectations. I, like all addicts, could and can mobilize from our own psychic resources a mood-altering "high" without actually being sexual. Just thinking about it can initiate a trance-like state of arousal that can blot out the current demands of real life.

Using obsession as a coping mechanism leads to low productivity and procrastination. In fact, most of the sex addict's time spent in the addictive cycle is spent in preoccupation. The exciting sexual feelings will be intensified when the addict seeks stimulation for his or her obsession. Addicts refer to the search for stimulation as "cruising," which means deliberately seeking an object or environment that is provocative or opportune. This has the quality of "teasing oneself." With this obsessive preoccupation, the addict has already lost control. For recovery, it is critical to identify the cues, time of day, place, situation, or other factors-which trigger the onset of the preoccupation stage. The *Sex Addicts Anonymous Big Book* calls this the Middle Circle. In Sex Addicts Anonymous (SAA) acting out can be defined as engaging in sexual behavior that we have put in our inner circle. Sexual sobriety, then, means abstaining from these inner-circle behaviors. By the same token, relapse (or loss of sexual sobriety) means engaging in an inner-circle behavior. The *Sexoholics Anonymous Big Book* (SA) would state that lust is the inner-circle activity that we must abstain from. It goes on to say that,

> "The addiction is thus to lust and not merely to the substance or physical act. Lust – the attitude itself – becomes the controlling factor in the addiction. This is why change of attitude is so crucial."

We can agree that most people who come to either SAA or SA don't really know what healthy sexuality is. They are usually uncertain about whether some behaviors are addictive or not. They place them in the middle circle until they can determine if they are compulsive or have negative consequences. If we put masturbation in the middle circle, for instance, we might look at how frequently we masturbate, what kinds of fantasies we use, whether we are masturbating in an appropriate location, and how we feel afterwards. If we put lust in the middle circle then we are forced to consider every fleeting sexual fantasy and negative attitude. If we become convinced that a thinking and behavior is addictive, we may then decide to move it to our Inner Circle.

The middle circle can be things we do and think that make us vulnerable to acting out. For some of us, examples may include driving places where we used to act out, flirting or intriguing, wearing revealing clothing, or watching TV for sexual content. We may fool ourselves into believing that we have a legitimate reason to be in a slippery situation, when in fact this is part of the addictive pattern that can lead to inner-circle behavior. Putting this thinking and behavior in our Middle Circle is a way of warning ourselves when we are in danger of acting out.

We may also put non-sexual behaviors in our Middle Circle that we know lead us to slippery states of mind—unhealthy behaviors that don't support our recovery. Examples may include isolating from people, overworking, and other potentially addictive behaviors, like drinking, gambling, or overeating.

If we engage in Middle-Circle behavior, it too does not mean that the addict has lost their sobriety, but it is a signal that they need to reach out and ask for help. The Middle Circle can be seen as a safety net, allowing us to walk the tightrope of abstinence without having to fear that a false step would necessarily be disastrous. We may also think of it as a warning track or a guard rail. If we climb over the guard rail, we haven't fallen off the cliff. However, we should recognize that we are in a dangerous place.

"The *SAA Big Book*" goes on to explain that the outer-circle behaviors encompass a wide range of healthy activities. They are frequently the things we didn't have time to do when we were acting out. Examples may include working our recovery program, rediscovering hobbies we once enjoyed, playing sports and exercising, spending time with family and friends, socializing and making new friends in a safe environment, participating in a local church, or engaging in any other activities which make our lives more enjoyable and meaningful.

Ritualization

Addicts enhance their mental preoccupation with rituals, which are regularly followed methods of preparing for sexual activity to take place. Anything can become a ritual for the addict. Rituals involve context. Certain places, especially cruising areas, focus the ritualization and trigger sexual obsession. Beaches, magazine stores, bars, porn shops, computers, alcohol, drugs, or even getting involved in activities that precipitate rejection or failure, and then proceed to act out again, feeling fully justified.

Work behavior too can become part of negative ritualization. This may mean routine overextension to the point of exhaustion, when addicts become so depleted (a) they can no longer make decisions for themselves, (b) they are in desperate need for nurturing at any price, and (c) they can use their vulnerability to manipulate others into taking care of them sexually.

Regular self-defeating behavior - living from disaster to disaster - is a consistent underpinning of addictive behavior. The sense of crisis adds energy to the rituals: "I need it to survive, or "I deserve it." In the early years of my daughter's medical condition I felt that I was in a constant state of crisis, normalcy and stability seemed to become a distant reality. At moments there appeared to be no end to the heartache and disappointment. I would work all day and sit in the ICU at night. This pattern existed not for days, or months but years. I began to feel like I was in some kind of altered state of reality for which I could no longer cope. Desperately wishing and praying for some kind of good news, only to hear yet another heart breaking prognosis. In those moments of anger, hurt and frustration I would tell myself, "I need it to survive," I am going to explode and lose complete control of my faculties." "I deserve it, after all God doesn't seem to be helping." As I have discovered over these last few years, that was faulty logic and with this kind of faulty logic, the addiction gains momentum and power.

However at the time, the ritual seems magically to bring order out of chaos. Think of it as a dance (certain steps, certain sounds, rhythm) which can be very elaborate but have only one purpose: to put addicts into another world so they can escape the conditions of real life over which they feel they have no control. Fantasy is compounded by delusion at this point, for the mood-altered state is a "world" in which the addicts no longer care about control in the same way. Sexual obsession is pursued to its peak regardless of risk, harm, or other consequences. There is only one kind of control that matters now-control of source of sexual pleasure. Once they start dancing, they rarely, if ever, can stop on their own. The next stage is sexually acting out. Some examples are:

-the exhibitionist driving regular "routes" or settings

-the professional speaker scanning the audience for potential partners

-the prostitute patron frequenting the noontime topless show

-the female addict showing up at the local hotel's cocktail hour

-the compulsive masturbator browsing in adult bookstores

-the fetishist or cross dresser shopping for clothes at a rummage sale

The third distinct and sequential component to the addictive cycle is sexual compulsivity.

Sexual Compulsivity

Compulsivity, essentially, is out-of-control behavior. Sexual compulsivity, then, is the inability to control one's sexual behavior, and the behavior is the cornerstone of the addiction. To be preoccupied and to ritualize are precursors to this stage, but without the acting out the addiction is not established, because the behavior is still under control. However, determining loss of control with sex addiction is difficult because of the wide variety of behaviors possible. Nor is frequency a valid criterion. For example, there is no fixed number of times a day a person masturbates or has affairs, etc., which can be used as a cutoff point.

The number of contacts will mean different things to different addicts:

-number of anonymous sexual contacts

-number of prostitutes

-number of people exposed to

-number of relationships

-number of child sex contacts

-number of nude people seen

-any combination or variation of the above plus many others

The number is important but not the critical factor in determining whether the addiction has reached the establishment phase. I will explain what that stage means in the next chapter. When the sexual behavior becomes the most important aspect of the addict's life, the addict now has a pathological relationship with a mood-altering behavior. People, job, family, values, the elements that give meaning to our lives, become secondary. The primary relationship, is with the behavior. Binge cycles also have a pattern. In the establishment phase, these binges cease to be irregular periods of acting out and become predictable. For me these cycles were weeks and months apart and even years in one case. Despite the space between my activities, despair and shame always followed, which brings us to the last stage and the connecting link of the addictive cycle.

Shame and Despair

The addict's intense emotional pain is transformed into pleasure during the preoccupation and ritualization stages, becoming euphoric during the fleeting moments of sexual release. However, following the climax experience, the addict plummets into shame and despair more deeply with each repetition of the cycle. Isolation also increases.

Despair becomes the connecting link in all addictive cycles, creating the need to begin the cycle again. The purpose of the cycle in the addict's life is to keep pain at bay. Often, addicts in the despair stage of the cycle appear to be depressed. At this point they may make efforts to curb or stop the sexual behavior. These efforts may account for the times of abstinence of the periodic binger. The despair often has to do with shame at the loss of control. (See Appendix III: Your Addictive Cycle)

Chapter 5
Growth of the Addictive System

One of the common perceptions both in the addictive community and elsewhere is that addiction is always progressive in nature. I think this comes from three phenomena that is common to all addicts: tolerance, abstinence, and withdrawal as I quoted earlier from Sexaholics Anonymous.

These phenomenon have led to an addictive process that begins with an overpowering desire for a high, relief, pleasure, or escape. It provides satisfaction that is sought repeatedly and compulsively. It then takes on a life of its own and becomes excessive. The satisfaction becomes diminished because of tolerance to the drug and distress and withdrawal is produced. Emotional control decreases and the ability to relate deteriorates. This begins to impact and disrupt daily living. Denial becomes necessary and it has the potential take over everything else. It becomes the main coping mechanism, but it to begins to stop working.

However the process, it is not necessarily progressive. We see that the practice of our addiction includes the whole range from sporadic or periodic to continuous acting out. I believe this can be a real trap to the addict because as long as we believe that the addict is someone on the street, has lost everything or spent time in jail we will not qualify ourselves as an addict and minimize our addiction.

Patrick Carnes states,

> "Given available empirical data, it can be said with considerable certainty that sex addiction is not inevitably progressive. Some addictive patterns are some are not. Some sex addicts' behavior remain relatively constant for their lifetimes. Others quickly escalate their addictive behaviors within a month of establishing a base line. Some escalate to such a degree that the illness becomes acute, governing every facet of their daily lives. Others de-escalate their behavior, controlling it for years. In most cases, these people are still addicts, in a stage comparable to what alcoholics call "white knuckle" sobriety, since fear and obsession continue to govern their lives. Another much smaller group of addicts escalate to chronic illness." He goes on to suggest that the Addictive Cycle within the larger addictive system may develop and grow through five phases.

The First Stage: Initiation Phase

In the earliest phase, sexual behavior that is a precursor to addiction is difficult, if not impossible, to distinguish from normal sexual behavior. Many people have intense sexual experiences as early as their grade-school years. Experimentation and curiosity are a natural part of psychosexual development. Guilt may result, but most are able to move beyond it. Many addicts however, report that the impact of these early activities was exceptionally intense. Sex seemed to be more important to them than to their peers. Also, addicts can often recall that self-stimulation was not merely experimentation; it was already a way to anesthetize emotional pain.

This was consistent with my first experience at around age 12. I can vividly recall the euphoria was so strong and the emotional release so pronounced that I could only imagine it would be likened to the cocaine addict having his first hit. The emotional potintency was so powerful and intense that I was changed for life. From that time forward I would find myself going back to the well, to recapture that moment of emotional and physical release that could never be matched again.

In general, much time in adolescent and young adult years is spent coping with emerging sexual desire. Normal development usually involves some trauma, frustration, anxiety, and disappointment. Often young people get involved in situations that have unfortunate consequences. These are used as learning experiences and simply are not done again.

Addicts often perceive their maturing years differently. They see this period as punctuated by a series of events in which their sexual behavior risked serious disapproval. This was very true in my late teens and early twenties. Instead of learning experiences to draw upon for wisdom, I acquired a string of shameful memories like masturbating by my window or at times in the back yard with the hope of being seen, which casted doubt on my normalcy. Another aspect of this time in addicts' lives is that sex becomes a way to get through life's difficulties and pressures.

One of these pressures is peer pressure and some settings intimidate people into doing what everyone else is doing. Each of us has a need to be accepted and to have some sense of belonging as I stated earlier. Using can reduce inhibitions and help one forget their problems and responsibilities. Our ability to stand against peer pressure and to resist the temptation to throw off our inhibitions is dependent on how secure we are and how our basic needs are being met. Less secure people can stand against peer pressure—if they have another group to accept them and to provide a sense of belonging to them.

We are all driven to have our needs met for acceptance and belonging as I quoted earlier from Larry Crabb, but this also becomes the psychological basis for temptation to meet legitimate needs. The question is: Are these needs going to be met in Christ who promised "to meet all our needs according to His riches in glory" (Philippians 4:19). Or, are we going to succumb to the temptation to turn to counterfeit attempts by the world, the flesh and the devil to meet our needs? Paul admonished, "Let our people also learn to engage in good deeds to meet pressing needs, that they may not be unfruitful" (Titus 3:14).

Most are driven to fulfill inner needs for acceptance and belonging. Many will compromise their own convictions to gain acceptance and to avoid feeling alone. Some people act out of rebellion to authority. They usually come from dysfunctional homes, or legalistic religious settings.

Some addicts report that their growing up was quite normal, as I stated mine was. No sexual abuse. Relatively normal family lives. No unusual sexual problems and very limited sexual experience. But given an extraordinary situation with great stress and intensely pleasurable sexual experiences pursued to excess, they will begin to form a potent pattern of sex as stress relief with lifelong consequences.

There are two catalysts for these patterns. Catalytic environments are characterized by extremes. For example, situations that combine high performance expectations with a low degree of structure seem to be particularly potent, i.e., when I attended graduate school, the stressor was my progressive self-doubt. Addicts say they never had much faith in themselves. Anxiety and control are common aspects of these experiences.

In addition to noting the catalytic environments that are often part of the initiation phase of sex, one must also identify the catalytic events. These events may be seen as falling into two major categories: abandonment events and sexual events. Abandonment only has to be perceived and it comes in many forms. Feeling unnecessary and uninvolved, they attempt to relieve their anger and distress by their excessive sexual behavior.

Identifying abandonment events allows clients to begin to replace faulty beliefs with accurate beliefs or to restructure those false conclusions addicts carry within them causing them to lose faith in themselves.

While abandonment events are unquestionably damaging, equally harmful in terms of igniting addiction are the sexual events. I believe we can learn to live by the grace of God in spite of our circumstances and events in our lives. Unfortunately some like me choose to believe their "hope" lies in altering their circumstances. We are supposed to "cast all our anxiety upon Him [Christ], because He cares for us" (1 Peter 5:7). Christ has our best interest in mind. Learning to cope with pain is a critical part of growing up.

Regardless of why people choose to use, each person with an addiction has at least two of the following three conditions. First, their basic needs are not being met in legitimate ways. Second, they have not learned how to cope with life's problems. Third, they can't seem to resolve their personal or spiritual conflicts in responsible ways. The drug of choice they become addicted to will not meet their needs, enable them to cope or resolve their conflicts. Their addictions only make matters worse. Nobody likes being addicted. And nobody plans to become addicted. And everyone is sure it will never happen to them. So how does it happen?

<u>Addictive Cycle: Symptomology and Criteria for the phase:</u>

- Preoccupation: Sexual obsession helps cope.
- Ritualization: Determination to find ways to maximize behavior opportunities.
- Behavior: Episodic periods of acting out, abusive behavior.
- Despair; Concerns, disappointments or unease about behavior.
- Belief System: Loss of faith in oneself, feelings of unworthiness and distrust in an extreme environment.
- Impaired Thinking: Incongruency between feelings of exhilaration and reality of danger or degradation between perception of behavior as experimental or short lived and reality of regularity or potential of continuing pattern.
- Unmanageability: Catalytic events correspond with first complications of behavioral excess.

Once a pattern of behavior is developed, the addict enters the establishment phase of the sexual addiction.

Second Stage: The Establishment Phase

Understanding sexual addiction has the effect of putting on a new set of lenses. New patterns emerge where none has been discernible before. The addictive cycle forms and is repeated: trance-like preoccupation intensified by rituals leads to compulsive sex behavior, which is followed by shame and despair. For descriptive purposes, addicts whose behavior stays more or less consistently at the base line of established addiction are said to remain in the establishment phase.

Addictive Cycle: Symptomology and Criteria for the phase:

- Preoccupation: Preoccupation becomes routine way to avoid life problems.
- Ritualization: Repetitive patterns emerge which usually precede behavior.
- Behavior: Regularity and priority of behavior establish a baseline.
- Despair: Periods of depression sometimes followed by efforts to curb or stop behavior.
- Belief System: Behavior and unmanageability begin to confirm destructive core beliefs about self.
- Impaired Thinking: Thought processes start to distort reality, creating unrealistic confidence and negating potential problems.
- Unmanageability: Reversal of life priorities causes complications in family, work, relationships, and values and addict starts to live double life.

The first two phases are the developmental phases. They describe the beginnings of addiction; the next four phases will describe growth.

Third Stage: Contingent Phase: Escalation Mode

The individual`s addictive system is now fully established and given certain events and environments, begins to escalate-more intensity, more frequency, more risk, more unmanageability, etc. One of the surest indicators of escalation is crossing into new, more clearly risky or dangerous sexual behaviour than had been practiced before and seeking greater excitement with increased risk. Changing levels may also indicate a degree of desperation. Behaviour may escalate at a varying rate, or it may de-escalate. Indications of increased intensity might include: Starting to seek out situations with multiple partners, picking up someone not once but two to three times a week. Finding serial affairs insufficient and starting multiple relationships. Going from night time exposing to daytime exposing. Going from cruising two to three hours twice a week to three to five hours each day. Viewing pornography when you're home alone to viewing when others are around.

The addict's preoccupation focuses on new ways to accommodate the increase of sexual energy or to achieve the latest fantasy, while minimizing risk. The paradoxical part of such preoccupation is that addicts become victims of their own frequent lapses of reality. In attempting to fulfill fantasies or objectives that have become more and more consuming, they abandon logic and caution and ignore values that once were important to them. They attempt sexual behaviour at great risk and cost. Their defence mechanisms of projection, blame, and denial increase along with this escalating behaviour. Dramatic unmanageability results. Severe family strain as well as work and financial problems appear. Legal complications and even physical symptoms, such as insomnia or hypertension, may indicate escalating addiction.

For many addicts, escalation causes further unmanageability through substantial changes in other addictions (i.e. alcoholism or overeating) or compulsive behaviours (shoplifting and working). Changes in these concurrent addictions may mean an increase or a decrease in the addictive behaviour.

The shame and despair that come from the powerlessness and unmanageability help crystallize the core beliefs about personal unworthiness that were part of the addict's initial addictive system. These are "I am basically a bad person, unworthy person, no one would love me as I am, my needs are never going to be met if I have to depend on others, and sex is my most important need.

Part of the addiction's strength lies in its flexibly. For as rapidly as it can escalate, it has the power to go underground, lie dormant, and re-emerge at its former strength. We call this the de-escalation mode of the contingent phase as I will describe next.

Addictive Cycle: Symptomology and Criteria for the phase:

- Preoccupation: Fantasy life expands, including new or different behaviours and a problem solving quality.
- Ritualization: Rituals become variations of a theme.
- Behaviour: Rapid escalation of behaviour may include changes of intensity, range, or levels of behaviour.

- Despair: Excitement is balanced by an ongoing desperation with peaks of depression and even suicidal feelings.
- Belief System: Dramatic surge of behaviour shifts core beliefs into dominance.
- Impaired Thinking: Reality lapses are frequent as logic and caution are abandoned and defence mechanisms increase.
- Unmanageability: Severe strain on family, work and finances are compounded with legal consequences, physical symptoms, and shifts in concurrent addictions.

Fourth Stage: Contingent Phase; De-escalation Mode

In this mode, the addiction is still fully established, but for various reasons, addictive behaviours are less frequent, less risky; in general, there is less unmanageability. Behaviour may de-escalate for the remainder of the addict`s life without the addict dismantling the internal addictive system and really recovering. Or behaviour may escalate and the addiction may progress to the acute phase.

Some addicts, shocked at their own behaviour and its consequences, make a radical shift in an effort to control their addiction. The shock may have come from finally coming face to face with the unmanageability of their lives. They may have been arrested or have had a near miss. Their behaviour almost became public, or did. Someone in their family find out. They have run out of money. Or they have lost a job. Sometimes they are simply overwhelmed by despair. Whatever the reason, they make a dramatic effort to change their lives. Those addicts who subscribe to the narrow model of good versus evil-essentially a model built on shame and control-may return to the church.

Having come face to face with my unmanageability has caused me to make some dramatic changes. However it has not been a return to the church. Personally, I see many churches to be moralistic in its battle to control the lust driven sinner and shares a common element with the addict: obsession. The battlefield becomes a narrow continuum in which the only options are to be good or to be bad, licence or legalism. I think it excludes spirituality because it is not able to hold these things in tension. At best it is soulish and is characterized more as judge than an agent of grace and love.

Joseph Chilton Pearce quotes William Blake by saying,

> "The word satan means "the accuser." Keeping this in mind, consider that the church becomes allied with satan when it becomes the accuser of sin. His claim is that accusation, a dark addendum to the gospel spread by the church, nullifies the light of the gospel given to us by that figure on the cross. You can't have both the darkness of accusation and the light of the gospel—the darkness dispels the light. Hence Paul's exhortation, let those who are spiritual among you restore him in a spirit of meekness, of gentleness, remembering yourselves...

In my case having experienced judgement and no gentle restoration, I have not been able to return to the church as I struggle with the pseudo-spirituality. Because of my status as fallen pastor, I feel deep shame and rejection along with the stigma attached to my addiction. I have made special effort to become part of a recovery group and meet with a group of Christian guys who are seeking intimacy with God. I continue to recognize room for further healing and forgiveness in this area of my life.

For other addicts whose religious experiences have at best been peripheral, it may be a time for conversion experiences. Their conversion significantly occurs immediately after a major unmanageability event such as an arrest. Unfortunately, they may adopt wholesale the belief system of their new community in place of a thoughtful, long-term spiritual pilgrimage that integrates a new understanding with integrity.

Identifying de-escalation is difficult since it may look like recovery. The addict makes every effort to make life manageable and to live an honourable life. If the addict does not get involved in the church, there is usually some special effort to become part of a respectable group. There may be a surge of responsible behaviour at work. There is even a honeymoon period with the family members, as the addict attempts to make up for the way he or she has complicated their lives.

Most importantly, there is a rapid de-escalation to safe or acceptable sexual behaviour. Addicts may go to extremes and try to obliterate all sexual feelings. Some keep a low level of behaviour going, e.g., masturbation to soft-core magazines instead of hardcore porn, or keeping just one meaningful relationship. Others return to activities typical of their establishment or initiation phases. Addicts in the de-escalation mode often are still isolated. They still feel precariously close to sexually compulsive behaviour, because reducing the addictive behaviour did not reduce their alienation. They continue to guard their secret world, either to hide their obsession (which convinces them that they are not curable) or to keep intact the web of lies they wove during the time they were acting out. Thus, de-escalation is not recovery. Honesty with oneself and others, self-acceptance that includes one's illness, and support for change by people who know the addiction's power to delude are prime determinants for recovery.

Addicts in the de-escalation mode have, due to some catastrophe brought on by a totally unmanageable life, been stunned into deciding that they must quit. Believing their only options are to be "good" or to be "evil," instead of well versus sick, they feel caught at every turn: they want to be good but cannot stop thinking about being evil. Their impaired thinking tells them that their only alternative to the continuing catastrophe of addiction is a grim determination and a life without happiness or sex. Hopelessness is added to despair.

However, because such a life looks untenable, addicts may continue to "play" with the addiction during the de-escalation phase. They test themselves by going through the ritual of the point of acting out, but then stopping:

- going to a bar, but then leaving
- flirting with someone, but stopping before anything can happen
- seeing old sex partners, just "as friends"
- driving the old routes and perhaps even masturbating but not letting anyone see
- going into the massage parlour, asking prices, and then leaving
- buying a pornographic item, and then throwing it away

Such toying with rituals reinforces the addicts' beliefs that they can control it, that they are in charge of their behaviour. They are in fact getting high while minimizing risk. Sooner or later, in all probability, they will have a slip that may reactivate the addictive cycle. In fact, in the de-escalation mode, the cycle is simply suspended. Its basic elements and its supporting system are intact, active, and ready to be fully engaged.

Addicts can remain in the de-escalation phase indefinitely with only an occasional slip to remind them of their vulnerability. However, when addiction escalates to the acute phase, everything changes.

Addictive Cycle: Symptomology and Criteria of this phase:

- Preoccupation: Fantasy life can remain intense but may diminish entirely for periods of time.
- Ritualization: Rituals may be restricted except to "play" with addiction by tempting self.
- Behaviour: Rapid de-escalation of behaviour to safe, marginal or acceptable behaviour.
- Despair: Obsession with guilt and shame over behaviour may replace or co-exist with addictive preoccupation.
- Belief System: Core beliefs do not abate, keeping addict isolated and acting "as if."
- Impaired Thinking: Reality of near catastrophes breaks through delusion, leaving addicts stunned and even hopeless.
- Unmanageability: Efforts to make life manageable and to live an honourable life may result in excessive religiosity, shifts in concurrent addictions, responsibility at work, and "honeymoon" periods at home.

Fifth Stage: Acute Phase

The individual breaks with reality, abandoning his or her value system, becoming alienated from significant others and isolated within him or herself. Typically, addiction plateaus at a high level of activity; behaviour patterns become rigid. The addiction cycle is played out despite obvious risks; preoccupation is almost constant while shame and despair are seldom, if ever, felt. The addiction may continue to an end stage, stopped only by physical or social consequences such as death or confinement. Or addiction may de-escalate.

Addictive Cycle: Symptomology and Criteria of this phase:

- Preoccupation: Sexualization of thought patterns take on a desperate quality.
- Ritualization: Rituals become rigid despite even obvious danger, risk, or cost.
- Behaviour: Constant twenty-four hour to seventy-two hour behaviour cycles.
- Despair: Awareness of personal pain as well as impact on others diminishes.
- Belief System: Massive acceptance of addictive belief system governs daily behaviour.
- Impaired Thinking: Breaks with reality generate predatory thought processes and signal abandonment of value system.
- Unmanageability: Significant life losses occur including job, family, and finances as well as legal, physical, and other addictive complications.

Sixth Stage: Chronic Phase

The use of the word chronic in connection with illness means that the condition resists treatment. Most chronic phase addicts are institutionalized. The addicts rituals are extremely predictable and rigid, the behaviour limited only by opportunity. Some addicts are unreachable. Events in early childhood, for example, may have been so destructive that the resulting character disorder is not easily treated.

For chronic addicts, the damage to the sense of self-the loss of faith in self and others-may be beyond repair. This damage betrays itself in impaired thinking: the addict sees him-or herself as a victim, blames everyone else for all his or her troubles, and admits no personal responsibility. While many addicts start therapy thinking that way, sooner or later their denial gives way to the overwhelming evidence of their powerlessness and the unmanageability of their lives. However, in a chronic case, the addict seems incapable of admitting denial, or even acknowledging the addictive sex acts.

Addictive Cycle: Symptomology and Criteria for this phase:

- Preoccupation: No life occurs beyond the obsession.
- Ritualization: Rigid rituals extremely predictable.
- Behaviour: Behaviour limited only by opportunity.
- Despair: No apparent awareness of personal pain.
- Belief System: Damage to sense of self may be beyond repair.
- Impaired Thinking: Personal responsibility never acknowledged.
- Unmanageability: Nothing to hold on to or to work for.

I believe that Patrick Carnes gives a very comprehensive understanding of the pathology of the sexual addiction, and his 12 step model of recovery is helpful, however I don't believe it goes far enough. Primarily because it leaves one to believe that once an addict always an addict and one then defines themselves and their identity by what they do, not who they were created to be. I don't discard the pathology of sexual addiction as it relates to the physiology (the body) and psychology (the soul) of the individual but it does not address the deeper part of our being and that is our spirit. Our spirit is where the real disastrous effect of sexual addiction and lust has distorted our true identity and caused us to live out of a false self.

It is for this reason that I want to leave the clinical pathology of addiction and take time to focus on the nature of man and who we were created to be and ultimately how God sees us in body, soul and spirit. As I alluded to in chapter 3, I believe in order to experience recovery we need to understand the fundamentals of who we are by nature. It raises the question, who am I? Simply an addict (my identity being defined by my behavior and the pathology of my actions) or am I a Saint (a child of God, who has addictive behaviors).

Please bare with me as I go quite deep into the theological well to explore our true nature. I believe it is paramount that we understand the source and cause of the spiritual disease that has plagued our lives before addressing the symptoms of the disease that manifest itself in our soul and body.

Part III

The Nature of Man

Chapter 6
The Image and Likeness of Man

The Nature of Man

There are some very clear keys in the Scripture that can guide us in our understanding of our nature but also aid in our recovery. Just as doctors begin their training by dissecting a body so that they will understand its workings, so should we begin by understanding what is in the Scriptures about the nature of man. We can do this by asking the question, "What is man?"

A clue to the nature of man can be seen in the Trinitarian nature of God. There is only one God, but within the Godhead there are three "persons"- God the Father, God the Son and God the Holy Spirit. It is not surprising, therefore, that man, who is made in the image and likeness of God, should have a reflection of this trinity in his own being.

When writing to the Thessalonians, Paul most clearly defined the trinity of man. He prayed that they might be whole in spirit, soul and body (1 Thessalonians 5:23). By so doing, he directly implied that man has three distinct dimensions to his creation. Ray Stedman in his sermon *The Glory and the Misery of Man* not only emphasizes this trinity within man but expands on the uniqueness of the phrase, "the image" and "likeness" of God. Notice that this was never said of any other creature, never said of any animal, bird, fish or plant. This is the glory and the dignity of man, that at the beginning he was made in the image and likeness of God. Peter Horrobin, one of the founders of Ellel Ministries and whose Theophostic Model I had some training in, states in his book *Healing through Deliverance*,

> "Not even the angels, as spiritual beings, were given the capacity "to come in the flesh" and be at one and the same time beings with a spirit, a soul and a body. The capacity "to come in the flesh" is unique to God and to those who are made in His image. That is why the phrase "He came in the flesh" is such a critical statement in the major Christian creeds.

So it raises the question, what is that image? How does it appear in us? Of what does the image of God in man consist? Is it visible or invisible? Is it physical or immaterial? Is it the body, the soul, or the spirit?

The Image of God in Man

The Mormons (among others) teach that the image of God in man is the body of man; that is what is made after the image of God. They base this upon certain anthropomorphic expressions in the Scripture, those expressions which seem to impute human features to God, e.g., the eyes of God, the fingers of God, the hands of God, etc. The Mormons take these literally and say they prove that God does indeed have a body like our body. This is fundamental to the teachings of the Mormon faith. They fail to see that they are really turning the whole issue around and saying that it is God who is made in the image of man.

If, in this sense, man is in the image of God, then it is also true that apes and monkeys are made in the image of God, because bodily they look very much like us.

But if we are saying that God has a body, we also must ask, what kind of a body? What does it look like? What color eyes does God have? What is the color of his skin? Is it black or yellow or brown or what? What does God look like? You only need to ask questions like this to see how absurd this whole proposition is that God has a body like ours.

Anyone who is acquainted at all with the Scripture in depth knows that it specifically denies this about God. He does not have a body.

Then what is the image of God in man? Is it the soul of man? Is it because we are able to function on the level of the rational that we are like God? Is it because we are able to feel, to sense, to have emotional reactions? Is it because we have the faculty of volition and can choose and make decisions? These are the functions of the soul; and it is true that God also does these things. He thinks, he reasons, he feels, he reacts, he chooses, he decides. But if this is also true of God, it is likewise true of the animals. As we have already seen, they function in the same way though to a lesser degree. There is nothing distinctive about his soul that marks man as different from the animals. We cannot find the image of God there.

The last choice is the spirit of man, and here we do find something unique. No other creature of God, in this earthly realm, has a spirit, or more accurately, *is* a spirit. We are told specifically by the Lord Jesus in that remarkable account of his meeting with the woman of Samaria at the well, "God is Spirit, and those who worship Him must worship in spirit and truth," (John 4:24). Here was a poor, worldly woman, who had no education and evidently was not trained in theological matters, yet to her He imparted this great truth. Again, after the resurrection, appearing to his disciples, he identified his resurrected body as the one that had been crucified and laid in the grave. Then He said to them, "a spirit does not have flesh and bones, as you see Me have," (Luke 24:39). That is, a spirit can exist without a body, and God is Spirit.

Thus it is this that marks the image of God in man. Man, likewise, is spirit. This is the basic, fundamental nature of man. I have a body in which I live, much as I would live in a tent or house. When the apostles speak of leaving the body they speak of departing from it as one would from a house. I also have a soul by which I function on the levels of rational, volitional and emotional experience. But I am a spirit. That is the fundamental me, the fundamental you; we are spirits. Because we are spirits, dwelling in bodies (at least in our present stage of existence), it is a mistake to identify ourselves with our bodies, or even our souls' reactions. Fundamentally, we are spirits, invisible, unseen by one another, and yet expressing ourselves through the avenues of the body and the soul.

Now what is Godlike about our spirit? The spirit is made in the image of God, and, if so, then it can do things that God can do but no animal can. What are those faculties of spirit? Let me suggest three of them, at least. Perhaps there are others but I want to mention three:

First, there is creativity. "God made... God created... God formed... God fashioned." That kind of activity involves imagination, the ability to think in conceptual terms, i.e., abstract thinking, the ability to see a thing with the eye of the mind and then fashion it with whatever powers are available. This great faculty man shares with God. Man too is creative. Not to the same degree that God is, for we cannot make things out of nothing, as God does, but we can fashion things, make things. Man can compose a symphony or design a computer, he can paint a picture and plan a building, and he can even devise a new recipe. A baby can stack blocks on the floor and make a playhouse and, in imagination, enter it and live in it. No animal can do this. Man has the function of creativity because he is made in the image of God. This is the dignity of mankind that separates him, by a vast gulf, from the whole animal creation.

Unlike the animal kingdom, creativity can involve a union of forces in both our creative passions and our quests through a process that functions the same regardless of the character or nature. Current research shows the human brain to be far more flexible then we thought, shifting and changing according to stimuli from the environment. This circuit is sparked by the passion of the right hemisphere and its connections to the emotional-limbic brain, which is itself the connection to the heart. It is through this connection of the two hemispheres that we may have our creative moment. The left hemisphere prepares itself to receive what it going to be transmitted from the right hemisphere. It is in this process that we can experience eureka, a moment of enlightenment or creativity.

> "Like Mozart's creative procedure, to suggest it was simply breathed through him as though he were simply a channel would at best be disservice. His own comment was, "No one knows how hard I have to work

> at this," referring to the difficult translation stage before all was ready for the easier part of pen and ink. For the "answer" to move through Mozart, the neural pathways had to be formed and constantly tended, the soil tilled continually, even though such control must eventually be released to allow another part of the self to manifest. Perhaps Mozart was given much because he could receive it. (Pearce)

This may explain varying degrees of creativity and enlightenment between each of us, but each person bearing no less than the other the uniqueness of being made in the image of God.

Secondly, God communicates. He speaks, and so does man. Man is the only creature that can talk. Perhaps some are saying that animals also can communicate with one another. Animals do make sounds, but they do not communicate, they do not speak, as we use that term. They do not use language. They have certain signals which they utter and which are mutually understandable. But they do not convey ideas, they do not discuss matters together, they do not talk over an issue as we do. This ability is reserved for man.

We have found that the universe sprang into being because God speaks. It is the word of God which forms the ages, says the writer to the Hebrews. God uses words as power, which alters, changes, and affects events and people. This too is the way man speaks. We alone of all created beings on the earth are able to appreciate the power of a word and to use it to alter lives or to shape history. Someone once asked, "What are the three sweetest words in the English language?" To this he received a reply, "I love you." We know how words can affect us and change us. Words can wreck lives, they can heal and harm, injure and restore. What an amazing faculty is speech! It is part of the image of God in man.

Thirdly, we see in the creation story that God is always pronouncing things good. He is therefore a moral being, and man shares that character as well. Man, too, is a moral being. He has the faculty of being able to distinguish between good and evil. Remarkably enough, even in societies where there is a denial of morals, as in the relativistic society of today, men still go on pronouncing things good or evil. The standards may vary but the result remains: some things are called good and other things bad. This practice is found universally among men. Everywhere man has a consciousness of moral values. We feel the gnawing of a bad conscience when it sits in judgment over us. Even though we try to stifle it, it keeps insinuating itself upon us and we cannot get away from it. We recognize moral choices and moral values, and this marks us as having been made in the image of God.

Now with these three remarkable faculties: the ability to create (with all man's wonderful inventiveness involved in that); the ability to communicate (to share ideas which affect, and infect, others), and the divine ability to treat certain things as bad and others as good, man was told to do two specific things. The command came, "Be fruitful and multiply and fill the earth" (that is one command, given in three different ways).

Secondly, he was told to subdue it; and have dominion over the fish of the sea and over the birds of the air and over every living thing that moves upon the earth. Man was given the task of filling up the earth. To rule it and govern it, by exercising dominion over everything within the earth to subdue its forces, to master them and bring them all under his control and direction. The whole course of history is simply the record of man's attempt to fulfill these divine injunctions. As a race we have never forgotten these commands and have been engaged in doing them ever since.

But what have been the results? The interesting thing is that the fulfilling of these divine commands, given to man at the earliest dawn of history, has produced results which are utterly disastrous. Man retains the image of God, but now the creature that is called "God's glory" has become God's shame. Men behave as children, without reason, irrationally. As someone has well put it, "Our problem seems to be that we're suffering from a prolonged adolescence merging into a premature senility."

Why is this? To understand how and why this is true, we must first look at the bigger picture. Again looking at the creation story at the risk of repeating myself, it is paramount that we understand these doctrinal truths if we want to understand the key fundamentals behind addiction.

In the beginning God said, "Let Us make man in Our image, according to Our likeness; and let them rule over the fish of the sea and over the birds of the sky and over the cattle and over all the earth" (Genesis 1:26). "Then the Lord God formed man of dust from the ground, and breathed into his nostrils the breath of life; and man became a living being" (Genesis 2:7). The Lord God said, "It is not good for the man to be alone; I will make him a helper suitable for him" (verse 18). "The man and his wife were both naked and were not ashamed" (verse 25).

As already stated God created humans in His own image. He breathed life into a hunk of clay and Adam became spiritually and physically alive. However, something was missing. It was not good for Adam to be alone, and no animal form of life could fulfill his need. So "God created a suitable helpmate for him" (verses 21-23). Together they were "naked and were not ashamed" (verse 25). Their bodies had no dirty parts. The sexual relationship between husband and wife was not separated from an intimate relationship with God. There was no sin, nothing to hide, therefore, no reason to cover up.

Adam and Eve's purpose and responsibility was to rule over the rest of God's creation. God placed them in the "Garden of Eden to cultivate it and keep it" (verse 15). By being fruitful and multiplying, they could fill the earth. As long as they remained in a dependent relationship with God, Adam and Eve were given tremendous freedom. They had a perfect life, and they could have lived forever in the presence of God. There was no need to either search for significance nor strive for acceptance, because they had a divine purpose. They were totally secure in the presence of God. They also had a sense of belonging to God and to each other. God provided for their every need.

The ability to think and make choices was inherent in Creation, because Adam and Eve were created in the image of God. It is apparent from Scripture that evil was in the universe (Isaiah. 14:12-14; Ezekiel 28:11-19). "The Lord, therefore, commanded Adam and Eve not to eat from the tree of the knowledge of good and evil" (Genesis. 2:17). He explained that if they ate the fruit, they would die. Satan was not going to silently sit by and let God's plan to rid the universe of evil go uncontested. So he questioned and twisted the Word of God and tempted Eve (Genesis 3:4-6). Satan used the same three channels that exist today:

"the lust of the flesh and the lust of the eyes and the boastful pride of life" (I John 2:16). Deceived by the craftiness of Satan, Adam and Eve made a choice, thus declaring their own independence. They died!

They did not die physically, they died spiritually, although physical death would also be a consequence of sin (Romans 5:12). The effect was immediate. All the inherent personal attributes of Creation (spiritual life, identity, acceptance, security, significance) were gone, and each became a glaring need.

Adam was overcome with shame and guilt. He covered his nakedness, and hid from God. But the Lord immediately took the initiative by confronting Adam. "Where are you?" "And he (Adam) said, 'I heard the sound of You in the garden, and I was afraid because I was naked; so I hid myself." And He said, "Who told you that you were naked? Have you eaten from the tree of which I commanded you not to eat?" " And the man said, 'The woman who You gave to be with me, she gave me from the tree, and I ate" (Genesis 3:9-12). The Lord knew the answers before He asked Adam the questions. So why did He ask? He wanted Adam to immediately become accountable for his actions.

Adam responded by blaming Eve and suggesting maybe even God had something to do with his downfall. He thought, after all God, You were the one who created this woman for me. Ever since Adam's first sin, we have resorted to defensive patterns of projecting blame for our own downfalls. Every addict must first get through his or her own denial of the problem before he or she can begin to address it.

Precedence was established for the degradation of humanity in the Creation and Fall of Adam and Eve. The gospel offers the only hope for a solution. When Adam and Eve lost their relationship with God, they were immediately overcome with fear and guilt. The first emotion expressed by fallen humanity was fear. Adam confessed, "I was afraid because I was naked, so I hid myself" (Genesis 3:10). Fear of being exposed drives many away from the light that reveals their sin. They run from the light or discredit its source because they do not understand God's unconditional love and acceptance. Satan raises up thoughts "against the knowledge of God" (2 Corinthians10:5), and a deceived humanity mocks His very existence. Unable to achieve God's eternal standards for morality, the fallen are left alone to deal with their fears, guilt and shame.

So although we did not lose what it is to be made in the image of God (to have the ability to rule and have dominion and the ability to create) we did lose the second part "our likeness of God."God made man in his image but also after his likeness. Well, you ask, what is the difference between image and likeness? Aren't these the same thing? No, they are closely related, but they are not the same thing.

The Likeness of God in Man

The image, as we have already seen, is the existence of man as a spirit. It is the equipment that God has given us, the capacity to be godlike. The likeness is the proper functioning of that equipment. It raises the question of whether man is actually godlike or merely has the capacity to be so. As he was made in the beginning, man was both in the image and after the likeness of God. Thus when Adam was formed by the Creator he stood before God as a spirit dwelling in a body, exercising the functions of a soul. He had the ability to be creative, to communicate, and to make moral choices. But he not only had the ability to do so, he was actually doing it. He was exercising the function of godlikeness.

The secret, as we learn from the rest of Scripture, lay in an inner dependence that continually repudiated self confidence. This is the hard lesson for us to learn. How confident we are in ourselves. How sure we are that if we set our mind on something we can do it. If we are motivated enough to obtain a thing, all we have to do is to mobilize our resources, set our jaws, clench our fists and move to it and we will get it done. That is the false self-confidence that has been the ruin of the human race. But the principle of godlikeness is the repudiation of that self-confidence and a resting on the working of another who dwells within. That is what Adam knew. That is the way he functioned, and thus fulfilled his manhood and manifested the likeness of God.

If you want to see this in history, read the record of the Gospels concerning the Lord Jesus. See him stilling the storm on the Sea of Galilee with but a word, "Peace, be still" (Mark 4:39). See him walking on the water in the middle of the storm, to the concern and fright of the disciples. Watch Him changing the water, instantly, into wine. How does He do these things? Is it because He is the Son of God? Is it because He is the Creator that He can do this? No, He Himself denied that. He said it was not because He was God the Son that He did these things. He said, "The Son can do nothing of Himself" (John 5:19). "The words that I speak unto you," He said repeatedly, "are not my words. The works that I do are not My works." "The Father who dwells in Me, He does the works" (John 14:10). All is done out of a reliance upon the work of the Father indwelling Him. He knew the secret of manhood, the lost secret of humanity.

What this world has forgotten and is vainly groping and seeking after, what every course in psychology is hoping to find, what every self-improvement program is attempting to realize but never can, this lost secret of how man was intended to operate, He knew. The likeness of God is lost. That is why man can create, but everything he creates has a twist toward evil. That is why he can communicate, but not only does he communicate truth and beauty, but also lust, hate, filth, bigotry and death. That is why, though he still knows moral values, he denies them and rationalizes them to exalt evil, just as the last verse of Romans 1 describes: "men who not only do evil things but delight in watching others do the same things" (Romans 1:32).

This is where the gospel comes in. The Apostle Paul shows us the plan of God to counteract the fall of man. In Colossians 3:9 and 10, he says to the Christians, "Do not lie to one another, seeing that you have put off the old nature with its practices and have put on the new nature, which is being renewed in knowledge after the image of its creator" (Colossians 3:9-10).

There is the likeness of God, being restored in man. The image of God has never been lost, for man still retains the capacity to be godlike but he has no longer the ability -- until Jesus Christ is restored to the human heart. When he enters there begins a process which, little by little, step by step, day by day, through trial and heartache, sorrow, disappointment, and judgment, through glory, and blessing, and thrilling experiences of grace, is changing us so as to reproduce in us the likeness of God once again. Thus we not only have the capacity to be Godlike, we are actually becoming Godlike. That is what God is after. Being renewed in knowledge is the restoration of the likeness of God.

This is why Jesus said to the woman at the well, "God is Spirit, and they that worship him must worship in spirit [in the image of God] and in truth" [in the likeness of God] (John 4:24). Remember also that verse in Second Corinthians where Paul says. "But we all, with open face beholding as in a glass the glory of the Lord [that is, seeing the face of the Lord Jesus through the experiences of our life, in the nitty-gritty of life, through the humdrum routines of life, in the high points and the low spots], are being changed from glory to glory into the same image, by the Spirit of the Lord" (2 Corinthians 3:18). That is the process of restoring the likeness of God in man.

It is not surprising, therefore, that man, who is made in the image and likeness of God, should have a reflection of God's trinity in his own being. That trinity within man consists of the body, soul and spirit. In this section it will be important to clarify not only the difference of these three areas of our being but to also shed light on how the enemy affects humans and interferes in our lives, in contrast to how God works in our lives.

Chapter 7
The Trinitarian Nature of Man

The Scriptures appeared to be quite clear in separating these three parts of being. I Thessalonians 5:23 states, "Now may the God of peace Himself sanctify you entirely; and may your **spirit** and **soul** and **body** be preserved complete without blame at the coming of our Lord Jesus Christ." And Hebrews 4:12 states, "For the word of God is living and active and sharper than any two-edged sword, and piercing as far as the division of **soul** and **spirit**, of both joints and marrow (**body**), and able to judge the thoughts and intentions of the heart."

The Word of God itself is structured with this nature in mind. The five poetical books: Job, Psalms, Proverbs, Ecclesiastes, and the Song of Solomon. Are a reflection of the rejoicing and the protests of man in response to life. They reflect all the changing, colorful passions of life; all the feelings of the heart, of the soul; the deep-seated, almost inexpressible yearnings and desires of men and women, all are found in these books. Because man is a threefold being, and these five books are bound to man, they reflect what man is -- what we are. They fall into three divisions which correspond to the makeup of man -- the spirit, the soul, and the body.

Bear with me as I take some liberty to expand on this to help you have a deeper appreciation for the Bible and help to make it more practical for you in your recovery. As a pastor I was often told by people that they want to read the Bible but didn't know where to start. As an addict I would suggest you begin with the book of Job, which addresses the needs of the spirit of man -- the song of the spirit. Job is the oldest of the books of the Bible and, in many ways, the most profound, because it is the deep protest of the spirit of man in the face of apparently senseless suffering.

The book of Job faces this problem squarely. It tells what the answer is, for here is the cry of a tortured man who cannot understand the ways of God. I have often heard this cry -- as does anyone who works with human beings to any extent at all -- this deep, almost unuttered, inexpressible protest from the very center of man's being, the spirit of man within him crying out in a tragic protest against the seemingly senseless suffering that life affords.

Most of us know the story of Job. It is a rather simple story. It begins in heaven with an encounter between God and Satan. Satan comes and challenges God, and God challenges Satan in return and calls his attention to a man named Job, a man of remarkable ability. It is difficult to place the land of Uz, where he lived, but we can logically fit the time of the book of Job between the eleventh and twelfth chapters of the book of Genesis -- way back in the history of man. God said to Satan (Job 1:8),

"Have you considered my servant Job, that there is none like him on the earth, a blameless and upright man, who fears God and turns away from evil?" (Job 1:8b)

Satan didn't challenge that statement, but he raised a question about it (verses 9b-12a):

"Does Job fear God for not? Hast thou not put a hedge about him and his house and all that he has, on every side? Thou hast blessed the work of his hands, and his possessions have increased in the land. But put forth thy hand now, and touch all that he has, and he will curse thee to thy face." And the Lord said to Satan, "Behold, all that he has is in your power; only upon himself do not put forth your hand" (Job 1:9b-12a).

You know the story -- how there came one tragic event after another. As soon as the message had arrived about one terrible catastrophe it was immediately followed by another. An invading army took away all of Job's wealth. A windstorm destroyed his house; his children had been gathered in it, and they were all killed. One by one, the tragic reports came to him -- until everything was swept away in one day. What a terribly shocking experience! But Job was absolutely unmoved. He bowed in sorrow before God, but his heart was open to him. God said to Satan, "You see, Job still serves me" (Job 2:3). And Satan made that famous statement, "All that a man has he will give for his life" (Job 2:4b). Then he went on to argue, "The trouble is, you haven't touched him deeply enough yet. Let me touch his body, and then you will see him turn and curse you to your face" (Job 2:5). God said, "He is in your power; only spare his life" (Job 4:6b).

The result was the outbreak of a terrible siege of boils on Job. The book tells us he was covered with boils from the top of his head to the soles of his feet. The closest I can relate to this was when I was around age twelve and had a severe outbreak of poison ivy. Without knowing it at the time, my sister and I were actually playing in a bush of it for several hours. Needless to say we were both covered from head to toe and both highly allergic. I had severe blisters from the bottom of my feet and all over my body including my face. The itching at times was unbearable and I might say torturous, my skin was so raw that it was beginning to fall off my feet. My only comfort was that my sister was suffering the same fate, and her face had swollen to the size of being unrecognizable.

Even one boil will keep a man well occupied as I recently discovered with a planters wart on my heel, when being treated with liquid nitrogen seemed only to increase the pain. But here was a man who had boils from the top of his head to the soles of his feet. So poor Job took a potsherd with which to scrape himself, and sat on ashes. In abject misery he faced the situation in which he found himself - the cry of a tortured man who cannot understand what life has done to him.

When you get to that place you discover what the whole book is all about. The book of Job is nothing more or less than Chapter 7 of the book of Romans. You will recall that the Apostle Paul ends that chapter by saying (verse 24),

"Wretched man that I am! Who will deliver me from this body of death?" (Romans 7:24)

This is exactly where God brings Job. Thus we learn that apparent punishment or suffering at God's hand is the way by which he teaches us that man by himself is helpless, that he can do nothing, and has nothing to stand upon. But God is sufficient for every circumstance of life. All man needs is God, and God only. When we come to this place in Job, or Romans 7, then we are ready to hear the great declaration of Romans 8 (verses 1, 4b, 2): "There is therefore now no condemnation for those who are in Christ Jesus ... who walk not according to the flesh but according to the Spirit... For the law of the Spirit of life in Christ Jesus has set me free from the law of sin and death." This is where Job ended up. As a result God, in tender grace and mercy, poured out blessing upon him. He entered into what is the equivalent of a 'Romans 8 experience.' If you would like to understand the book of Job, read Romans 7 and 8. Conversely, if you want to understand Romans 7 and 8, read the book of Job.

Then we come to the second division in the books of Psalms, Proverbs and Ecclesiastes. Here we have the songs of the soul. The soul of man is made up of three faculties as I stated earlier: the intelligence, the emotions and the will - or, to put them in the order in which these books address them, the emotions, the intelligence and the will. In the book of Psalms we have all that the soul ever experiences in terms of emotional responses to circumstances. In the book of Proverbs we have the intelligence at work, working out through experience the best way to react to situations - all the accumulated wisdom of man, guided by divine light. In the book of Ecclesiastes we have the will of man expressed - the deliberate investigation and exploration by the will of various areas of knowledge and experience.

The book of Psalms is intended to express every possible facet of human emotion. The longing of hope is expressed in the Messianic Psalms; the burning of anger in the Imprecatory Psalms - those Psalms which seem to call down fire from heaven on everything which opposes God. The expression of sorrow is found in the Penitential Psalms; the glorying in grace in those Psalms which rejoice in victory. Whatever your feeling is, turn to the Psalms! All the expressions of the heart are found reflected in the Psalms. As a recovering addict I have found myself going back to Psalms 51 more than any other Psalm and asking God to be gracious to me according to His loving kindness and according to the greatness of His compassion and echoing the words of David as he confessed his sexual sin to God.

The book of Proverbs follows. It is the expression of the intelligence of man guided by divine wisdom. Here you have the logical, reasonable approach to life -- the discovery of the laws of heaven for life on earth. It is a very simple book and begins with a wonderful introduction explaining why it was written. I love these words (verses 1-6):

The proverbs of Solomon, son of David, king of Israel:

> "That men may know wisdom and instruction,
> understanding words of insight,
> receive instruction in wise dealing,
> righteousness, justice, and equity;
> that prudence may be given to the simple,
> knowledge and discretion to the youth --
> the wise man also may hear and increase in learning,
> and the man of understanding acquire skill,
> to understand a proverb and a figure,
> the words of the wise and their
> riddles" (Proverbs 1:1-6).

"And then the secret of it all:

> The fear of the Lord is the beginning of knowledge;
> fools despise wisdom and instruc-
> tion" (Proverbs 1:7).

There follows a series of remarkable discourses on wisdom, given from a father to a son. Ten times in this section we find words to this effect: "Hear, my son..." The discourses begin with the child in the home, and then follow the youth out into the busy streets of the city as he encounters various circumstances of life. These proverbs teach him how to choose and make friends; then they follow him as he becomes a man facing some of the perils which are at work to destroy his life; and, finally, they help him to discover some of the forces which will make him strong.

Ecclesiastes (the title means "The Preacher") is the protest of man's will against the monotony and emptiness of life. It is a deliberate investigation by a man with unlimited resources and money, and wholly unhindered in the expenditure of his time. Solomon had everything it took, and he deliberately set himself to answer these questions: Can life be satisfying apart from God? Can the things found under the sun satisfy the human heart? He set himself systematically and deliberately, by the choice of his will, to investigate these areas. He first tried knowledge, and he said that the result was nothing but emptiness - vanity. Then he tried pleasure; he gave free reign to his passions - he did whatever he felt like doing. He says it was all vanity. Then he tried wealth, and he found that great amounts of money gave a man no more than poverty. It was all emptiness and vanity. Then he tried philosophy as a means of facing life with its various problems, and the mystery of death, and the inexplicable tragedies of sin. His whole conclusion was, "It is all vanity."

Then his final conclusion, near the end of Chapter 12 (verse 13):

"The end of the matter; all has been heard. Fear God, and keep his commandments; for this is the whole ... of man" (Ecclesiastes 12:13).

Most translations read "the whole duty of man." But the word "duty" is not in the Hebrew: "This is the whole of man."

This man has finally stumbled upon a brilliant truth! He has discovered, after years of searching, that there is nothing which makes man complete except God, and at the conclusion of the book he says so.

The last of the poetical books is the Song of Solomon. In many ways this is probably the least understood and most neglected of all the books of the Bible - probably because it is the expression of the ideal for the human body. It is a flagrantly sensuous book in many ways, for it is a song of the perfection of bodily grace and love. Therefore it has been regarded as shameful - as even the human body itself is oftentimes thought to be shameful, though, of course, it isn't - it is only its abuse which is shameful. It puts bodily life in proper perspective.

The story of the book is a bit difficult to trace, but in general it is the story of a young maiden whose family evidently rented attractive land from King Solomon in the north country of Israel. She is the Cinderella of the family. She has two brothers and two sisters, but she has been left to tend the flocks and to work in the vineyard. She spends her time out in the open sun all day, so she is sunburned. "I am very dark, but comely," she says. She watches the beautiful ladies of the court riding in their carriages up and down the road, and envies them, but is willing to remain in her quiet, humble life. One day she looks up to see a handsome stranger, a shepherd, looking at her very intently. She is a bit disturbed by his gaze, but he says to her, "You are all fair, my love; there is no flaw in you." That goes a long way to establish a friendship, and they soon draw closer to one another. Then he suddenly leaves. But before he goes he promises that he will return, and she believes him. Through the night she dreams of him and wishes for him, remembering what he looks like, and describing him to her friends. Then one day there is a great commotion in the valley. She looks out, and there is the royal carriage of the king, and the entire valley is excited. To the amazement of everyone, the king sends his riders to her house with the message that he desires to see her. She comes out, shy and afraid, and is brought to the royal carriage. When she looks inside she sees that the king is none other than her shepherd lover. He carries her away to the palace, and they enter into a blissful state of wonderful communion together.

As we read the book we can see in it the wonderful old story of God's redeeming grace to man. We are that maiden, and he is the great King who has come down - in disguise, as it were - to manifest his love for us and has gone away, but he shall come again to take us away. In the meantime, there is the expectation of his coming and a yearning for his presence. There is the memory of his preciousness and the rejoicing in his nobility of manhood and the remembrance of his expression of love, as well. When we get through we can see that it is nothing less than what the Apostle Paul describes in Ephesians 5, Verses 25-27:

"Husbands, love your wives, as Christ loved the church and gave himself up for her, that he might sanctify her, having cleansed her by the washing of water with the word, that the church might be presented before him without spot or wrinkle or any such thing, that she might be holy and without blemish" (Ephesians 5:25-27).

This entire section makes it obvious that the Bible is the book that goes with man. It is a description, divinely given, entering into every detail of our lives - spelled out for us - of man as God intended him to be.

I hope this gives you even a deeper appreciation for the Word of God by showing you how it structurally separates the three parts of man in his triune nature. It is exciting and there is so much more I could say to reveal these concepts as I navigate through it and seek to make it active and living for my own recovery. I now want to discuss the distinct parts of man and his triune nature. I will start with the body and end with the spirit.

The Body

The body is the easiest part of our created realm for us to understand and define, primarily because it is a solid and visible reality. The body is our world-consciousness. Through the five senses, we are aware of what goes on around us. There is the physiological aspect. Medical practitioners have made huge strides in their ability to treat physical disorders. But the body is so incredibly complex that even with the enormous advances that scientists have made there are still huge holes in our understanding. Only the sheer genius of God could have conceived and put together hundreds of mutually dependent and perfectly balanced organs to create the human body.

Listen to what Glenn R. Schiraldi in his *Self-Esteem Workbook* says about the human body.

> "At conception, a sperm and egg combine in a way that is only partially understood. From this union is formed a single cell that will multiply countless times according to a unique, unmatchable genetic code that is inherited-the sum of all of one's ancestors. The cells multiply according to the genetic code consisting of six billion steps of DNA. Though it could stretch the length of the adult's body, this genetic code is coiled

within each cell's nucleus to a length of only 1/2500 inch. Soon after conception, cells are producing over 50,000 proteins needed for life. Although each cell contains the same genetic blueprint for the body, and could turn into any kind of cell in the body, cells specialize by activating and repressing certain genes. Thus, some cells become cells of the eye, others become heart cells, others become needed blood vessels or nerves that appear in their proper places at the proper times. Over the course of a lifetime, the cells of the body will manufacture five tons of protein. Each day the mature body produces three hundred billion cells, to maintain the body's total of seventy-five trillion cells. Placed end to end, the cells of the body would stretch 1,180,000 miles!

The heart brings life to every cell. Weighing only eleven ounces, this magnificent muscle tirelessly pumps three thousand gallons of blood each day, beating 2.5 billion times over a course of a lifetime—a pace that would tire other muscles in minutes. The heart actually is two pumps side by side. One propels blood forcefully enough to circulate through the body's seventy-five thousand miles of blood vessels. The other sends blood to the lungs so gently that it does not damage the delicate air sacs there. When separated, cells of the heart beat with different rhythms. Together, however, they beat with the unison and synchrony of an exquisite symphony orchestra. Technology cannot replicate the heart's durability. The force of blood hurled against the aorta would quickly damage rigid metal pipes, while the flexible, tissue-thin valves of the heart are sturdier than any man-made materials.

The 206 bones in the body are ounce for ounce stronger than solid steel or reinforced concrete. Unlike these man-made materials, they become denser and stronger with weight lifting. Sixty-eight constantly lubricated joints allow for incredible continual movement. For example, the thirty-three vertebrae of the spine, supported by four hundred muscles and one thousand ligaments, permit an infinite variety of head and body positions. Or consider the vast capacities of the hand—to powerfully turn the lid of a jar, or delicately remove a splinter. For durability, precision, and complexity, science cannot duplicate the thumb, whose rotation requires thousands of messages from the brain. The hand will tirelessly extend and flex the joints of the fingers—twenty-five million times over a lifetime. Incredibly efficient utilization of space, the marrow of the bones will manufacture 2.5 million red blood cells each second, replenishing a supply of twenty-five trillion red blood cells—which laid end to end would reach thirty – one thousand miles into the sky. Ponder also the role of the body's 650 muscles. A simple step takes two hundred muscles: forty leg muscles lift the leg, while muscles in the back maintain balance, and abdominal muscles keep you from falling backward.

Our senses are also an incredible wonder. You see multicolored flowers, people strolling, clouds lazily rolling, and feel the wind on your face. In less than a blink of an eye, complicated neural circuitry and countless signals in the brain allow you to sense the world around you. Let's consider the wonder of these capacities.

The eyes, ears and nose are truly marvels of miniaturization. When you look at yourself in the mirror, you see in three dimensions though the image is entirely flat. Constant movement of the eyes, equivalent to walking fifty miles a day, and tens of millions of receptors in the retina that perform billions of calculations each second, make the eye more sensitive and priceless than any camera. Unlike the camera, the eyes are self-cleansing.

Conversation displaces the eardrum a distance equal to the diameter of a hydrogen atom. Yet the exquisitely sensitive ears enable us to distinguish individual voices and turn toward the source of the sound. In addition, the ears inform the brain of the slightest postural imbalance.

Compressed into an area smaller than a postage stamp, each nostril has ten million receptors for odors, enabling the brain to distinguish and remember up to ten thousand different scents.

Could you imagine a finer covering for the body than skin? Under the average square centimeter (the size of the little finger's nail) are hundreds of nerve endings that detect touch, temperature, and pain. Not to mention one hundred sweat glands to cool and numerous melanocytes to protect from the sun's rays.

Each moment, the body defends against an army of potent invaders with a defense system that is more sophisticated than any nation's. The skin forms the first line of protection. Its salty, acidic makeup kills many microbes and keeps many other impurities from entering the body. Each day we inhale seventeen thousand pints of air, the equivalent of a small roomful of air, containing twenty billion foreign particles. The nose, airways, and lungs constitute a remarkable, self-contained air-conditioning and humidifying system. Lysozyme in the nose and throat destroys most bacteria and viruses. Mucus traps particles in the airways, and millions of tiny hairs, called cilia, vigorously seep mucus back to the throat for swallowing. Powerful acid in the stomach neutralizes potent microbes, which is why a child can drink water from a puddle and usually remain healthy. In the nose, incoming air is conditioned to a constant seventy-five to eighty percent humidity.

On cold days, additional blood is sent to the nose to warm the air.

Those microbes that evade destruction trigger a most remarkable flurry of activity. Billions of white cells relentlessly ingest or slay invaders that have entered the body. Other cells of the immune system multiply and summon antibody-producing cells. (A million different antibodies can be produced, each specific to a single microbe.) When needed, white cells can trigger fever that helps to defeat invaders, and shut down fever when the battle is over. The lessons of the battle are preserved, as the immune system remembers the invader and the way to defend against it in the future.

Near the digestive tract, which absorbs needed nutrients, is the liver. In addition to five hundred other vital processes, this vital organ processes all nutrients absorbed by the intestines and neutralizes toxins. For example, in the eight seconds it takes for blood to flow through it, the liver greatly detoxifies caffeine or nicotine, which could be deadly if sent directly to the heart.

Overseeing the myriad complexities of the body is the brain. Weighing but three pounds and containing one hundred billion nerve cells, this organ makes even the finest computer seem crude by comparison. Since each nerve cell can connect with thousands of others, each in turn connecting to thousands of others, the flexibility, complexity, and potential of the brain is truly awe inspiring.

The brain, for example, keeps the interior of the body remarkably constant to preserve life. If a person is living in the desert in 120-degree weather, the brain directs more blood to the skin to release heat and increases perspiration. In the Arctic, blood is diverted from the skin to critical internal organs, while shivering

> generates heat. If a person bleeds, water is pulled from tissue into the blood vessels and nonessential blood vessels constrict to keep blood pressure adequate. While maintaining internal equilibrium, the brain also makes decisions, solves problems, dreams, retrieves stored memories, recognizes faces, and affords unlimited capacity for wisdom and personality.
>
> Appreciate for a moment the three hundred million alveoli, or air sacs, in the lungs, which exchange oxygen from the air we breathe for carbon dioxide from the body's cells. Spread flat, these alveoli would almost cover a tennis court."
>
> Ponder the body's ability to repair itself. Unlike a table leg or a pipe, bones, blood vessel, skin, and other parts of the body can self-repair. Many organs have a backup system: two eyes, two kidneys, two lungs. The single, vital liver, however, has an extraordinary capacity for regeneration. It will function if eighty percent is destroyed or cut away, and can rebuild itself in just a few months to its original size.

I did not write to bore you on the human anatomy but to help you see that the way you view your body influences the way you feel about yourself, body, soul and spirit.

This is not the place to get too involved in the whole evolution/creation debate, except to say that the more I learn about the intricacies of the created realm and the more I see of a decaying world, the less credible seem the highly theoretical and totally unproven arguments of the evolutionists.

However one interprets the various theories of the origin of man, God is ultimately the Creator, and I stand by the scriptural assertion that "in the beginning, God created." The body that each of us has is an incredible commentary on the wonder of the created realms. However, as everyone knows, the body does not always function perfectly, and irrespective of how God created man in the first place, his body is now subject to sickness, disease, malformation and accident and is often in need of healing.

It is only when the built-in systems fail, or the injury is so bad that additional help becomes essential, that most people think in terms of medical treatment. Unless one understands something of God's creation of man the working together of body, soul and spirit, it is not always easy to pinpoint the source of the problem and bring healing to the one who is suffering.

The body is a metaphor for our soul and spirit in the way we experience the body is often the way we experience our core selves. For the body, for example, is one way that we can receive and experience love. Consider the feeling of a hug or a gentle touch from someone who genuinely cares. The feeling that the body senses is also perceived by the inner core. As you cultivate appreciation for the body, it becomes easier to experience the core self more kindly.

As sex addicts, we have often come to have a very distorted perception of our bodies and fail to see the correlation between the soul and the spirit. Although I didn't talk about how the body is biologically and physically affected by our sexual addiction in this section, I will in a later chapter.

The Soul

The second distinction of the trinity of man is the soul. The soul can be defined as our self-consciousness, our awareness of who we are and how we relate to other people. This is the psychological aspect of man. When it comes to the soul, one is venturing into territory that cannot be measured by scientists; it is often referred to as soft science, but can be understood in the light of Scriptures and experience. When God created the human race, He gave to each person a living soul. The soul is that dimension of our flesh-life that is eternal. The physical part of our being is unarguably temporary, limited to a tiny span - a time capsule within the realms of eternity.

When the body dies, its period of usefulness is over. The soul, however, is not restricted to the dimensions of time and the limitations of three score years and ten. It is our eternal destiny beyond the grave that gives urgency to evangelism and emphasizes the need to be born again. Each one of us is a spiritual being to whom God gave a soul, and together spirit and soul reside within the body and are the personality that we are.

Most commentators would agree that the soul itself has three principal dimensions- the mind, the emotions and the will, all of which need to be clearly understood if we are to have a doctrine of man that is an adequate foundation on which to build a theology of healing. It is important to realize that the mind, the emotions and the will are not physical organs that can be removed in an operation or given pills, however the body can be given pills and treatment, which can, in turn, have a profound effect on the soul. I want to take a moment to break down each of these functions of the soul because it is paramount that we understand how it functions so that we are better able to put ourselves, God and the enemy in their proper place.

The Mind. The mind is that part of the soul that processes all incoming information through the physical senses, thinks and provides a rational basis on which to make the day-to-day decisions of life. The mind is not the brain but it is a function of the brain. The brain is a biological part of the body and is a large physical organ that acts very much like a computer, storing much information and carrying out many routine functions that control the body without the mind having to think about what needs to be done next. Researcher and neuroscientist Paul D MacLean from the National Institute of Health after a half a century of work presents a complex model of the brain that I think helps us understand how it evolves through the developmental stages of life and how it is impacted by trauma.

McLean describes the brain as "triune or three-parted" which again I see as being consistent with the triune nature of man and his soul. McLean states,

> "The most primitive part of the brain within our brain is the reptilian or visceral, brain. This brain contains our primitive strategy for safety and survival: repetition."

An example of this would be a mammal who wears a path to water and once determined safe, will continue to take this path until it dies. The visceral brain also maintains our body's automatic physical functions, such as breathing.

The next brain within our brain is the paleomammalian, or feeling, brain. This is technically called the limbic system. The limbic system houses our feelings of excitement, pleasure, anger, fear, sadness, joy, shame, disgust amongst all of our other emotions.

The most sophisticated brain system within our brain is the neocortex, or thinking, brain. It gives us our human abilities to reason, use language, plan ahead, and solve complex problems, and so on. Although I don't agree with his evolutionary development theory of the brain, I do believe these three brain systems are independent but they also work together to maintain the equilibrium of the whole brain. The brain system's equilibrium is governed by the need to keep painful distress at a minimum.

The brain has no trouble with life's occasional distress. It uses the expression of emotion to maintain balance. When our distress reaches a certain peak, we storm with anger, weep with sadness, or perspire and tremble with fear. Scientists have shown that tears actually remove stressful chemicals that build up during emotional upset. The brain will naturally be moved to equilibrium by means of the expression of emotion unless we are taught to inhibit it.

The mind or thinking can also, however, override some of the brain's standard bodily instructions or the visceral part of the brain (such as breathing—for a limited period of time it is possible to hold one's breath and suspend the intake of oxygen), but fortunately most of the brain's functional control of the body is totally involuntary. We cannot choose, for example, to make our hearts stop beating. Voluntary control of such vital mechanisms was not programmed into the computer by its Designer!

Also with the mind we can choose whether or not to store important information in the brain, and then we can recall the information when we need it. With the mind we can think through ideas, create pictures, generate schemes and work out plans of action without moving our body an inch. The ability to conceptualize and be creative is one of the strongest evidences that man truly is made in the image of God, who is the Creator.

When a person's mind and brain are dislocated so that there are no longer rational thought processes or consequentially sane bodily behavior, we say that person is mentally ill. The Greek origin of the word psychiatrist, is "doctor of the soul." Modern psychiatry depends heavily on drug treatments that affect chemical processes in the brain (the body). These are undoubtedly effective in suppressing behavior that is both antisocial and damaging, both to the individuals who are unfortunate enough to be suffering and to those who have to care for and live with them. But few psychiatrists would go so far as to claim that such medication is a cure, and many would freely admit that they have little idea as to why the chemicals they give act in the way they do!

Regrettably, the side effects of much medication are considerable, and in psychiatry a balance has to be maintained between destroying either the quality of life of the patients, or that of those who would otherwise have to cope with their bizarre extremes of human behavior.

I am not in any way questioning the integrity or commitment of the psychiatrists. I believe that most of them are dedicated individuals who are operating to the very best of their ability within the parameters that have been laid down for them by their profession. But these parameters inevitably exclude the spiritual dimensions to mental health.

Without a doubt, just as the body can be sick, so can the mind. Coming from a holistic approach I believe we must be aware that the root cause of a person's condition could lie in any one of these areas that I have mentioned. I have some concerns with a one dimensional approach that either is purely biological, psychological or spiritual. I see things to be much more systemic and integrative for example children growing up in dysfunctional families are taught to inhibit the expression of emotion in three ways: first, by not being responded to or mirrored, literally not being seen; secondly, by having no healthy models for naming and expressing emotion; and thirdly, by actually being shamed and/or punished for expressing emotion. Children from dysfunctional families commonly hear things like: "I'll give you something to cry about," they are often actually spanked for being afraid, mad, or sad. But when emotions are inhibited, or when stress becomes overwhelming and chronic, the brain has difficulty. When traumatic stress occurs, the brain system takes extraordinary measures, which is called the "ego defenses", which I will describe later.

With regards to thoughts themselves, I believe thoughts can only come from three possible sources. God can give me a thought. I can choose to think a thought, or the enemy can impose a thought. There is no other source from where thoughts come. For example, I can give you an idea, but I cannot project a thought into your mind and make you believe that you are thinking it. God has limited Himself by giving us a free will, not to impose thoughts. God communicates directly to our spirit. Our mind is an inappropriate tool for understanding God because He is so far beyond our mind's capability.

I Corinthians 2:13-14 drives home this point by stating, "which things we also speak, not in words taught by human wisdom, but in those taught by the Spirit, combining spiritual thoughts with spiritual words. But a natural man does not accept the things of the Spirit of God; for they are foolishness to him, and he cannot understand them, because they are spiritually appraised. Spiritual things are spiritually discerned. We cannot use our minds to understand the things of God directly. The Holy Spirit, through our spirit, must reveal them to us."

We have a clear example of this notion in Scripture when Jesus told the disciples He was going to die on the cross. "And Peter took Jesus aside and began to rebuke Him, saying, "God forbid it, Lord!" This shall never happen to you. But Jesus turned and said to Peter, "Get behind Me, Satan! You are a stumbling block to me; for you are not setting your mind on God's interests, but man's."

Peter said it and thought that it was his own thought, but Jesus recognized that it was not his own thought, but that it was the devil giving him those words, and so commanded the devil, instead of Peter. If the devil could speak through Peter, then he can speak through us.

The Enemy uses thoughts of inferiority to make us believe in his lies; we strive to compensate, withdraw, or make a host of other attempts to cope and coexist with our problem. Therefore we need to learn to discern what the lies are and what truth is. We need to identify the source of our thoughts.

Here lies the key: we need to identify the source of our thoughts. Most are very naive and some give the devil too much credit, however he is opportunistic and does take full advantage when he can. I believe this happens every time when we are growing up and we are given a distorted perception of love. The earlier the emotions are inhibited, the deeper the damage. There is growing evidence that there is a sequence in brain maturation. Neuroscientists have shown that the visceral brain predominates in the later stages of pregnancy and in the first postnatal period.

The limbic brain system or the emotional part of our soul begins to operate during the first six months of life. This emotional brain allows for the important early bonding to take place.

The neocortex is still developing during our early years, and the thinking brain needs a proper environment and proper stimulation in order to develop healthily. In his research on children's cognitive growth, Piaget did not find true logical thinking until approximately six or seven years of age.

When we reflect on the fact that the visceral brain is concerned with survival issues and is governed by repetition, the idea of permanent imprint makes sense. Neuroscientist Robert Isaacson has argued that traumatic memories are difficult to root out because they are memories of life-saving responses. Since the visceral brain learns and remembers, but is poor at forgetting, it imprints the trauma with a permanence that will dominate its future. Whatever a child survives in the first years of life, a time of intense vulnerability, will be registered with survival benefits in mind.

Much of this neurological research supports what every psychotherapist from Freud until now knows firsthand: that neurotic people have a compulsion to repeat. There is also a neurological explanation for the severe over reactive responses I mentioned earlier. Brain researchers have suggested that enlarged neuronal imprints from stressful experience distort how the organism reacts to stimuli as an adult. Ongoing painful experiences actually engrave new circuits in the brain, so that it becomes more and more prepared to recognize as painful stimuli that another person might not notice.

This supports the theory that once the core material is set up in childhood, it acts as an overly sensitive filter shaping subsequent events. The contaminations of the wounded child fall into this category. When an adult with a wounded inner child experiences a current situation which is similar to a prototypic painful event, the original response is triggered as well. Harvey Jackins describes this as "a tape recorder whose on button is stuck." Something which is actually trivial or quite innocuous is reacted to with intense emotion. This is a case of responding to what isn't there on the outside because it is still there on the inside.

John Bradshaw suggests that "original pain feeling work" rests on the hypothesis that the early emotional pain is numbed out and inhibited. We act it out, because it has never been worked out. It can't be worked out because our inhibiting mechanism (ego defenses) keeps us from knowing the emotional pain is there.

We act the feelings out, we act them in, or we project them on to others. Since we can't feel them, and since they are unfinished business, they need expression. Acting out, acting in and projecting these feelings are the only ways our wounded child knows to express them. But acting out, acting in, and projecting are not permanent solutions. My compulsivity (a core wounded child issue) did not end when I quit using. I simply changed it to exercise or work and school.

Until I work out my wounded child's original pain, I would continue to act it out in my insatiable need for excitement and mood alteration. My ego defenses kept the emotions inhibited.

The brain research work of Ronald Melzack may help to explain how ego defenses work. Melzack discovered an adaptive biological response for inhibiting pain which he calls "neuronal gating." He states,

> "That the three separate brain systems within the triune brain have interconnecting fibers that perform both a facilitating and an inhibiting function. Neuronal gating is the way information between the three systems is controlled. What we call repression may take place primarily at the gate between the thinking and feeling brain."

To put it in the simplest way possible, when the emotional pain in the limbic system reaches overwhelming, an automatic mechanism shuts the gate into the neocortex. It's as if there were some loud noise streaming in from another room and you walked over and shut the door. Freud believed that the primary ego defenses are integrated into more sophisticated secondary defenses as the human being matures. These secondary defenses take on a thinking quality. For example: rationalizing, analyzing, explaining away, and minimizing.

R.L. Isaacson supports this theory with the work that he has done. He reports that the gating system of the neocortex (the thinking brain) functions "to overcome the habits and memories of the past...the neocortex is profoundly concerned with suppressing the past." These habits and memories include the deeply grooved imprints (neuronal pathways) created by overwhelming stress and trauma. Our thinking brain can thus function unhindered by the noise and signals generated in our internal world.

But the signals don't go away. Instead, researchers theorize that they continue to travel around and around closed circuits of nerve fibers within the limbic system. So the ego defenses bypass the tension and pain, but the tension and pain remain unresolved.

John Bradshaw, in his book *Homecoming* states, that original pain work involves actually experiencing the original repressed feelings. He calls it the "uncovery process." It is the only thing that will bring about "second-order change," the kind of deep change that truly resolves feelings. In first order change, you change from one compulsion to another compulsion. In second-order change, you stop being compulsive. I believe it is paramount to know the source of our thoughts and subsequently the lies we have come to believe because we have never come to terms with the original distress of our wounded inner child.

As I stated in the beginning of this book, I went to 12 Step programs, but kept acting out, I worked as a Therapist and a Pastor, but kept acting out. I read lots of books and discussed my problems in therapy, but I kept acting out. I studied a course in Miracles; meditated and prayed (sometimes for hours); but I kept acting out. I was compulsive even about higher consciousness. What I didn't know was that I needed to embrace my heartbroken little boy's loneliness and unresolved grief.

This is Soul work and I have come to understand that the Inner Child forms your core beliefs. Christ can play a significant part in healing this, but not until we understand the source of our thoughts and the lies we have come to believe will make us feel loved and accepted.

This brings me back to my original point that as we consider our thoughts there are two ways to discern the origin of a thought and determine whether the thought is a voluntary one. Thoughts that originate from yourself you can control and change them at will. For example I can choose to think about my house or not. However if someone does something to threaten my house I may have thoughts of revenge and decide to stop thinking that way but five minutes later it is back again and I don't seem to be able to stop obsessing on the thought of revenge. Trauma will leave an indelible impression on our thinking and distort our perception of reality which leads to self defeating learned behaviors and obsessive thoughts.

A second way of discerning the lies imposed by the enemy himself, Satan, is to recognize when negative thoughts regarding myself come with the personal pronoun "You," such as, "You're stupid!" The devil cannot read our thoughts because he is not all-powerful (omnipotent) or all-knowing (omniscient). However he can see by our actions and by our speech whether or not we believe what he has told us. He will take full advantage of the negative messages that were given to you as a child and seek to reinforce them at every opportunity. He is called the "accuser of the brethren," for a reason. Like a good prosecutor he builds a case to use against you, to remind you all the reasons why you are stupid and why it is true.

The Emotions. The second function of the soul is the emotions. Although I have spent time talking about the Limbic System as it relates to the brain and our development we do know that emotions are feelings that we experience inside ourselves as a response to events that are going on around us. They are neither good nor bad; they are simply a barometer of our belief system. Those events may affect us through our bodily organs-such as a sudden loud noise to which our response may be fear or through our minds. A bad decision can lead to anguish and distress. I believe that the highest expression of our emotions is experienced when our spirit, soul and body are working in perfect harmony and in relationship with God.

Much of the Church has despised emotional experience as being irrelevant to real spirituality. But that attitude denies the fact that God created us with emotions for a purpose. Instead of denying a precious part of God's creation, it would be far more honest to recognize emotional reality and bring our emotions to the Lord for healing. Indeed, if damaged emotions are not healed, the potential for making shipwrecks of our lives, and the lives of those with whom we relate on a day-to-day basis, is enormous. Emotions need healing as much as physical wounds.

It was perhaps a reaction against this possibility that made some people equate sensitive and responsive emotions with superficiality and produced accusations of emotionalism against all evangelical initiatives. There is a world of difference between a genuine reaction in the emotions to being in the presence of God and whipped-up feelings that bear no relationship whatsoever to the real thing. For most people, the experience of conversion, being born again, is a rightfully emotional moment, and I would never want to deny people the privilege of responding to God with their feelings when He comes into their lives or on any other occasion in their spiritual journey.

Similar comments apply to many of the experiences that Christians go through in their personal journeys. The damage done to countless Christians who have been forced to bury their emotional pain thus shutting the gate to their Limbic System has left us with a generation that is scarred and hurting in this area. There are few people whom I have counseled in the past twenty-five years who have not needed deep emotional healing, in addition to ministry for the obvious presenting symptoms that prompted the original request for counseling.

There are many different sources of emotional pain—experiences such as sexual abuse or physical violence and any kind of trauma which is ultimately determined by the individual not some kind of criteria for trauma. For example two of my children growing up with a special needs sister frequently saw rescue crews rushing into our home and whisking her away by ambulance hooked up to machines and wires to the ICU at the Children's Hospital. Also experiencing her violent rages has been very traumatic. That has not only left scarring in the lives of all three of my children but also in my wife and me. Most recently I too had seizures with no prior medical history that has further deepened the wounds for my wife and children who witnessed the medical emergency. It is in these experiences and others that we experience very painful emotions and yet rarely in our culture are they ever addressed or allowed to be expressed. Mankind has become quite expert at putting on a mask to hide these real feelings. Nowhere more so, it seems, than in the Body of Christ, where "feeling fine," irrespective of the real situation, is almost a hallmark of certain brands of stoical Christianity!

I truly believe that God wants to heal our damaged emotions, whether caused by trauma or those areas of our lives that have been damaged by the lack of consideration or even the plain ignorance of those we have had to associate with in the past. I believe it is in the area of damaged emotions that Satan can have a tremendous negative impact on our lives. Because not only does the devil impose thoughts directly into our intellect, but he often imposes feelings on our emotions as well. Some people are gripped with the spirit of fear and are almost incapacitated and they don't even know why. Imposed feelings are very convincing because they happen right inside the emotional part of our being. Coupled with the fact that the world tells us to trust our feelings, we are easily fooled.

For example, if a hiker goes into the bush and sees a bear, he will experience fear. This is a healthy God-given fear because it is purposed to keep him safe. On the other hand, when the hiker goes into the bush when it is getting dark and sees a dark object that he believes is a bear, it produces the same fear. If someone shines a light on that dark object and the hiker sees that it is only a tree stump, the fear no longer has power over him. This helps us to understand John 8:32 "And ye shall know the truth, and the truth shall make you free." As long as that hiker believes that the tree stump is a bear, it might as well be. A lie believed as truth has the same power as if it were true.

The first sin in the Garden of Eden was not the eating of the fruit. The first sin was believing the devil's lies. The devil said God knows that in the day you eat from it your eyes will be opened, and you will be like God, knowing good and evil. When Eve believed she could have something good for herself apart from God, she rejected what God had said and believed the devil's lie. That was her sin. This belief gave the devil power in her life, and she then looked at the fruit and desired it. It was after she believed the lie that she felt desire towards the fruit.

If you can recognize that the thoughts or feelings are not coming from you, then you can get a handle on the problem.

The Will. The third function of the soul is the will, or volition. Scripture talks about the spirit is willing, but the flesh being weak. The meaning of this phrase, which has become part of the language of temptation, is simply that if the flesh has not been crucified, then the will gets out of control.

Satan will use every trick in the book to make our will subject to the flesh, instead of the other way around. A person who is walking in wholeness and obedience before God is one whose will is under the Lordship of Jesus Christ and whose flesh life, as a consequence, is under His control. This is not an area that many people will freely talk about—for if the real truth about all our lives were made public, there would be some very embarrassed and red faces in the church each Sunday! For the sex addict it equates to total humiliation.

Crucifying the flesh is not the most popular of Paul's graphic spiritual phrases, but it is a road to wholeness (holiness-Christ likeness) that, if followed, will have enormous benefits in every dimension of our lives. There are many people who are so sick in this area of their lives that they are incapable of making rightful decisions-temptation is always too strong for them. One of Satan's major tactics with all Christians is to gain control of this area. If he wins here, he has won everywhere. The healing in this area comes back to what I have talked about in this book earlier.

I'm not talking about willpower here, but about making choices whether to believe a lie or the truth. If we want to change something and can't change it with willpower, then we are up against a different power, namely, Enemy-power. If we choose to believe it is ourselves and are not able to change our situation with willpower, then we will feel defeated, discouraged, and in bondage. Romans 8:2 teaches, "for the law of the Spirit of life in Christ Jesus has set you free from the law of sin and of death." In understanding this verse, we see we are not trying to fight to get victory. Rather, we are fighting from the position of victory. When we fight to get victory, we've already lost victory. We've lost it because we've failed to recognize that in the particular area we're struggling with, Christ has already been victorious, and we have failed to see that He lives in us. When we fight from the position of victory, we then rely on the fact that the enemy is already defeated, and we can stand on that truth. If we say, "The devil made me do it," we are incorrect because the devil can only have power if we believe the lie he fed to us. We are still responsible.

The Bible consistently challenges us to choose to exercise our will: "Choose this day, who you will serve" (Joshua 24:15). The choice is ours, but if we believe the devil's lies and see the situation through his perspective, we are in bondage. However, if we choose to believe God's truth and choose to see it through His perspective, we are free. Romans 6:16 states; "Do you not know that when you present yourselves to someone as slaves for obedience, you are slaves of the one whom you obey, either of sin resulting in death, or of obedience resulting in righteousness?" To yield ourselves is a decision, which is an exercise of the will.

We have the choice to see any circumstance through either the Enemy's perspective or through God's. We're not a victim; "we are more than a conqueror!" (Romans 8:37). The story of God throwing the devil out of Heaven is in Isaiah 14. The devil hates God in the worst way. Since God is all-powerful, the devil can't fight God directly (although he is very powerful in his own right), and so instead, he torments God's children. In that way, he gets back at God because he knows it hurts God when His children reject His truth and instead believe the devil's lies. The devil does not ignore us, but takes advantage of the fact that we ignore him.

The Spirit

This brings me to the third distinction in the trinity of man, the spirit. The spirit is our God-consciousness, our awareness that we answer to a divine Creator. The spirit is the vehicle to communicate with God. Many are unable to distinguish between soul and spirit.

In some versions of the Scriptures, there is confusion over the correct translation of the words for soul and spirit, in spite of the fact that there are perfectly good Greek words for both soul and spirit that make the distinction clear. In various places the same Greek word is translated as either soul or spirit according to the understanding of the translator. The writer of Hebrews that I just quoted, emphasizes the distinction by saying "division of soul and spirit" (Hebrews 4:12).The spirit and the soul are not one and the same thing. The soul is very much part of our flesh life. Failure to recognize this and distinguish between the spirit and the soul leads many people into condemnation and leaves them wide open to Satan coming as the "accuser of the brethren" and undermining the security that they should have in God.

Without this understanding, those who are alive to God in the spirit, following conversion, are tempted to discount the reality of their new life in Christ because of problems they are experiencing in their soul. Satan loves to have us confused on this issue and keep us in defeat.

Over these past few years I have come to realize that this has been my Achilles heel. I have not been able to distinguish between the two and the result has been devastating. I was unable to distinguish who I really was in spirit because of what Christ had done and who I was in soul because of what I did. This is why I am going to such great lengths to try to explain this not only for your sake but mine. Not understanding the distinctions has left me under constant condemnation as a perfectionist and confused as to why recovery and healing always seemed to be elusive. So let me explain further the trinity of man and its distinctions and implications.

I Thessalonians 5:23 states, "And may the very God of peace sanctify you wholly; and I pray to God your whole spirit and soul and body be preserved blameless unto the coming of our Lord Jesus Christ." Again most people actually believe that they're only made up of body and soul. They confuse soul and spirit as being basically the same thing. Therefore, on a day-to-day level, they only acknowledge a physical part and an emotional, mental part known as personality.

Wommack states,

> "That even *Strong's Concordance* fails to distinguish all three! The Greek word for "spirit" is "pneuma" and is defined as being "immortal soul." He would suggest that it means "inner most part" not your, "immortal soul." Most people don't recognize the fact that their spirits are the core of their beings. They function primarily out of their soulish realm, believing what they think and feel is reality. They may perceive their souls to be the core of who they are, but God's Word says differently.

It is difficult to explain to you the strange relationship between the soul and the spirit. We only know it from what Scripture tells us. You can't feel that difference. We can feel the difference between our souls and our bodies. You can say, "I feel weak, or weary", or "I feel great today". What part of your being are you referring to? Yes, your body. Your glands, your blood pressure, your heart are in good shape, and you feel great. You will notice we refer to this part of our being with the first person pronoun. You may say "I feel wonderful", and then later you may say, "I feel sad." Is your body sad? No, it's your soul. You may feel happy, or emotionally drained. You're no longer talking about your body; you've made a quick shift to a third part of your being, your soul. And every now and then the most primitive, or least religious person, will say something like "I want something, but I don't know what it is." "I feel a desire to do something or be someone." We have difficulty putting this into words. But what are we talking about is the spirit, the spirit that is longing for something beyond what we already have. This is unique to man, and we can switch between these three with no effort. We understand this about one another; we all have these sensations.

When the spirit enters the body it creates the soul, and the soul exists only existentially – only as long as the spirit is in the body. The best illustration I've heard is from Ray Stedman who states,

> "You can liken it unto a light bulb. Whether a light bulb is a fluorescent or incandescent light, you know that a light bulb is made up of two major parts. Metal and glass combine to make the material aspect of a light bulb. Then there is a second essential, and that is a stream of electrons, called electricity, that has to flow through that mass of metal and glass. When it does, a third entity is created, called light. The light is there only as long as the energy is flowing through the metal and the glass. As soon as the stream of electrons is interrupted, the light goes out but the metal and the glass remain, and the electricity remains available but not in contact.

That seems to be about as close as we can come to understand how humans function.

In the book of James it says "as the body without the spirit is dead, so faith without works is dead." James uses the analogy of the body and the spirit. So what happens when we die? According to Ecclesiastes, the body goes into the grave, but the spirit returns to God who gave it, and the soul goes out. It no longer continues in that sense.

As I stated earlier, Psychologists work with the soul, but they do not work with the spirit. The weakness of psychology is that they do not understand that there is a spirit. The closest I have seen secular psychologists understanding the spirit is in the work of Victor Frankel, the Jewish psychologist who survived the holocaust in Germany, and was in a prisoner of war camp there for a long time. He went through terrible tortures before he was freed. He developed a system of thought he called "logo therapy". He so named it because he saw there was a function in man beyond the soul. He didn't know what to call it, so he called it "logos", the word, or the spirit. He couldn't define it, describe it, or work with it. He had no access to it, other than to know that it existed. This is the limit of the secular mind.

That's why Hebrews 4:12, states: "For the Word of God is living and active, sharper than any two-edged sword, piercing to the division of soul and spirit..." So only the Word of God can tell us the difference between the soul and the spirit. That is why it takes revelation to understand man as he really is. Hebrews continues, "of joints and marrow (these are symbolic divisions of these major areas of life) and discerning the thoughts and intentions of the heart."

The term "heart", in this text is making reference to the spirit, but sometimes it is referencing the physiological heart; however usually, it is a reference to the spirit. When we say, "I did it with my whole heart", we're talking about our spirit, which is the deepest part of our humanity, the most important part of our being. It's the major part of man, which reflects the image of God.

However the physiological heart draws some wonderful comparisons to the function of the spirit and perhaps we should not be surprised that the heart and the spirit are often used as synonymous terms. Science research in the field of neuro-cardiology is beginning to help us understand that the heart as an organ is more than just a pump. Pearce, in his book *The Biology of Transcendence, A Blue Print of the Human Spirit* suggests that the heart also is triune. Just as the brain is triune in nature with three functions so too is the heart. It is electromagnetic, neural and hormonal in function.

> "He goes on to say that the heart's neural system has no structures for perceiving or analyzing the context, nature, details, or logic of our emotional reports like the neurons of the brain can. Thus, the heart can't judge the validity of or reason for these reports and responds to them as basic facts. However the heart responds on all levels: electromagnetically, through the unmediated neural connections to the limbic brain, and through neural connections to a myriad of body functions. Additional responses include hormonal shifts between the heart and the body and the heart and the brain."

In other words, without the heart nothing else works.

The dialogue between our heart and brain is an interactive dynamic where each pole of our experience, heart and brain, gives rise to and shapes the other to an indeterminable extent. No cause-effect relationship can be implied in such an organic and infinitely contingent process. He concludes that this mirroring is another vital example of the creator-created dynamic. Perhaps this organic relationship can best be summarized in Jesus words: "Not I but the Father within me does these things." That is the relationship of the heart and the brain and the heart and the body. So it is with our spirit. "Apart from Him we can do nothing, and yet in Him all things are possible."

Meister Eckhart adds to this by stating,

> "The heart is the primary mode of being and all else in our life springs from it. The end result is a heart that generates species-specific characteristics that we all share, yet reflect the personal characteristics of each brain and its experiences to make for a unique expression of a shared form. The interaction of these two aspects-the universal and individual, unity and diversity, creator and created-results in a human being that is the same as all others but different too.
>
> In this way what is broad, generic and universal is expressed on an intimate, personal level, making each of us, even " the least of these our brothers,' equal expressions of the totality. Thus, if we have the vision, we will see God in each other or find God in the "least of these our brothers," as Jesus did.

So as we differentiate between the Soul and the Spirit we understand our soul to be like the brain but our spirit (heart) is what connects us to the heart of God.

The Apostle Paul states, "which things we also speak, not in words taught by human wisdom, but in those taught by the Spirit, combining spiritual thoughts with spiritual words. But a natural man does not accept the things of the Spirit of God; for they are foolishness to him, and he cannot understand them, because they are spiritually discerned"

(I Corinthians 2:13-14). God is a Spirit: and they that worship him must worship him in spirit and truth (John 4:24).

When God desires to speak into our lives, He chooses to do so directly through our spirit: "Spiritual things are spiritually discerned" (I Corinthians 2:14). It is heart to heart. God doesn't come through the same avenue as the devil, which is through our soul as I explained earlier. It is not that our soul is useless, but it has to be governed through our spirit, and not vice versa.

I believe God speaks his desires into our spirit and we are able to understand them because we have been given the mind of Christ in our spirit. To be honest I have not heard much preaching on this subject and I have to confess I have never preached on it or even thought about the implications of such a passage. "For who hath known the mind of the Lord, that he may instruct him? But we have the mind of Christ" (I Corinthians 2:16). I think Wommack does a good job in explaining the meaning of this truth by stating,

> "That when you were born again, you received the mind of Christ in your spirit. However, your spirit mind doesn't have to be developed, trained, or taught because it was born again in perfect knowledge.
>
> He goes on to say that this may appear contradictory to I Corinthians 13:9-10, which talks about only "knowing in part until that which is perfect is come." That however is referring to your natural mind in your soulish realm. Right now, you don't understand everything with your physical mind. You are in the process of renewing it, which won't be complete until you receive that which is perfect—your glorified body. But in your spirit, you have the mind of Christ, which is already complete.
>
> Your spirit mind and physical mind are two separate entities within you. When they don't agree, double-mindedness occurs. "Purify your hearts, ye double minded" (James 4:8). The key to the Christian life and

> recovery is training our physical mind to agree with our spirit mind, which is the mind of Christ.
>
> You are spirit, soul, and body. Your born again spirit always agrees with God. However your body is under the influence of what it can see, taste, hear, smell, and feel. When your natural mind thinks the same way as your spirit mind, you're single-minded. That's when you believe with all your heart and see God's power in recovery. Your spirit mind always thinks the way God thinks. The Word perfectly represents what you think in your spirit. Hence God speaks to us in our spirit because it is one with His Spirit and mind.
>
> In your spirit you know all things! "But you have an unction from the Holy One, and you know all things" (I John 2:20). "Unction" simply means "a special endowment with power, or ability." The Holy One is Jesus.

This passage makes it quite clear that we know all things. Right about now your natural mind is saying no I don't, because I couldn't even remember where I put the car keys last night. That is yet more evidence that we need to grab this concept of body, soul and spirit. Because it is your spirit, that knows all things because it has the mind of Christ, not our natural mind. The Greek word for "all" means "to the exclusion of nothing." This means you not only know some things or many things but all things. In your spiritual mind, you know everything Jesus knows. If you're at all like me your immediate response may be WOW!! Your second response is probably, okay that is great but what good does it do me? How is this going to help me in my recovery over my addiction?

The first step is you must believe that you have the mind of Christ in your born-again spirit, even if you mess up and relapse. Secondly you need to learn how to release the mind of Christ. There are several scriptures that reveal this inner witness. "The Spirit itself bears witness with your spirit, that we are children of God" (Romans 8:16). First John 5:6-10 also describes this, specifically verse 10, which says, "He that believes on the Son of God hath the witness in himself."

Before I move on, I want to address a scripture that may seem to contradict the very thing that I am talking about. I Corinthians 2:9 says, "But as it is written, Things which eye has not seen and ear has not heard, and which have not entered the heart of man all that God has prepared for those who love him." This passage seems to be saying that you can't really know the things of God.

If we don't stop reading there and read the next several verses I think it will bring some clarity and understanding. "But for us God revealed them through the Spirit; for the Spirit searches all things, even the depths of God. For who among men knows the thoughts of a man except the spirit of the man, which is in him? Even so the thoughts of God no one knows except the Spirit of God. Now we have received, not the spirit of the world, but the Spirit from God, that we might know the things freely given to us by God…But a natural man does not accept the things of the Spirit of God; for they are foolishness to him, and he cannot understand them, because they are spiritually appraised. For who has known the mind of the Lord, that he should instruct him? But we have the mind of Christ"(I Corinthians 2:10-16).

I Corinthians 2:9 contrasts Old Testament saints, who couldn't understand, with New Covenant believers, who know all things in their spirits! In this verse, Paul quoted an Old Testament scripture, Isaiah 64:4. Old Covenant people weren't born again, so they didn't have born-again spirits. Because of this, it's totally accurate to say that they couldn't understand the things of God. To them it was foolishness because they have to be spiritually discerned (I Corinthians 2:14). However, it's inaccurate to say the same thing about a New Testament believer who has the mind of Christ in their born again spirit. You can understand the things of God!

This brings me back to the question that I proposed earlier. So what? How is this going to help me in my recovery over my addiction? If you believe this as truth that you have the mind of Christ then that is the first step. The second step is applying this truth to your life and recovery. I will discuss this in more detail in Chapter 11 under the subject of Soul recovery.

I will say this however: one-third of your salvation is already complete! Your spirit isn't in the process of growing or maturing. Right now in your spirit, you are exactly the way you'll be throughout eternity (I John 4:17). You have a physical body and soul that haven't been changed yet. They are subject to change and can change, but it's not automatic. However, the change of your spirit at salvation was total, complete and automatic.

So let me get back to the function of the spirit within us. Much like the soul, the spirit also has three functions: Intuition, conscience, and communion.

The intuition. This is not speaking of a woman's intuition but rather, what is God's revelation to us. Revelation comes to us when we by faith accept Biblical truth, and then God reveals it to our spirit. When we receive something by revelation, we don't need to defend it. For example, you can know that you are saved. "We don't need to wrangle about words and argue over the point of your salvation" (2 Timothy 2:16), for we know the truth in our spirit. The Spirit itself bears witness with our spirit, that we are His children.

Our part is to believe God's Word. God's part is to reveal it to our spirit and give us the faith. Hebrews 11:1 tells us, "Now faith is the assurance of things hoped for, the conviction (evidence) of things not seen." Faith is substance. It does not just believe something is real, but knowing it is real. When God reveals something to our spirits, and our minds immediately grasp it as well, it may seem to us that it came through the mind, but this is not the case. Sometimes we know that God is saying something to our spirit—we sense it—but our minds don't yet grasp it. It may take days or years before we hear or read something that allows our minds to grasp it.

So our part again is to read the Word of God and choose to believe it. Then God makes it real to us. Our choosing to believe the Word frees God to reveal it to us without imposing on our free will. Sometimes people will say, "I want to forgive somebody," or "I want to trust God," and they will even express their prayers in this way. Wanting is not enough; we have to choose to trust and allow God to work on our behalf, without violating our free will. If we wait until we feel like forgiving somebody, the Enemy will make sure the feeling will never come. However, after we choose to forgive, God can work out the rest in our lives. We are so used to going by feelings and accepting that all the feelings we are aware of are originating from us, that it hinders us from believing the truth of God that would set us free.

The Conscience. The second function of the spirit is conscience. Most people believe that guilt feelings come through the conscience, but this is incorrect. Romans 8:1 states, "There is therefore now no condemnation (guilt) to them which are in Christ Jesus, who walk not after the flesh, (the soul) but after the Spirit."

This verse shows us that God does not use guilt or condemnation. Romans 2:4 tells us what God does use: "Or do you think lightly of the riches of His kindness and forbearance and patience, not knowing that the kindness of God leads you to repentance?"

The devil is the one who comes with guilt and condemnation, and that comes through the soul via our intellect and emotions. This happens when he succeeds in having us focus on self. He imposes thoughts on us like, we shouldn't have done a certain thing, or that we should have done another thing or that God can't forgive a sin that is so horrible, etc. If we believe those thoughts, then guilt stays with us. We may confess them, but when the feelings of guilt from the Enemy remain, we don't feel forgiven and, therefore, believe that God has not really forgiven us. So, again, we go by the feelings and not by the fact given to us in I John 1:9 which says: "If we confess our sins, He (God) is faithful and just to forgive us our sins, and to cleanse us from all unrighteousness." We need to choose to believe the Word of God rather than the feelings that we are aware of, rather than, "This is the way I feel." We should take ownership of imposed feelings. If we acknowledge them as ours, we are giving the Enemy power in our lives.

"For as high as the heavens are above the earth, so great is His lovingkindness toward those who fear Him. As far as the east is from the west, so far has He removed our transgressions from us" (Psalm 103:11-12). So often, instead of trusting God's forgiveness when we confess our sin, we look at our feelings as evidence as to whether or not we are forgiven. Since the devil hinders us from feeling forgiven, we continue to carry the guilt of our sins and believe that God has not forgiven us.

If God does not use guilt feelings or condemnation, how does He deal with us? God comes with conviction and with the conviction, He gives us repentance, and this happens when we focus on God and not on self. When Isaiah saw the Lord, he said, "Woe is me, for I am ruined! Because I am a man of unclean lips, and I live among a people of unclean lips; for my eyes have seen the King, the Lord of hosts" (Isaiah 6:5).

When we focus on God, we come into the light, and light exposes the darkness. The light will expose areas of darkness in our heart: "The heart is more deceitful than all else and is desperately sick (wicked); who can understand it? I, the Lord, search the heart; I test the mind, even to give to each man according to his ways, according to the results of his deeds" (Jeremiah 17:9-10). It is both the Word of God and the Spirit of God that will expose our selfishness and sinfulness. We need to ask God to expose our heart instead of trying to search it ourselves. If we do the latter, the Enemy will accuse us of all sorts of things and will condemn us. The Psalmist emphasizes God searching rather than "I" searching.

"Search me, O God, and know my heart: try me, and know my thoughts: And see if there is any wicked way in me, and lead me in the way everlasting" (Psalm 139:23-24). There is a simple way to differentiate between guilt feelings, which come from the enemy, and conviction, which comes from God. Guilt feelings are depressing, discouraging and we feel down. Conviction on the other hand lifts us up to a higher ground and is encouraging. As we see our sinfulness, we also see the forgiveness, and this brings true joy.

Communion. This brings me to the third function of the spirit, communion. Communion means fellowship and the way we have fellowship with God is through prayer-not just asking God for things, but waiting for Him to speak to us as well. We also have fellowship with Him through praise, through reading and meditating on His Word, and through seeing God's hand in trials. Job, after he went through his trials said, "until now I heard about you, but now, I am seeing you!" (Job 42:5)

Through communion, we get to know God and who He is, how much He loves us, how much He is concerned about us, and since He is Almighty, how much more He will take care of us. And we know that "all things work together for good to them that love God, to them that are called according to His purpose" (Romans 8:28). Therefore, if we worry, it shows that we have taken our eyes off God and put them on ourselves. We may not understand all that is happening, but we can always choose to trust.

If we operate in the soul, where the Enemy imposes lies, it will be a downward spiral. We will become discouraged, distressed, and despondent. But if we are functioning in the spirit, we will spiral upwards with God. As we have greater communion with Him, we will get more revelation in our intuition from Him. As we have more revelation from God, we will see more of our own sinfulness because we are coming into the light. We will be convicted in our conscience because of our sinfulness. Because we don't want anything between God and ourselves, we will repent, and He will forgive and cleanse us. This makes our fellowship closer than ever.

I have taken some time to explore and unpack what I believe to be the nature of man and who we were created to be and ultimately how God sees and relates to us, body, soul and spirit. Now, I believe in order to experience recovery we need not just understand these doctrinal truths but we need to appropriate it by faith. Faith is the key to becoming spiritually alive; without faith in God our spirit remains dead. To Quote Martin Luther, "nothing we do helps us spiritually. Only faith helps-only what we believe." It's not that we can't believe but what we believe. Patrick Carnes, in his research has made it quite clear that we have believed the wrong thing: that we are innately bad and unlovable, which has led to self defeating addictive behaviors. This naturally brings me to the question what should I believe and what is faith?

Part IV

Recovery from Addictive Behaviors

Chapter 8
Faith

I have had the privilege of preaching on this subject a couple times in the past and I want to extrapolate from those messages to bring some clarity to this whole subject of faith. The common conception of faith which prevails today is that it is a confidence in some kind of magical potion or power, and that if we could work up enough of this remarkable substance, or feeling, or whatever it is, we could do anything. Unfortunately, this widespread misconception prevails not only among non-Christians.

"Faith" is a very important word in the Christian life and is evident to anyone who reads the Bible at all. The word is found on almost every page of Scripture from Genesis to Revelation, because faith is the means by which man receives anything at all from God. Without faith, as the book of Hebrews tells us, it is simply impossible to please God. It is not difficult - it is impossible! It can't be done. Without faith we can receive nothing from God. Without faith all the promises of the Scriptures are absolutely invalid so far as we are concerned. So faith becomes a tremendous power and force to reckon with and to count upon as we consider our recovery.

I want to introduce this subject by reflecting on many of the questions which have been raised on the subject of faith:

How can people really believe that God cares about them as individuals?

I met a friend in recovery about three and a half years ago who I have come to love dearly. He calls himself a self professing atheist and would say that the fundamental tenets of the Christian faith seemingly are founded upon flimsy speculations, not facts. I wish that I could believe the bases were facts; yet I find that even some Christians are as torn by confusion, self doubt, and as conflicted as everyone else. How much can we really believe about this elusive power of love? This is the paramount problem.

This is the position which many people have in regard to faith. The problem with my friend, as with many of us, is that we are looking at our faith and trying to analyze it, thinking that if we can understand exactly what faith is, we somehow can produce it. Here is where the problem lies. For the strange thing about faith is that, though it is absolutely essential to experiencing anything from God, yet when you begin to examine it in your own life, it disappears. It flies out the window. You can't find it anywhere. You can't get your fingers on it. You can't pin it down. It seems impossible to define. The reason is that faith, in itself, is of no value whatsoever. In fact, it cannot even exist in itself. So the minute we try to look at it, it isn't there.

The reason for this is that faith is produced only as we set our eyes upon the facts on which it rests. When we look at the facts, faith comes very naturally. The amazing thing is that the easiest thing in the entire world for a human being to do is to believe. The proof of this is found in the letter to the Hebrews, the Hall of fame of Faith; "And without faith it is impossible to please Him [God]. For whoever would draw near to God must believe that he exists and that he regards those who seek Him" (Hebrews 11:6).

In other words, that is the minimum level of faith. That is the one thing necessary for human life, for the development of human fulfillment -- in other words, for salvation. If we do not draw near to God we cannot be saved. Therefore, if faith is not possible to any human being, he is outside the bounds of salvation and redemption. But this is not true. Every human being can believe. That is what he is made for. Human nature is made to believe. We were made to be dependent creatures. We were made to be continually drawing upon another's resources. We are continually relying on something else. That is belief. Thus, the one characteristic which we have as human beings is the capacity to believe. We automatically do it. All day long we believe. If you are sitting in a chair, you believe it will continue to hold you up. If you are under a roof, you believe it is adequately supported and is not going to crumble and fall on you. All through our lives we continually believe and therefore, faith is the most automatic response of the human spirit.

The problem is that we need to fix our attention upon facts, because the process of human activity always follows the same channel, no matter what realm of life is involved. It is impossible for us to prove anything completely before we experience it. Therefore, some people state that they are not going to believe until they see the proof of Christian faith. This is totally ridiculous, because it is simply impossible to prove any fact without experiencing it. Apart from experience there is nothing we can prove, even to our own satisfaction. All we can do is come to as good an evaluation by reason as we possibly can and then plunge in and try it: test it, leap out on it, put our weight upon it. This we do continually all day long. This is the process of believing. I like what a little child said to their parents on a recent Christmas movie, "seeing isn't believing, believing is seeing."

What is Faith?

In the letter to the Hebrews, the subject is "What Is Faith?" It is illustrated positively for us in the Old Testament through the lives of Moses, Joshua, Melchizedek and Aaron. And the negative is brought forth as well, so that we see what faith is not, and what the results of not believing are. In the book of Hebrews we discover that faith is simply awareness that there exist certain invisible realities which we cannot perceive with our five senses, but which we are nevertheless convinced exist by the evidence brought before us. After we have come to a certain level of knowledge concerning these facts, we are expected then to test them and try them. Our only other alternative is to draw back. The whole book of Hebrews is written to warn us what happens if we draw back and don't make the test, don't take the plunge. All through this letter warnings are interspersed about what happened when men drew back after they had had all the evidence they needed that a fact existed upon which they could rest their faith.

In chapter eleven, you have this great record of men and women who did exercise faith. And they always did it in rather simple terms. There is nothing very dramatic about them. Only a few of them are what we would call "leaders of men," or "outstanding" characters. Many of them are obscure personalities: common, ordinary people, like you and me. But in every case they were aware of certain facts which were propounded to them, but which they could not prove completely. Nobody could. But they finally became so convinced by the evidence being presented to them that they were willing at least to venture out and put it to the test. We see this in verse 8:

"By faith Abraham obeyed when he was called to go out to a place which he was to receive as an inheritance; and he went out, not knowing where he was to go" (Hebrews 11:8).

He couldn't prove where he was going. But, having received the word which he could not deny came from God - certain evidence which was overpowering to him, which he had at least to accept as being there, and undeniable - he ventured out upon the call. And the journey took him into the experience by which all that had been promised became available to him. That is all that faith is. We strengthen our faith not by looking at it but by concerning ourselves again with the facts upon which faith must rest.

That is why the Scripture says, "... faith cometh by hearing, and hearing by the word of God" (Romans 10:17). The word of God has a quality about it that awakens faith. That is the amazing thing about this book. As you read it through and reread it and study it and think about it and meditate upon it, there comes a quiet conviction to the heart, "This must be true!" This is the basis upon which faith then is invited to act.

There also comes with faith, immediately, a doubt. All of us experience this. There is nothing wrong with it, nothing abnormal about it. We say, "Yes, this must be true." And then a voice says, "Ah, yes, but maybe it isn't, too." So we are put in the place where we can have no further evidence until we venture. Faith is simply that willingness to venture; to reckon upon what God has said, to step out upon it. And then the answer comes, the proof follows, invariably. That is the entire record of Scripture.

Now, I have dwelt upon the subject of faith at length in order to help us see more clearly what faith is. Faith, as the book of Hebrews tells us, is "the assurance of things hoped for" - what you long to be, what you long to see in your life - based upon "the conviction of things not seen" (Hebrews 1:1). What brings you to that conviction? Simply the remarkable quality about the word of God that rings a bell in our hearts and says, "This is true;" that is all.

We have, of course, the evidence of those who have ventured before us and have given testimony to us that what they ventured upon was found trustworthy. That is what Hebrews12:1 means: "Therefore, since we are surrounded by so great a cloud of witnesses ..." They are all talking to us, telling us, "Come on in, the water's fine! It works. Try it and see." We are continually being exhorted to venture out in faith.

So don't try to examine your faith to see how much or how little you have.

The epistle of James is a practical book and the key to the letter is found in chapter 2, verse 26:

"For as the body apart from the spirit is dead, so faith apart from works is dead" (James 2:26).

All that James is telling us is that it really isn't faith until you have ventured. That is what he is saying. We are so prone to say. "Well, yes, I do believe that such and such is true, but don't ask me to try it or to do anything on that basis." We call that faith, but it is not faith. It is not faith for me to say, "I know that chair will hold me." I can stand here all night and say, "I know that chair will hold me. I believe that it will. I have confidence that it will. I am certain that it will." But that is not faith. It is only mental conviction. Faith is when I go over and sit down on it. This is what James is saying. It is not faith until you have tried it, until you have ventured on it. Faith that does not venture, he says, is dead. Therefore, when faith does venture, it will accomplish certain things and one of those things is that it will stand up under temptation.

Peter in his two letters weighs in on the subject of faith. Peter the disciple who, in his impulsive brashness, declared that he would never deny the Lord. He was perfectly sincere when he said, "Lord, the others may fail you, but you can count on me." That very night, as Jesus had warned him, he betrayed the Lord with a curse and denied Him three times before the cock crowed. He went away into the night with Jesus' words ringing in his ears, "When you have turned again, strengthen your brethren" (Luke 22:32b).

When you read Peter's letters, you find that this is what he is doing. He is strengthening his brethren in the midst of the trial of faith. For the things which make faith tremble are trial and testing, hardship and suffering, strange things which happen to us, unusual catastrophes which come into our lives out of the blue and yes even the battle of addiction. These things make us fearful, and we ask, "Why?" Peter answers that question. Why do these things happen? Because faith makes us a part of the life of Jesus Christ and to reach the people of a lost and rebellious world costs pain, and suffering, and heartache, and the willingness of love to put up with rebuff and rebuke, and still to follow after them. We become part of that. Peter is simply saying that in the hand of the Lord we are the instruments by which he is fulfilling the work that he does in this world. As Paul put it in Colossians 1:24: "Now I rejoice in my sufferings for your sake, and in my flesh I complete what is lacking in Christ's afflictions for the sake of his body, that is, the church" (Colossians 1:24). That is the reason for the trials of faith, the answer to why faith suffers.

John teaches us how faith works. The key verse is in chapter 3, verse 23, of his first letter: And this is his commandment, "that we should believe in the name of his Son Jesus Christ and love one another, just as He has commanded us" (1 John 3:23). That is how faith works. It believes continually and is continually venturing. Today one venture, tomorrow another; this moment a step of faith, the next moment another step of faith. As the 12 step program states, one day at a time, one step at a time. This is the walk of faith.

Jude discusses the subtle perils which will undermine faith and keep it from venturing upon the promises of God. As we read it through we learn what they are. There is the desire to have your own way. There is immorality. There is greed. There is false authority, divisiveness, and all the other perils upon the pathway of life. But Jude closes his letter with these admonitions (Verses 20-21):

"But you, beloved, build yourselves up on your most holy faith [that is the key; that is the operative word]; pray in the Holy Spirit [that is the exercise of faith]; keep yourselves in the love of God [that, again, is the exercise of faith]; wait for the mercy of our Lord Jesus Christ unto eternal life" (Jude 1:20-21).

All this is the continual exercise of faith. Now, it is possible for us to have great possessions in Christ without any or very little experience of exercising faith. That is why the continual exhortation is to be strong in faith; not by looking at our faith, but by looking at the great facts which God has set before us. As we contemplate these facts which God himself has uttered - a God who cannot lie - and we think about them, and as we remember how many others have stepped out upon these promises and have found they work, we find there is an urge to venture. That is the test. That is strength of the spiritual 12 Step Programs that are based on biblical principles that remind us that we are not alone, that others have gone before us and battled with the same issues and have found recovery, it worked! When you feel a sense of being led to try it, to dare it, then respond!

The book of Hebrews also tells us of the great complaint which God had against his people. It is recorded for us in the fourth chapter, verse 2: "For good news came to us just as to them; but the message which they heard did not benefit them, because it did not meet with faith in the hearers" (Hebrews 4:2).

It didn't do any good because they didn't respond -- they didn't venture out upon it. On more than one occasion, the Lord has said, "Be it done to you according to how you believe." There is no greater sin than the sin of unbelief. "Everything that does not come from faith is sin" (14:23). If we choose to believe a lie, we will live a lie; but if we choose to believe the truth, we will live a victorious life by faith in the same way that we were saved. If we wake up in the morning and based on our feelings, we say, "I'm an addict who is hopeless. I need to "use" to cope with life. What would we do next?

What is the right response? As we consider our triune nature of body, soul and spirit and consider appropriating faith in these areas, what does that look like? What is our responsibility and what is God's. In this last section it is my hope to break down practically and positionally how to experience recovery in all areas of our lives. I want to start by considering the spirit because I see this to be the foundation on which everything else is built.

At this point in the book it is obvious that I advocate the foundation of recovery starts in the healing of the deepest part of our being, our spirit. Just as the 12 Steps start with the Spirit and works outward, so must we as we consider the process of recovery from the inside out. I have also been advocating that this requires having a personal relationship with Christ as not only Savior but Lord. Let me take some time to explain this at the risk of repeating myself.

Chapter 9
My Spirit

I want to take a few minutes to review some of the concepts that I introduced earlier in the book and tie them together as we consider the Spirit's role in our recovery.

I have made the point in this book that working harder doesn't bring about recovery and freedom from sexual addiction. There are two verses in the Bible that succinctly state what must happen in order to experience sexual sobriety and spiritual freedom. "The reason the Son of God appeared was to destroy the devil's work. No one who is born of God will continue to sin, because God's seed remains in him" (I John 3:9). If we are going to be set free from sexual bondage and walk in that freedom, our basic nature must be changed, and we must have a means for overcoming the enemy.

For those of us who are Christians, these conditions have already been met. "God has made us partakers of His divine nature" (2 Peter 1:4) and provided the means by which we can live in victory over sin and addictive behaviors and thinking.

Before spiritual conversion at the cross, the following words described all of us: "You were dead in your trespasses and sins, in which you formerly walked according to the course of this world, according to the prince of the power of the air, of the spirit that is now working in the sons of disobedience. Among them we too all formerly lived in the lust of our flesh, indulging the desires of the flesh and of the mind, and were by nature children of wrath" (Ephesians 2:1-3).

But change took place at salvation. Paul wrote, "You were once darkness, but now you are light in the Lord" (Ephesians 5:8). Our old nature in Adam was darkness; our new nature in Christ is light. We have been transformed at the core of our being. We are no longer "in the flesh"; we are "in Christ." Paul wrote those who are in the flesh cannot please God. However you are not in the flesh but in the Spirit, if indeed the Spirit of God dwells in you" (Romans 8:8-9).

At salvation God "rescued us from the dominion of darkness and brought us into the kingdom of the Son he loves, in whom we have redemption, the forgiveness of sins" (Colossians 1:13, 14). We no longer have to give in to prompting and triggers of society, the flesh and the devil. We "have been given fullness in Christ, who is the head over every power and authority" (Colossians 2:10). We are free to obey God and walk in righteousness and purity.

None of us can fix our past failures, but by the grace of God we can be free from it. God's Word promises, "If anyone is in Christ, he is a new creation; the old has gone, the new has come!" (2 Corinthians 5:17). Furthermore "we are seated with Christ in the heavenlies, far above Satan's authority" (Ephesians 2:4-6; Colossians 2:10, 11), paving the way for us to live in victory of sin and more specifically, addictions.

But this comes down to what I just stated in the last chapter, faith. We must believe the truth of who we are in Christ and change how we walk as children of God to conform to what is true.

Paul writes in Ephesians 1:18,19, "I pray also that the eyes of your heart may be enlightened in order that you may know the hope to which he has called you, the riches of his glorious inheritance in the saints, and His incomparably great power for us who believe."

As you work through the last section of this book it is my prayer that the eyes of your heart will be opened to see the inheritance and power God has provided for you in Christ. It is also my personal prayer as I have discovered how deceitful and wicked my own heart has been.

It's my hope that you will discover and believe in order to find freedom from sexual addiction. Before examining my own position in

Christ from the book of Romans let me make one thing clear to quote Neil Anderson, "When you come to a command in the Bible, the only proper response is to obey it. But when Scripture is expressing something that is true, the only proper response is to believe it." It sounds like a simple concept but I have spent most of my Christian life trying to do something God only expected me to believe and accept it as truth before trying to live according by faith.

Nowhere is this truer than in Romans 6:1-11. This passage is not about what you can do; it's only something you can believe. But believing it will totally affect your walk by faith. It is the critical first step to finding the way of escape from sexual addiction. We also discover specific truths that we are called to believe about ourselves, sin and God.

Dead to Sin

"What shall we say, then? Shall we go on sinning so that grace may increase? By no means! We died to sin; how can we live in it any longer? (Romans 6:1, 2). How do I do that? How do I die to sexual addiction? Because Lord knows if you're anything like me, you have tried and tried and tried some more. The answer is you can't do it! Why not? Because you have already died to sin at salvation. "We died to sin" is past tense; it has already been done. This is something we must believe, not something you must do"

Your spirit is the part of you that's dead to sin. Your body and soul can still do sinful things, but the born again part of you cannot. Notice how being baptized into His death is automatic, but walking in newness of life isn't. "Therefore we are buried with him by baptism into death: that like as Christ was raised up from the dead by the glory of the Father, even so we also should walk in newness of life" (Romans 6:4).

But it depends on how you renew your mind. "For if we have been planted together in the likeness of his death, we shall be also in the likeness of his resurrection" (Romans 6:5, 6). Your spirit died to sin, cannot sin, and has no desire for sin, but this doesn't automatically mean that your soul and body will reflect that change. Your walking in resurrection life depends upon you "knowing this, that our old man is crucified with him, that the body of sin might be destroyed, that henceforth, we should not serve sin" (Romans 6:6).

"Old man" refers to the spirit you had prior to salvation. It's your spirit realm that was dead in trespasses and sins (Ephesians 2:1). Your old man no longer exists because it's been crucified, has died, and was buried with Christ. Most Christians today believe they have an old nature and a new nature. That's wrong because your old man died, and your new man is now who you are in the spirit. I won't go into any more detail on this because I unpacked it in an earlier chapter and my focus is showing you how to overcome the flesh.

At the new birth, your old nature is crucified, dead, and gone. In its place, God gives you a brand new spirit, and you become a new creature. That spirit is so united with Christ that there is actually no difference between your born again spirit and the Spirit of Christ, which was sent into your heart. You literally became one with Him (I Corinthians 6:17). Your born again spirit is identical to Jesus. The two of you have become one, making a brand-new person. Then, your spirit was sealed, surrounded, and encased by the Holy Spirit!

People embrace this concept of having an old nature that drives them to sin and lust because it logically explains their continued propensity for it. But Romans 6:6 explains what you need to know to be free. "Your old man was crucified with Him." Then, the body of sin has to be destroyed.

I kept thinking, "I can't be dead to sin," because I don't feel dead to sin." Like me you're going to have to set your feelings aside, because it's what you believe that sets you free not what you feel. God's Word is true whether you choose to believe it or not. Believing the Word of God doesn't make it true; His Word is true, therefore you must believe it even if your emotions don't cooperate.

I think Colossians 3:3 is the key, "For you died, and your life is now hidden with Christ in God." It is stating I am already dead, past tense, so I don't have to keep trying to die. As I stated in the earlier chapters, over the years as a Pastor and being a Christian Counselor I have come to realize that there are many people like me who have been desperately trying to do something that has already been done and trying to become something they already are.

"Don't you know that all of us who were baptized into Christ Jesus were baptized into death?" (Romans 6:3). Again I want you to note that it doesn't say or imply that there is something we have to do. We were already baptized if we have confessed with our mouth that Jesus Christ is Lord and believed in our hearts that God raised Him from the dead. Ephesians 2:8, 9 states that, "it's by grace that we have been saved through faith and that it is not of our selves (or anything that we have done), lest any of us should ever boast." It is futile to seek something which the Bible affirms we already have: "We were all baptized by one Spirit into one body" (1Corinthians 12:13). "We were" is past tense. It's done, so it must be believed.

This passage is dealing with our spiritual baptism into Christ, not to be confused with the external ordinance of water baptism which is only a symbol. Augustine called baptism a visible form of an invisible grace. As a pastor I have had the privilege of baptizing people of all ages who wanted to obey the Lord's Command by publically indentifying with the death, burial, and resurrection of the Lord Jesus Christ.

When Christ died on the cross and was buried, as pictured by a baptismal candidate being immersed in water, you died and were buried to sin. And when or if you place your faith in Jesus Christ as Savior and Lord, your death and burial was activated. You died then; you can't do it again. You can only believe it.

New Life in Christ

"We were therefore buried with him through baptism into death in order that, just as Christ was raised from the dead through the glory of the Father, we too may live a new life. If we have been united with him like this in his death, we will certainly also be united with him in his resurrection" (Romans 6:4, 5). Paul's argument is twofold. You cannot identify with the death and burial of Christ without also identifying with His resurrection and ascension. As I have proven in my life you will live in defeat if you only believe half of the gospel. "You have died with Christ, and you have been raised with Him and seated in the heavenlies "(Ephesians 2:6). Every child of God is spiritually alive and therefore "in Christ."

Because we are in Christ, we have the spirit of God within us. We must learn how to live our lives in total dependence upon God. Before we were in Christ, we depended on our parents, ourselves, doctors or counselors and our drug of choice, whatever that is, to help us survive and cope; and we can continue to do so after salvation, as I did. The enemy is very subtle and gets us to put all our confidence in our programs, strategies, others or even ourselves. Apart from Christ, we are not handicapped. Apart from Christ, we are not limited in what we can do. "Apart from Christ, we can do nothing" (John 15:5), "but because we are in Christ, we have the assurance that He will meet all our needs" (Philippians 4:19). Our "being" needs, i.e., life, identity, acceptance, security and significance.

I believe it is crucial that we know who we are in spirit and in truth. This is the hinge of my thesis for this book. Am I an addict or a saint? I came to understand and believe through this process of research and writing this book, that I am a saint, who is addicted. I don't believe that our Spirit is addicted however I do believe that our soul (our mind, emotions and will) can become psychologically and biologically dependent just as we can become physiologically dependent. Without this distinction the best we can hope for is once an addict always an addict. It is paramount that we not only understand that there are three parts to our humanity but that recovery is three fold. If we do not become dependent on Christ in Spirit by recognizing that "apart from Christ we can do nothing," then we will become dependent upon someone or something in body and soul which has the potential to be addictive in nature and very self destructive.

Let me conclude this chapter by stating that the last verse reveals the critical reason we should have faith and know our true identity in Christ. People cannot consistently behave in a manner inconsistent with their self-perceptions. If we define ourselves by our soul and call ourselves addicts, these pronouncements can become self-fulfilling prophecies. Our performance-based culture promotes the tendency to identify ourselves by the things we do (body and soul). So when we sin, we conclude we are sinners. However I believe the Bible makes it quite clear that we are saints (positional in spirit) who choose to sin (body and soul). Just as "having" an addiction and "being" an addict are two different issues. We have sin and we need to admit it, but we are not sin. "Having" sin and "being" sin are two totally different issues. We don't call a person "cancer" because he or she has cancer or some physical disease. However the human soul is still tragically diseased. Like disease corrupts the body so sin corrupts the soul to become evil. All men and women, no matter how "good or great" things they have done have been corrupted by sin.

Sin, is a disease of the soul. Like leprosy or cancer and yes even addiction, SIN slowly eats away until it kills. Like these diseases, some people succumb in a few short years. Others individuals it takes decades. Sin even after a lifetime may not be "That Bad' or "Criminal" but all have come short of the Glory of God. Again, like Cancer, It cares not how good you've been, what you've done or who you are or even how religious you've been. Sin without a cure will destroy your soul.

Christians have problems, but they are not the problems. If they were the problems, the problems could not be resolved. There is no question that as a Christian I created a lot of problems for myself by living in denial and not appropriating who I am by faith. As a Christian I can appropriately say, "I am child of God and right now I am struggling with self-defeating learned behaviors. I know that I can resolve this issue and live free in Christ because I am "dead to sin, but alive to God in Christ Jesus"(Romans 6:11). How can I be assured of that? Because, "the Spirit himself testifies with my spirit that I am God's child" (Romans 8:16). Also, in I Corinthians 6: "...but he who unites himself with the Lord is one with him in spirit." So there is the melding, the union of the two. Spirit with spirit meet, and it is at that level that regeneration takes place. That is why it is called, this new impartation of life, God re-inhabiting the human spirit to be born again and have new life in Jesus Christ.

Now that is true in the spirit, but it is not true of the soul. You see, it's been living a number of years, perhaps twenty or thirty, sometimes sixty or seventy years, governed by the flesh; therefore, all its habits are flesh-centered, habits of selfishness that run our lives. It is still twisted with our distorted belief system that we thought would meet our need for significance and security, that sense of self-worth. Therefore, the soul, the will, emotions and mind, are still under the domination of the flesh (remember I gave definition to the flesh in chapter 7), though the spirit is now born again. You can know it, feel the joy and peace of it, but still be governed by the flesh. You can still get involved in some of the old sins, but actually be born again. That is what is called in I Corinthians 3 "carnal", fleshly Christians. It's true of the soul, but not of the spirit. It was very hard for me to see that I was carnal when I was working so hard to be spiritual, and yet because of my addiction in the soul, by definition I was carnal. However as John tells us, the spirit cannot sin. I John 3:9: "No one born of God commits sin; for God's nature abides in him, and he cannot sin because he is born of God." (RSV) He is born of God, and therefore the Spirit in us cannot sin. But the soul can sin, and that is where much of our struggle comes from as Christians and addicts.

Listen to what Andrew Wommack states about carnality.

> "For to be carnally minded is death; but to be spiritually minded is life and peace" (Romans 8:6). Carnal mindedness doesn't necessarily mean "sinful" mindedness. All sin is carnal, but not all carnality is sin. "Carnal" literally means "of the five senses," or "sensual." Carnal mindedness is allowing your mind to be dominated by what you can see, taste, hear, smell, and feel. You are carnally minded when your thoughts center primarily on the physical realm.
>
> It is the business of the Holy Spirit coming into the human spirit to re-possess the soul. There may be clean areas where the Spirit of God has begun to assert the Lordship of Jesus over the soul. But in other areas it may still very much be a day to day battle and struggle, especially when it comes to areas of addiction and having to address deeper, biological, psychological, and physiological areas of our lives. We fight the Lord at

> that point. We drag our heels, delay, play mind games, and tell him we are yielding but we are not. But the Spirit keeps insisting that we submit this area of our lives to Jesus' Lordship.

It is what we call denial. It is what I alluded to earlier in Chapter 7 and what Freud defined as minimizing, rationalizing, justifying and analyzing. I am sure we are all aware of the meaning of that word; I hear it all the time, especially in the counseling office when I am dealing with couples. It is simply when an individual dismisses from their awareness the negative consequences of their behavior. Denial can be a very effective method for someone who wants to focus on the benefits of their self-defeating behavior (sin) or addiction, at the same time, keeping problems that their harmful behavior is causing them out of their conscious awareness. In order for the Spirit of God to impact the soul, and for us to arrest that harmful behavior, the denial must be deactivated. Identifying and acknowledging the problems that our behavior or addiction has resulted in for ourselves and others brings these problems into conscious awareness and consequently can go a long way in helping to neutralize denial and allow the Spirit to heal a sin sick soul, especially if this is done on an ongoing basis over time. (See Appendix II Denial & Self Defense Mechanisms)

I believe a prime example of this is found in 2 Samuel 12 and 13, where David lived in the sin of both adultery with Bathsheba and murder of her husband Uriah the Hittite, and the secret cover up. God, who is in the business of denial busting, was about to give David a big wake-up call and bring to his conscious awareness what his behaviors really meant. In chapter 12 God sends Nathan to rebuke David and to reveal to him that He saw it all. All of David's minimizing, rationalizing, justifying that came with denial was up; God called a spade a spade. "David you sinned", and David's denial was busted and in verse 13 David's response is, "yes I have sinned." Do note however David's response could have been more denial which would have simply drawn out this process of self-defeating behavior, lies, secrecy, guilt and shame described in Psalm 32. But like David because our soul can be very convoluted with lies and deception, we have to face the consequences, to bring home the impact of our behavior and bring true godly sorrow and repentance. We need to remember that grace and forgiveness is free but it is not cheap.

We all live our lives in segments, like an orange. There's our family life, our sex life, our personal life, and we keep switching back and forth among these throughout the day. Usually the Spirit of God will pick one of those areas and begin to talk with you about it. He'll say, "Look, this isn't right. You can't go on like this. You're a believer; you have to change at this point." And he will bring all sorts of pressures and influences upon it, and probably precipitate a crisis where we find ourselves at last knocked off our feet, or flat on our backs, and he gets our attention. Then he brings it up again and says, "See, this is the area I'm talking about. Now I want you to yield that to the Lord. Give it back to him and let him be Lord in that area. One of the principles you see repeated in the Word of God is that He will always bring individuals and nations full circle to the place of defeat, often to face their worst fears.

That is what is beautifully described for us in II Corinthians 3:17-18: "Now the Lord is the Spirit, and where the Spirit of the Lord is, there is freedom." We begin to get freed up in these areas. "And we, who with unveiled faces all reflect (contemplate is probably a better term) the Lord's glory (you're thinking of Jesus and seeing him as Lord of your life), "are being transformed into his likeness (this is what we call Christian growth. Gradually the soul begins to correspond to what is true with the spirit, and you begin to take on the likeness of Christ) "with ever increasing glory, (normally, in the course of the Christian life, the older we grow the more like Christ we ought to be becoming. Not because your spirit is more like Christ. It is made instantly like Christ, from the beginning, the moment you are born again. The soul, the conscious life, begins to reflect him), which comes from the Lord, who is the Spirit."

He drives the flesh out of your spirit, but it remains in your soul. And it may be you will work at this the rest of your life, until you receive increasing degrees of likeness to Christ. You can however relapse or you can give over an area to the Lordship of Christ and then take it back, and have to give it over again. It would be likened unto what Carnes calls the Coningent Phase in the addictive process.

So our responsibility is simple, "Submit therefore to God. Resist the devil and he will flee from you" (James 4:7). If you try to resist the devil without first submitting to God, you will have a fight on your hands. Submitting to God gives us the right to live like children of God. This is a winnable war if we know who we are and the tremendous position we have in Christ and understand the nature of the spiritual battle we have in our body and soul. (See Appendix IX Spiritual Battle)

Now let's consider what we are finally like when God finishes his work with us, which is at the resurrection of the body. The last part of our being to be redeemed is the body. It remains under the control of the flesh, and inheriting the weakness of sin all our lives. That's why we age and get weak, and why our minds falter, why we stumble, lose our way and our eyesight dims. All of this is part of a body not yet redeemed. Spirit is instantly redeemed when we are born again. It never changes. The soul is being redeemed as we grow in our relationship to our Lord and submit to his Lordship over areas of our lives. The body is redeemed at the resurrection.

This is the three tenses of salvation, such as you find in Scripture. Some passages speak of "we have been saved". That is referring to the spirit. Other verses describe us as "being saved". That's the soul. And we shall be saved: "now is our salvation nearer than when we first believed", Paul says. That is a reference to the resurrection.

The soul accompanies the spirit at all times, and goes to God. I believe that the moment we die we are instantly, body, soul and spirit, with the Lord, in a redeemed body. Our eternal security comes from the assurance that "he that is born of God cannot sin." That is the spirit part of our being. Nor can it lose its life. That's how Paul gets to that wonderful passage in Romans 8. "Who shall separate us from the love of Christ? Nothing! Neither in heaven, earth, hell or anywhere else; no power, no force, no being can separate us from the love of Christ.

I Corinthians 3:12-15: "If any man builds on this foundation (that is, faith in Christ) using gold, silver, costly stones, (these are symbols of the work of the Spirit in our lives) wood, hay or straw (symbols of the flesh at work), his work will be shown for what it is, because the Day will bring it to light. It will be revealed with fire, and the fire will test the quality of each man's work. If what he has built survives, (that is the gold, silver and costly stones, and not wood, hay or straw) he will receive his reward. If it is burned up, (if it is the flesh) he will suffer loss; he himself will be saved, but only as one escaping through the flames."

This brings me to the next chapter as to how we can win the battle that rages in our body and soul (our mind, emotions and will), and experience on going recovery and victory.

Chapter 10
My Body

Hardware & Software Impact

Scripture refers to the outer man and inner man (I Corinthians 4:16). As a point of review the outer man is our physical body, that includes the Peripheral Nervous System, the Autonomic Nervous System, the Central Nervous System, the Somatic Nervous System and of course the Brain that I spoke about in earlier chapters. Our minds are a part of the inner man (soul) and our brains are fundamentally different (body).

God created the outer man to correlate with the inner man. The correlation between the mind and the brain is obvious. The brain functions much like a digital computer. Every neuron operates like a little switch that turns on and off. Each has many inputs (dendrites) and only one output that channels the neurotransmitters to other dendrites. The computer hardware is made up of millions of these. Our minds, on the other hand, represent the software. The brain can be mindlessly programmed by the world, because the brain receives data from the external world through the five senses of the body. The mind, however, is the compiler and chooses to interpret the data by whatever means it has been programmed. Until we come to know the truth in God, it has been programmed by external sources (family, trauma, religion, culture, and personality bias, etc.) but now by faith we can make internal choices with the knowledge of God and the benefits of His presence.

The tendency of our Western world is to assume that mental problems are primarily caused by faulty hardware. Clearly, organic brain syndrome, Alzheimer's disease, or lesser organic problems such as chemical imbalances can impede our abilities to function. The best program will not work if the computer is turned off or in disrepair. However, our primary problem is not the hardware, it is the software.

The hardware consisting of the brain and spinal cord make up the central nervous system. It splits off into a peripheral nervous system. The peripheral nervous system has two channels: the autonomic and somatic nervous systems. The somatic nervous system regulates our muscular and skeletal movements such as speech, gestures, etc., in other words, that which we can volitionally (behaviorally) control. It obviously correlates with our wills that other part of our soul.

Our autonomic nervous system regulates our glands. We have no volitional control over our glands. We don't say to our heart, "beat, beat, beat" because they function automatically.

Let's apply this to the problem of stress. When external pressures put demands on our physical systems, our adrenal glands respond by secreting cortisone-like hormones into our physical bodies. Our bodies automatically respond to external pressures. If the pressures persist for too long, our adrenal glands cannot keep up, so stress becomes distress. The result can be physical illness, or we may become irritated with things that were not previously irritating to us.

Why can two people respond differently to the same stressful situation? Some actually seize the opportunity and thrive under the pressure while others fall apart. What is the difference between the two? Does one have superior adrenal glands? I don't think so. Although we differ considerably in our hardware, the major difference exits in the software. The degree of stress we experience is determined by more than external factor. We all face the pressures of deadlines, schedules, trauma and temptations. The major difference is in how we mentally interpret the external world and process the data our brains receive.

What we know of addicts is that there higher than average anxiety along with poor coping strategies to manage stress often leads them to self medication. Wendy and Larry Maltz in their book *The Porn Trap* tell us,

> "That when pornography use is combined with masturbation, the end result is orgasm. We all know the power of orgasm to create pleasure, numb pain, and generate a state of deep relaxation. It has the same effect as a sedative and opiate on the brain. What makes this a poor coping strategy for stress and highly addictive is the fact that powerful human bonding hormones such as oxytocin and vasopressin are released with the orgasm. They contribute to establishing a lasting emotional attachment with whomever, or whatever, you happen to be with or thinking about at the time. The more orgasms you have with porn, for example the more sexually and emotionally attached to it you'll become.

So the question is how we manage stress and anxiety in a healthy way. The mind can either choose to respond by trusting God with the assurance of victory, or choose to see itself as the helpless victim of circumstances, thus causing further stress and anxiety. Each personality has its own way of dealing with stress and I would dare say that there are many who do not even believe or trust in God, yet as an optimist are able to see difficulties as opportunities because of their natural positive mindset.

Arnold Schwarzenegger is one of those people that come to mind as an eternal optimist and choleric. After just recently reading his book *Total Recall My Unbelievably True Life Story* he states,

> "It is not always obvious what you should celebrate. Sometimes you have to appreciate the very people and circumstances that traumatized you. Today I hail the strictness of my father, and my whole upbringing, and the fact that I didn't have anything that I wanted in Austria, because those were the very factors that made me hungry. Every time he hit me. Every time he said my weight training was garbage, that I should do something useful and go out and chop wood. Every time he

> disapproved of me or embarrassed me, it put fuel on the fire in my belly. It drove me and motivated me." He goes on to say "that your parents have done their best and if they left you with problems, those problems are now yours to solve, so don't blame them."

He is a true optimist rarely letting life's stress dictate his outcome in a negative way. Always seeing it as something to conquer and defeat rather than be defeated and avoid. However I will note that in his book he self confesses that as positive and accomplished as he has been, it has been at the cost of not being able to develop trust and intimacy in his relationships. There has been a disconnect between his soul and spirit. He concludes his book by stating that in a week moment he slept with his house keeper which consequently brought a baby boy into the world. For the next decade he kept it a secret and eventually cost him his marriage. Even the true optimist personality when managing life's stress and temptations solely dependent on its own resources and not trusting God can end in disaster, because it is not just a personality issue. It is a Trinitarian issue (Body, Soul & Spirit).

Let me further drive home this point, Sex glands are part of the autonomic nervous system. For example, a woman has no volitional control over her menstrual cycle. A man can wake up in the middle of the night with an erection, and it may have nothing to do with lust. It is just part of a rhythmic cycle all men go through about every 90 minutes. That is the way God created us. If we have no control over our sex glands, then how can God expect us to have any sexual self-control?

The good news is we don't need to have any volitional control over our sex glands to have self-control. We have control over what we think. Our sex glands are not the cause of sexual immorality. They will "naturally" function in their God given way to ensure our sexuality. However, if we load our brains with pornography, we will drive our autonomic nervous systems beyond the stops. We may not have any control over what comes out, but we do have control over what we put in. Just like a computer, garbage in – garbage out!

What we see in the world comes through the eye gate. We can stop it by closing our eyes, but even then our imaginations can run wild. If we look at objects of temptation, the signals will be recorded in our brains.

At the moment, we have a choice. If we choose to let our minds dwell on these unwholesome images, we can expect an almost instantaneous physiological response, because the peripheral nervous system is fed by the central nervous system. I heard it said recently in regards to women, although men will struggle with lust through the eyes, women struggle with the temptation of being lusted after, just the opposite side of the same coin.

Have you ever wondered why it is so difficult to remember some things and forget others? I have. I could spend hours studying for an exam and pray that by the next morning that the register didn't clear before I took the exam. But if I saw one pornographic image, it seemed to stay in my mind for years. Why? When we are visually stimulated, a signal is sent to our adrenal glands. A hormone called epinephrine is secreted into the bloodstream when we become emotionally excited. Dopamine production spikes and researchers tell us dramatic spikes are likened unto the high received by crack cocaine use. There is also the increased production of other "feel-good" chemicals such as adrenaline, endorphins, and serotonin. Epinephrine goes to the brain and locks in the visual or audio stimulus present at the time of the emotional excitement. It caused us to involuntarily remember traumatic as well as emotionally positive events.

We can become emotionally excited and sexually stimulated by simply entertaining thoughts of sexual activity. That is why men and women will have an emotional rush before any sexual contact ever takes place. The man going to the store where pornography is sold will be sexually stimulated long before he sees the magazines. It began in his thoughts that triggered his nervous system that responded by secreting epinephrine into the bloodstream.

Our autonomic nervous systems obviously correlate to the emotional parts of our inner man. Just as we can't control our glands, we can't control our emotions. If you think you can, give it a try! Try liking someone right now that you previously couldn't stand. We can't order our emotions to feel-no instruction in Scripture suggests that we do that. We must, however, acknowledge our emotions, because we can't be right with God and not be real. What we do have control over is what we think, so Scripture tells us to take responsibility for our thoughts.

"Brothers, stop thinking like children. In regard to evil be infants, but in your thinking be adults" (I Corinthians14:20).

I need to repeat this point again, we have no control over how we feel, and therefore, I encourage you to eliminate the following line from your vocabulary in reference to yourself and others: "You shouldn't feel that way." It is a subtle form of rejection, and no addict needs any more of that. What can people do about how they feel? Nothing! The real issue is what we think, or how we perceive ourselves and the events around us. Perhaps we haven't fully understood the whole situation, maybe we have wrongly judged someone or maybe we just need to trust God.

Our feelings are primarily products of our thought lives. Our tendency is to believe something or somebody made us feel a certain way, but that isn't true. All external data is processed through our minds, and we have control over them. It logically follows that our feelings can be distorted by what we choose to think or believe. If what we choose to believe does not reflect truth, then what we feel will not reflect reality. If what we see or mentally visualize is morally wrong, then our emotions will be violated.

Before I get ahead of myself by looking at the soul at length, I want to look at the body from Paul's perspective in Romans 6:12. "Therefore do not let sin reign in your mortal body so that you obey its evil desires." Here lies the practical reality that I introduced in the last chapter.

Whose responsibility is it not to allow sin to reign in our mortal bodies or for our sex drive to drive the bus? Clearly it is our own personal responsibility. As much as I would have liked to believe that the devil-made-me-do-it, unfortunately I know that I am and always have been responsible for my actions and attitudes. What must we do to prevent sin from reigning in our mortal bodies? Paul provides the answer in verse 13, "Do not offer the parts of your body to sin, as instruments of wickedness, but rather offer yourselves to God, as those who have been brought from death to life; and offer the parts of your body to him as instruments of righteousness."

We are not to use our bodies in ways that would serve our sexual addiction. If we do, we allow our addiction to reign (rule) in our physical bodies. Here lies the pathology of addiction and the cycle that

Patrick Carnes so clearly presents in his research and I gave you a quick snapshot earlier in the book. (See Appendix III)

This perhaps raises the question, are our body evil? I know there are some that would suggest that it is, however, to the contrary, I believe they are amoral or neutral. So what are we to do with the neutral disposition of our bodies? We are told to present them as instruments of righteousness. "Present" means "to put at the disposal of." The Lord is commanding us to be good stewards of our bodies and to use them only as instruments of righteousness.

You may think that is not true because we are not all the same biologically. You are right, I was assessed and it was determined that I was at the ninety-eight percentile for sex drive. As an addiction counsellor and having taken "Bio-Psycho-Social Aspects of Addictions as part of my formal training, my answer is that there are indeed predisposing factors that contribute to any addiction. However that does not mean that the body itself is evil nor does it mean that having a high sex drive will lead to sexual addiction. These same hormones have allowed me to have lots of energy and do very constructive things. The choice has still been mine, for everyone who has a high sex drive are not sex addicts and the opposite is also true, every sex addict does not have a high sex drive. I will go into more detail of the biology of sexual addiction in chapter 11 as it relates to our hardwiring.

Let's continue to apply this line of reasoning and read from Paul in I Corinthians 6:13-20 "The body is not meant for sexual immorality, but for the Lord, and the Lord for the body. By his power God raised the Lord from the dead, and he will raise us also. Do you not know that your bodies are members of Christ himself? Shall I then take the members of Christ and unite them with a prostitute? Never! Do you not know that he who unites himself with a prostitute is one with her in body? For it is said, "The two shall become on flesh." But he who unites himself with the Lord is one with him in spirit. Flee from sexual immorality. All other sins a man commits are outside his body, but he who sins sexually sins against his own body. Do you not know that your body is a temple of the Holy Spirit, who is in you, whom you received from God? You are not your own; you were bought at a price. Therefore honor God with your body."

This passage teaches that we have more than a spiritual union with God. Our "bodies are members of Christ Himself" (verse 15). Romans 8:11 says, "If the Spirit of him who raised Jesus from the dead is living in you, he who raised Christ from the dead will also give life to your mortal bodies through his Spirit, who lives in you." Our bodies are actually temples of God, because His spirit dwells in us. If we use our bodies for sexual immorality, we defile the temple of God. In further support of the Trinitarian nature of man, if we consider the Temple in the Book of Exodus that was introduced to us as God's dwelling place amongst Israel, it is a wonderful picture of our bodies (I Corinthians 3:16). The Outer Court represents our bodies, the Holy Place represents our Soul and the Holy of Holies represents our Spirit which is the dwelling place of the living God. If I had the time I would go into more detail because this in and of itself is a tremendous study. Christ himself became the fulfillment of this temple in the New Testament, when He told the Pharisees that he could rebuild the Temple in three days if they destroyed it, meaning His own body. Now by faith and being in Christ we have become the fulfillment of that temple, "therefore we are exhorted to glorify God in your body and your spirit which are God's" (I Corinthians 6:20).

In considering Christ, I believe He was fully God and also fully man. I believe He was sexually a man and although I don't know what his hormone levels were at, I do know that the Scriptures states that He was tempted in the same way that we are tempted. But Christ never sinned. His earthly body was not meant for sexual immorality-neither is ours. If our eyes were fully open to the reality of the spiritual world and we completely understood the consequences of sinning against our own bodies, we would "flee from sexual immorality" (verse 18).

If we commit sexual sins, we allow sin to reign in our mortal bodies! We will still be united with the Lord? Yes, because He will never leave us nor forsake us. We don't lose our salvation, and our spiritual position, but our soul and body can lose their freedom. To the point that when the addiction says "jump", we jump and when it says "sit," we sit. Our spirit can be quenched and rob us of love, joy, peace and all the fruit that comes with living in the spirit, including life itself.

That being said, we can break the addictive behaviors by complete repentance. You know the old cliché, "confession is good for the soul." How profoundly true that is. There is no secret formula; we simply start the process by praying. We ask the Lord to mentally reveal every sexual use of our bodies as instruments of unrighteousness. As the Lord brings every sexual sin into the mind, we need to renounce the use of our body in that sexual act and ask the Lord to break our bond with each use. We then need to commit our bodies to God, as living sacrifices, wholly and acceptable to Him. If we are married we need to reserve the sexual use of our bodies only for our spouses.

Repentance means we turn away from something wrong and turn to something right. It is not enough to acknowledge the lie, we must choose the truth. To renounce or admit that something is wrong amounts to only the first half of repentance. We must announce or choose what is right to make it complete. We need to commit ourselves and our bodies as instruments of righteousness.

To put this into context, we must examine the bigger picture starting with the Old Testament. The sin offering was a blood offering. The blood was drained from the carcass, and then the carcass was taken out and disposed of. Only the blood was sacrificed for the sin offering.

Who is our sin offering? The Lord Jesus Christ. "Without shedding of blood there is no forgiveness" (Hebrews 9:22). After He shed His blood for us on the cross, His body was taken down and buried. But not for long, praise the Lord.

The Old Testament sacrificial system also required a burnt offering. In Hebrew "burnt offering, unlike the sin offering, was totally consumed on the altar-blood, carcass and all.

This raises the second question, who is the burnt offering? We are! Paul wrote, "Therefore, I urge you, brothers, in view of God's mercy, to offer your bodies as living sacrifice, holy and pleasing to God-this is our spiritual act of worship" (Romans 12:1). It is great to know our sins are forgiven-Christ did that for you and me. But if we want to live victoriously in Christ, then we must present ourselves to God and our body as an instrument of righteousness. We need to be filled with the Holy Spirit.

Paul not only urges us to present our bodies to God as a living sacrifice in Romans 12:1 but goes on in verse 2 to state, "we do this by the renewing of our minds." This is the Soul work that I want to discuss in the next chapter. I want to discuss how we must reprogram our minds, because they were programmed to live independently from God.

Chapter 11
The Soul

Like a computer, our brains have recorded every experience we have ever had. These impressions have a lasting impact on our physical bodies. I have seen adults recoil in physical pain as they get in touch with childhood memories of abuse. Because of the trauma, lies, fears, and incorrect beliefs about themselves it has affected how they see God, and has affected their temperaments and altered their personalities. It takes time to renew their minds, and to replace the lies they have believed with the truth of God's Word.

As I spoke in earlier chapters, these lies are formed at different stages of development and maturation. A basic agreement exists among all developmental theorists that our attitudes are primarily assimilated from the environment in which we are raised. The major programming of our minds took place during our early childhood in several ways.

First, through prevailing experiences such as the families we were raised in, the churches we did or did not attend, the neighbourhoods where we grew up, the communities where we lived, the friends that we did or did not have, etc. Every experience had an effect upon the development of our minds, our world views, and even our addictions, but out of all those environmental and sociological factors, family has the biggest impact.

Family Impact

Let me take a few moments to expound on how our family of origin impacts our world view and our addictions. The last fifty years have ushered in a new awareness about the impact of families on personality formation. While it's always been known that our families influence us, we're now discovering that the influence is beyond what we had imagined. We now understand that families are dynamic social systems, having structural laws, components and rules.

The most important family rules are those that determine what it means to be a human being. These rules embrace the most fundamental beliefs about raising children. What parents believe about human life and human fulfillment govern their ways of raising children. Parenting does form children's core beliefs about themselves.

John Bradshaw in his book, *The Family* states that there is a crisis in the family today. It has to do with our parenting rules and the multigenerational process by which families perpetuate these rules. Our parenting rules primarily shame children through abandonment. He goes on to say that parents abandon their children in the following ways:

- By actually physically leaving them.
- By not modeling their own emotions for their children.
- By not being there to affirm their children's expressions of emotion.
- By not providing for their children's developmental dependency needs.
- By physically, sexually, emotionally and spiritually abusing them.
- By using children to take care of their own unmet dependency needs.
- By using children to take care of their marriages.
- By hiding and denying their shame secrets to the outside world so that the children have to protect these covert issues in order to keep the family balance.
- By not giving them their time, attention and direction.
- By acting shamelessly.

In abandonment the order of nature is reversed. Children have to take care of their parents. There is no one to take care of them.

Abandonment creates a shame-based inner core. To compensate, one develops a false self in order to survive. The false self forms a defensive mask which distracts from the pain and the inner loneliness of the true self. After years of acting and performing and pretending—one loses contact with who one really is.

So as we relate this to our addiction we must examine these rules in order to come to terms with our compulsiveness. Shame with its accompanying loneliness fuels our addiction. Shame is like a hole in the cup of our soul. Since the child in the adult has insatiable needs, the cup cannot be filled. We are driven. We want more sex, more food, more money, more drugs...it doesn't matter what it is we just want more. Our dis-ease is about the things of everyday life. Our troubles are focused on what we eat, drink, work, how we are intimate, how we play and even how we worship. We stay so busy and distracted that we never feel how lonely, hurt, mad and sad we really are.

Our families are the places where we have our source relationships. In families we learn about emotional intimacy. We learn what feelings are and how to express them. Our parents model what feelings are acceptable and family authorized and what feelings are prohibited. In our families we adapt to the needs of our family system. We take on roles necessitated by the dynamics of the system. Such roles demand that we learn certain feelings and we give up certain feelings.

Alice Miller, in her book *For Your Own Good* has grouped these parenting rules under the title "poisonous pedagogy". The subtitle of the book is, *Hidden Cruelty in Child-Rearing and the Roots of Violence.* She argues that the poisonous pedagogy is a form of violence which violates the rights of children. Such violation is then re-enacted when these children become parents.

> "The "poisonous pedagogy" concept exalts obedience as its highest value. Following obedience are orderliness, cleanliness and the control of emotions and desires. Children are considered "good" when they think and behave the way they are taught to think and behave. Children are virtuous when they are meek, agreeable, considerate and unselfish. The more a child is "seen and not heard" and "speaks only when spoken to" the better

> that child is. This system imparts to the child from the beginning, false information and beliefs that are not only unproven, but in some cases, demonstrably false. These beliefs are passed on from generation to generation ("sins of the fathers").
>
> The great paradox in child-parent relationships is that children's belief about parents comes from the parents. Parents teach their children the meaning of the world around them. For the first ten years of life, the parents are the most important part of the child's world. If a child is taught to honor his parents no matter what they do, why would a child argue with this?"

In the first eight years of life, according to the cognitive psychologists, such as Jean Piaget, children think magically, non-logically and egocentrically. The magical part of the child's thinking deifies the parents. They are gods, all-powerful, almighty and all-protecting. No harm can come to the child as long as he has parents. For a child at this stage to realize the inadequacies of parents would produce unbearable anxiety. So the child must idealize the parent(s); but this idealization also creates a potential for a shame-binding predicament for the child.

For example, if the parents are abusive and hurt the child through physical, sexual, emotional or mental pain, the child will assume the blame, make himself bad, in order to keep the all-powerful protection against the fears of the night. No child, because of his helplessness, dependency and fear, wants to accept the belief that his parents are inadequate, sick, crazy or otherwise imperfect. So by blaming themselves, they interject the parent's voices. This means that the child continues to hear internally the shame dialogue he originally had with the parent(s), hence the birth of negative self-talk.

The child parents himself the way he was parented. If the child got shamed for feeling angry, sad or sexual, he will shame himself each time he feels angry, sad or sexual. We adopt our parent's words as our own and they become the new negative voice of authority in our head. All of his feeling, needs and drives become shame-bound. The inner self-rupture is so painful, the child must develop a "false self". This false self is manifested in a mask or rigid role which is either determined by the culture or by the family system's need for balance. Over time the child identifies with the false self and becomes totally unconscious of his own true feelings, needs and wants. The shame is internalized. Shame is no longer a feeling, it is an identity. The real self has withdrawn from conscious contact. The soul has become so loaded with self rejection and fear that it can no longer hear words and actions of love and acceptance, they are always met and filtered with a 'ya but...' The more one feels worthless the more one feels powerless to change. The more one feels powerless—the fewer choices one feels he or she has. To have one's feelings, body, desires and thoughts controlled is to lose one's self. To lose one's self is to have one's soul murdered.

"To live and never know who I really am" is a great tragedy. The rage, crimes and violence are symptoms of our soul sickness demonstrated in our world today. It is also directed against ourselves as the shame fuels our addiction. We learn to defend ourselves with our defense mechanisms. We repress feelings; we deny what is going on; we displace our rage onto our possessions or our friends; we create illusions of love and connectedness; we idealize and minimize; some will dissociate so that we no longer feel anything at all. Our addiction is the way we alter our mood. It helps us to numb out emotionally. They are ways of being alive and our ways of managing feelings. This is most apparent in experiences that are euphoric, like using drugs, alcohol and sex.

When I first started in the field of counseling I heard that statistically most families in North America are dysfunctional; so should it be any surprise that addiction has become our national lifestyle and not solely relegated to alcohol, drugs, or sexual addiction? It is a death style based on the relinquishment of the self as a worthwhile being to a self who must achieve and perform or use something outside of self in order to be lovable and happy. Addictions are pain-killing substitutes for legitimate feelings.

That being said, sexual addiction is the fastest-growing problem in our society and eating disorders are a close second. I shared in the preamble of this book some startling statistics and those numbers have grown exponentially since being recorded. As individuals and as a society it appears that our wills have run riot. Bradshaw calls this the "disabled will." Once our will is disabled, we lose our freedom. Since shame binds all emotions, everyone in a dysfunctional family has their freedom greatly impaired. Harvey Jackins' presentation of blocked emotion in his book *The Human Side of Human Beings* states,

> "The will needs the eyes of perception, judgment, imagination and reasoning. Without this source, the will is blinded. The mind cannot use its perception, judgment, reasoning and imagination when it is under the impact of heavy emotion. The particular emotion, which is a form of energy, has to be discharged before the mind can function effectively. When the emotion is repressed, it forms a frozen block which chronically mars the effective use of reasoning. Anyone who has had an outbreak of temper or been depressed has experienced how difficult it is to think under the power of these emotions."

Such contamination seriously lessens one's decision-making process, since the will needs perception, intelligence and imagination in order to make decisions. The human will become 'disabled.' Since the will is blind, it has no resource for its choice making. The only object left for the will to use is itself. As one wills to will, one becomes willful.

Leslie Farber points out in *The Ways of the Will,*

> "The will becomes the self. With each act of willing for the sake of willing, one feels whole and complete. This is the basis of impulsiveness. To act on impulse is to will just because you can. In every 'act of will' the person feels complete. When one can only will to will, one has become grandiose. One plays God. Self-will has run riot. There is an attempt to control what can't be controlled."

For example the addict believes he can control his addiction, the spouse believes she can cure the addict. Parents believe they can control their children. We believe we can control our emotions. Other examples are to be always driven and compulsive, always looking for a grand experience, the perfect something, everything is extreme, black and white, good or bad, they are for me or against me, etc.

Control results from the disabled will and is one of the major defenses for shame. A shame-based person will attempt to control all the relationships they are in. Shame is the feeling of being flawed and worthless. It demands that one hide and live in secret. One must guard never to be unguarded. In a moment of being unguarded, one could be exposed. This is too painful to bear. Shame-based parents control their children. Children in shame-based families play their rigid roles as a way of controlling their parents. Always being Helpful, always being a Hero, a Rebel, a Perfect Child, a Scapegoat, etc (See Appendix X ----for definition of each role). This controlled madness is another way to show why dysfunctional families set their members up for an addiction. Addictions are ways to be out of control. Addictions provide relief.

Co-dependency is the major outcome of dysfunctional family systems. Suffice it to say that co-dependants no longer have their own feelings, needs and wants. They live in reaction to the family distress.

It breaks my heart when I consider how my own shame and addiction has created dysfunction in my family and was only compounded by the distress of Stephanie's ongoing medical crisis. As the spiritual head of the home my heart breaks and is burdened with guilt as I see my own children and wife who I love very much suffer an ill fate. Playing such roles as Scapegoat, Lost Child, Hero and Caregiver Roles. Compounding all this has been the fact that each of them has been deeply wounded by the dysfunctional church family in their own way. My wife would say, that as a pastor's wife, she received no emotional and spiritual support and each of our kids were dropped immediately with no follow up or support. This has not only reinforced the shame but also deepened the feelings of rejection, hurt and confusion.

Of course none of this happens over night, I have spent my adult life believing that I was accurately assessing and adequately supplying the physical, emotional and spiritual needs of my wife and children. When the denial is lifted, it has been very painful to see their own pain and how far short I have come.

Perhaps nothing so accurately characterizes dysfunctional families as denial. This denial is often referred to as the delusional thinking of the dysfunctional family trance. The delusion is to keep believing the myths and vital lies in spite of the facts, or to keep expecting that the same behaviors will bring about different results. Of course in the12 Step Program we call this insanity.

This delusion and denial also applies to false self roles. We become so identified with each others' role that we could pass a lie detector test. Our true self has been buried so long in the unconscious that we think the role is who we really are. We not only act outside of what we were wired to be in personality and soul, but we are also in conflict to who we are in spirit.

This will often lead us to Act Out or Act In. In order to understand this we need to acknowledge the primary motivating force in our lives is emotion. Emotions are the fuel that moves us to defend ourselves and get our basic needs met. For example anger may move us to defend ourselves (fight response), fear moves us to (flight response) and sadness can move us to tears. If we are not able to express our emotions in healthy ways because they were repressed, it will be expressed in abnormal behavior. This is called "acting out". For example a person who was abused as a child may as an adult re-enact the abuse by going from one abusive partner to another, trying this time to make it right, I will show him I love him and he will show me affection.

Unresolved emotions can also lead to "Acting In" which is acting out on ourselves. We punish ourselves the way we were punished as children. Some will say things like, "you're such an idiot, how can you be so dumb, can't you do anything right." Emotional energy that is acted in can cause severe physical problems including gastrointestinal disorders, headaches, backaches, neck aches, severe muscle tension amongst other things.

Bradshaw suggests that,

> "It is also important to note that if a child cannot get his age-appropriate developmental needs met, he will be emotionally arrested at that stage of development. Children who fail to get their infancy needs met become fixated on oral gratification. This may manifest sexually with a fixation on oral sex. Children arrested in the toddler stage are often fascinated by buttocks. Fascination with a genital part is called "sexual

> objectification," and it reduces others to genital objects. (see Appendix X "Wounded Child Questionnaire")
>
> Sexual objectification is the scourge of true intimacy. Intimacy requires two whole persons who value each other as individuals. Many co-dependent couples engage in intensely objectified and addicted sex."

It is not hard to see that my people-pleasing and approval seeking, my overly developed sense of responsibility, and drive, are not just personality quirks but characteristic of my role in a dysfunctional family and ultimately became my character defects. My compulsivity was a problem that was having life-damaging consequences: Remembering that an addiction according to the World Health Organization is a pathological relationship to any form of mood altering that has life-damaging consequences. In my own journey of recovery I have come to realize the addictive nature of my personality (soul), and the self defeating learned behavior of both "Acting Out" and "Acting In."

I want to summarize the impact of dysfunctional families with a poem originally written by Leo Booth and reworked by Bradshaw in his book *Healing the Shame That Binds You.*

My Name is Toxic Shame

I was there at your conception
In the epinephrine of your mother's shame
You felt me in the fluid of your mother's womb
I came upon you before you could speak
Before you understood
Before you had any way of knowing
I came upon you when you were learning to walk
When you were unprotected and exposed
When you were vulnerable and needy
Before you had any boundaries
MY NAME IS TOXIC SHAME

I came upon you when you were magical
Before you could know I was there
I severed your soul
I pierced you to the core
I brought you feelings of being flawed and defective
I brought you feelings of distrust, ugliness, stupidity, doubt, worthlessness, inferiority, and unworthiness
I made you feel different
I told you there was something wrong with you
I soiled your Godlikeness
MY NAME IS TOXIC SHAME

I existed before conscience
Before guilt
Before morality
I am the master emotion
I am the internal voice that whispers words of condemnation
I am the internal shudder that courses through you without any mental preparation
MY NAME IS TOXIC SHAME

I live in secrecy
In the deep moist banks of darkness, depression and despair
Always I sneak up on you I catch you off guard I come through the back door
Uninvited unwanted
The first to arrive
I was there at the beginning of time
With Father Adam, Mother Eve
Brother Cain
I was at the Tower of Babel the Slaughter of the Innocents
MY NAME IS TOXIC SHAME

I come from "shameless" caretakers, abandonment, ridicule, abuse, neglect—perfectionistic systems
I am empowered by the shocking intensity of a parent's rage
The cruel remarks of siblings

The jeering humiliation of other children
The awkward reflection in the mirrors
The touch that feels icky and frightening
The slap, the pinch, the jerk that ruptures trust
I am intensified by
A racist, sexist culture
The righteous condemnation of religious bigots
The fears and pressures of schooling
The hypocrisy of politicians
The multigenerational shame of dysfunctional family systems
MY NAME IS TOXIC SHAME

I bring pain that is chronic
A pain that will not go away
I am the hunter that stalks you night and day
Every day everywhere
I have no boundaries
You try to hide from me
But you cannot
Because I live inside of you
I make you feel hopeless
Like there is no way out
MY NAME IS TOXIC SHAME

My pain is so unbearable that you must pass me on to others through control, perfectionism, contempt, criticism, blame, envy, judgment, power, and rage.
My pain is intense
You must cover me up with addiction, rigid roles, re-enactment, and unconscious defenses
My pain is so intense
That you must numb out and no longer feel me.
I convinced you that I am gone—that I do not exist—you experience absence and emptiness.
MY NAME IS TOXIC SHAME

I am the core of co-dependency
I am spiritual bankruptcy
The logic of absurdity
The repetition compulsion
I am crime, violence, incest, rape
I am the voracious hole that fuels all addictions
I am insatiability and lust
I twist who you are into what you do and have
I murder your soul and you pass me on for generations
MY NAME IS TOXIC SHAME

This poem sums up the significant ways that our false beliefs were formed. The spiritual bankruptcy that occurs when we become disconnected to our real identity. The loss of our primary needs of significance and security not being met, leaving us to feel abandoned and all alone. It is quite clear that so many of the predisposing factors to our addiction are laid down at an early age.

Consider what John Hopkins University researcher John Money hypothesized in the early 1980s.

> "The sexual neuropathways could be the ``prototype`` of all addictions. Access to the neuropathaways comes through what Money termed a ``lovemap`` that every one of us carries inside. Between the ages of five and eight, most of us already have formed this map about what is sexually arousing to us. It serves as a template with which we decide whether a specific situation is arousing—and then we act on that template.
>
> Problems occur when that template or map becomes distorted. Minimal distortion occurs when a family will not talk about sex or casts a negative judgment about anything sexual. Early sexual experiences, especially if they involve shame or fear, can also distort beliefs about sex. Physical and sexual abuse can have a profound effect on what Money termed a ``vandalization`` of a person`s lovemap. The tragic result can be that

> the person may become aroused in ways that are self-destructive or not functional."

As an example, I had a female client who while growing up sought after her father's love and attention. Around the age of 7 or 8 she spent much of her time at the garage that her father owned. It was there that she was subjected to pictures of pin up girls that lined all the walls of her father`s shop. She listened to the mechanics in the shop make many sexually exploitive comments when well figured women came in to have work done on their cars. As she grew into her teen years she was noted as being underdeveloped and often teased by her peers and at times by the men in the shop and even her father. By her late teens she spent thousands of dollars getting breast implants, braces, Botox among many other things. She found herself with a whole new sense of self-confidence that solely hinged upon her sex appeal. She eventually met the guy of her dreams; he worshipped his cars and objectified his women. Despite her new found beauty he always found something to criticize about her looks. She found herself watching hours of pornography weekly, to learn new things so she could please him and keep him. Sex became the bond as she felt accepted and loved as long as she could please him. Like millions of other young ladies, the inevitable happened, she became pregnant, her body changed and he rejected both her and the baby. Today, along with her beautiful baby and despite all the pain and grief she continues to move forward. She is finishing her degree and challenging her false beliefs with the truth of who she really is in body, soul and spirit.

A second example is a boy who learns about sex looking at women wearing lingerie in department store catalogs. He becomes fixated on lingerie and discovers lingerie Web sites. He also becomes sexually involved with a woman who works for a lingerie company. He eventually breaks into a home and steals lingerie and is caught and arrested.

Notice in these examples that these incidents became incorporated into what was arousing for these children as adults. These experiences were integrated into the arousal template. When sex becomes addictive, it`s often because this template, as well as the total belief system of the addict, is distorted.

The family and the environment that we grew up in are not the only factors that determines how we develop. Two children can be raised in the same home, have the same parents, eat the same food, have the same friends, go to the same church and respond differently. So it raises the question, "were we born this way?" This question has had sociologists working on figuring it out for decades. They have tried to show us that environment is more important than heredity, that we are born as little blank pages for Fate to write upon. We've been told that if you change a person's dwelling place or standard of living, or put money in his pocket, you will change him. In spite of millions of dollars spent in moving people into new buildings, the experiment has failed. When I was the co-ordinator of a Housing First Program, I got the concept of dignity and the basic human right that people should be housed, yet changing their environment did not change the person. We are not all the same; God created each one of us as a unique individual, a blending from our parents whether we are observing hair and eye color or analyzing personality.

To further drive home the point that our personalities pre-exist, in 1979 Dr. Thomas J. Boauchard, Jr., started a study in Minnesota of "Twins Reared Apart." Since then the researchers have examined thirty-eight identical and sixteen fraternal sets of twins reared apart. The tests measured the physical, psychological, and intellectual abilities. The results showed amazing similarities in choices of clothing, food, and names, not to mention parallels in medical, behavioral, and intelligence traits.

> Dr. David Lykken, a research team member observer concluded, "Much of what we think as human individuality—temperament and pace and all the idiosyncrasies that make you different from your friends—may relate a lot more to your particular genetic individuality than we thought...The capacity for happiness seems to be more strongly genetically wired in than I had thought... Little Mary's sunny disposition may be part of her genetic makeup, enhanced by - but not the result of - her adoring parents' care.

Since that time there have been thousands of sets of twins studied and the results have strongly indicated that we are not just products of our family. Every individual can and does interpret the world they live in differently because they have their own unique personalities. Scripture is clear in stating that God uniquely created each of us in our mother's womb and has known us from the foundations of the world (Ephesians. 2:10).

Personality Impact

So I believe it is fair to say that the first contributing factor to our false beliefs is the bias of our own personalities and how we interpret our world, our environment and the experiences that happen to us. As I stated earlier in the book, even trauma is not defined by the event but by the interpretation of the event. There is much written about personalities and many of the personality theories suggest they fall into four categories. For the sake of choosing one, I will pick the oldest theory that was developed over two thousand years ago by Hippocrates. His terms have been modified and relabeled many times, but their usefulness and validity remain the same today as they were in ancient Greece.

Temperament is a term from the Latin meaning "a mixing in due proportion." What they were mixing were fluids, or humors, from the Latin word for moisture. A person with a lot of red blood coursing through his veins was Sanguine: cheerful, outgoing and optimistic but not very serious or organized. The original Choleric had too much yellow bile making him "bilious," short-tempered and ill-natured, but giving him a dynamic desire for action. As his hole, Greek for "bile," was "mixed in due proportion," he charged into leadership positions. Too much melas, Greek for "black," and chole added up to Melancholy; deep, genius. Phlegm was a cold, moist humor which caused people to be slow and sluggish but enabled them to stay calm, cool, and collected under pressure and heat.

According to Michael Gartner, writing about the original concept, "If you had too much of any one humor you were considered unbalanced, a little odd or eccentric. Sometimes, normal folks would laugh at their friends with too much of a humor, and that's how the word humor got its present-day meaning of ludicrous, comical or absurd."

Although we can conclude that family is not powerful enough to make our personality, it does have the ability to alter our personality and cause us dis-ease or ill-at-ease. This is what *Diagnostic and Statistical Manual of Mental Disorders (DSM-IV-TR)* would call a Personality Disorders. I stated under family systems, that shame can cause splitting in our personalities which will often mean that we will begin to wear masks, and seek to perform and be someone that we were not really created to be. I don't want to go into each of the personality characteristics in this section but have listed them in Appendix XI. However I will quickly summarize some of the differences and their biases.

Four Types of Personalities

When we think of someone who has "personality" we are usually referring to a Sanguine even though we may not know the term. They are often the ones who appear confident in groups, life-of-the-party, and ingest an instant sense of humor. However before you get too envious, as charming as they are they also lack discipline and they seldom reach their full potential.

When we consider someone of "power" we are more than likely thinking of a choleric. If you have listen to and seen a motivational speaker you will begin to see that the seminars are conceived by Cholerics, written by Cholerics, taught by Cholerics and only the Cholerics can catch the vision. They relate to the speaker, charge forth, and meet the challenge. The Sanguine will show up late, forget the syllabus at home because they can't remember where they put it and will take it as a sign from the Lord that they didn't need it anyways. The Melancholy personality comes prepared with their own notebook, assorted pens and 3X5 cards and can become bogged down in the details of the message, or lose interest in the speaker because he comes across as insincere. The Phlegmatic personality didn't want to go to the seminar in the first place, and has no intention of changing his way of life. They measure all activities by how much energy it will take to succeed, and this is all too much like work. He can't believe they are for real and he plans to leave at the next coffee break.

I think you're probably getting the picture. When we think of "Perfectionist" you will often hear the phrase "can't you ever do anything right?" For the Melancholy there is no other way. They can't understand why someone would want to do less than their best. We will often use the term "anal retentive" to describe this person. The people around them often feel like they can do nothing right. They are constantly tying up loose ends of life and they wonder, since they are right, why the rest of us don't see it their way. The Choleric is more interested in getting things done quickly than perfectly. The Sanguines don't realize they haven't done it right and the Phlegmtic just don't care that much. The world needs Melancholy to keep the rest of us on track, but sometimes the standards are set so high that no one can achieve them and then we all get depressed.

While the Sanguine is running around spreading joy and the Choleric is trying to get things under control, the Melancholy is dusting off the details and the Phlegmatic is trying to keep peace among us all. The heart of the Phlegmatic is peaceful and he will do anything, including compromising his principles, if he can avoid a potential problem. They will always choose relationship over principle. Other personalities admire the phlegmatics' ability to keep their heads when all around other temperaments are losing theirs.

Personality Masks

So again I ask the question, "who am I?" What is the clue that I may be wearing a mask? One of the first clues is when you complete the Personality Profile and it comes out relatively even split between Sanguine (outgoing- optimistic) and Melancholy (Introverted-pessimistic) or half Choleric (aggressive-active) with Phlegmatic (passive-peaceful). Because these are diametrically opposed sets of traits, these combinations indicate there may be a masking. God didn't create us with antagonistic personalities in one body. "A double-minded man is unstable in all his ways" (James 1:8).

The person who functions as a Sanguine/Melancholy split has happy highs alternating with deep periods of depression. The Choleric/Phlegmatic, on the other hand, swings in and out of controlling and submissive responses. Many studies of the four basic temperaments, no matter what labels are used, show the Sanguine/Melancholy and Choleric/Phlegmatic combinations to be normal blends of people who have fluctuating extremes in their natures. They have also found these conflicting traits to represent an adaptation to adverse circumstances of the past.

So when do these masks first appear? Usually we find that a child who lives in a stressful environment where their natural personality is not acceptable for one of many reasons will try to adapt to what is expected of them. They will take on a family role to keep the balance, they may have pain they cannot express or the expression of feelings are not permitted. For example, trauma shocks them out of their true nature, molestation floods them with guilt and shame, an oppressive parent grinds down their personality, a well-meaning but dictatorial parent plans out their life, a favored sibling they are encouraged to emulate, unrealistic goals suited to their ability, crisis situations where they have to adapt to survive, rigid or religious families where conformity equals righteousness, or chaotic and enmeshed families where the child is denied feelings of their own, or the unrealistic rules of a dysfunctional family.

So many of us have a false front when we meet up with circumstances we can't control or relationships we can't handle. We wear masks that so gradually become a part of us that we no longer know where the mask ends and we begin. As I type these words my mind instantly goes to Daphne Evans, who I have had the privilege of knowing since our teen years. She recently wrote her powerful and impactful true story in a recent book called *With the Stroke of a Match*. In the book she shares being the youngest of six kids, that is until a seventh child came along five years later. I will let her tell you first person the account and the personal impact it had on her.

"When I was five years old, my little sister was born. The day she came home, I ran down the hill from the neighbour's house and looked at her in the crib-enthralled and curious. She was the first baby I had ever seen up close! Of course, this meant I was no longer the baby of the family and I lost the limelight. Being a very quiet child, I was then generally overlooked and ignored, consequently becoming very shy and insecure, trying hard to please everyone, but never feeling successful. I looked down a lot, not wanting to meet the eyes of anyone for fear they would see how wretched this cute little girl with the blond curls really was (the beginning of a false belief and shamed-based system). There was no abuse in the family, but neither was there a display of love. My mother was quite critical of me throughout my life, likely because of my shyness. I don't hold this against her, since she was an extrovert and maybe couldn't understand why someone would be so quiet, and perhaps she thought that since I didn't speak much, there wasn't much going on in my mind; which couldn't have been farther from the truth.

As I proceeded through elementary school, my life was a bit of a paradox. On the one hand, I was very shy, but on the other hand, I was drawn to risky situations (Evidence of role playing and personality splitting). I was the one who generally suggested things like trying to smoke and flirting with guys we didn't know. There was a personality trying to show itself, but not quite knowing how to set itself free. There was a carefully constructed wall rising up around me, as impenetrable as a stone fortress to protect my fragile emotions" (defence mechanism).

Daphne goes on to share about her marriage, "two beautiful children and a very successful business and yet there remained a "but" through it all. In her words

> she states, my self-esteem should have been at an all-time high, but it was at an all-time low. The man who should adore me was expressing more and more disdain for me. As I looked around and listened to people talk, I believed that if I just work harder, if I became even more successful, maybe people would love me. I became ever more distressed and experienced panic attacks. To deal with the internal conflict and stress she took up running and used it as a method to dispel some of the tension, but it too became extreme.
>
> By nature she states that, I was still always an introvert. I learned to put on a smile and pretend to be outgoing. It was a mask, and as people responded to this facade, I began to use alcohol to bolster my courage. When I drank I became another person. I could talk with anyone and everyone and not feel intimidated. I slowly began to use alcohol as my source of strength.
>
> She goes on to say that "I had been so busy trying to be someone I wasn't that I had done a very bad job of being myself (She had lost her I AMness body, soul and spirit). I couldn't seem to find someone who would love me for myself and who cared enough to make me feel that love. I felt totally unloved and unlovable.

Despite her pursuit of love, significance and security her world came to a head on July 21, 2009, when she decided she could no longer live with the pain of rejection, loneliness , unworthiness and loss of identity. Knowing that it didn't matter how hard she tried, it was never good enough. It was on that day, with unbearable feelings of hopelessness and despair that she ended her life in a fiery grave. After drinking a copious amount of alcohol to dull the pain she ignited her vehicle with herself entombed inside. Minutes after being in golfed by flames like a human torch, she was pulled out of the burning vehicle unconscious. In that moment was she not only resuscitated but resurrected to a new life. A life that would now include several years of very painful skin graphs and re-constructive surgery to her face, body and throat as a to be able to speak again. It is not only a story of God's grace, but the courage of a young lady to find hope and strength in God. It is a story of women embracing her spiritual rebirth, accepting her new body with all its changes and reconnecting with her soul, her personality, her mind, emotions and will. The day that she accepted the Trinitarian Nature of who she was created to be, her true identity (body, soul and spirit) was the day she began a new life of wholeness (holiness), maturity towards Christ likeness and a peace that surpasses comprehension that now guards her heart (spirit) and mind(soul) in Christ.

If you're Personality Profile shows an unusual split, if you feel uncomfortable about your identity, or have a constant under tone of depression, begin to question these conflicting patterns.

The person who puts on the Sanguine mask of personality is usually one who learned early in life that his parents valued a happy face beyond any other attribute and that being "on stage" brought approval and applause. A child does not need to know his own name before he can sense what brings affirmation from his parents.

The difference between a born Sanguine and one masquerading is how natural the personality is. Anyone can learn to say cute lines and memorize jokes, but any astute person can tell when it's strained. The real Sanguine has a sense of humor that bubbles out easily, and can take any ordinary event of life and turn it into a hilarious story. The one wearing the mask, doesn't have the innate sense of timing and can fail to be funny when repeating a story exactly as he heard it.

The Melancholy mask is one of attempting perfection and frequent pain. Those who put the Melancholy mask on as children were often ones with parents who demanded perfection either because they were Melancholy and know no other way or because their status couldn't accommodate a frisky child. You will often see this with Pastors' kids, the father will feel that his whole ministry depends upon the proper behavior of his children.

Besides the Melancholy mask of perfection, there is the very common Melancholy mask of pain. When the Personality Profile comes out with Sanguine strengths and Melancholy weaknesses this is a clue that the person is either a melancholy wearing a Sanguine mask or a Sanguine that has somewhere along the line put on a mask of pain and become depressed. Phlegmatics and Cholerics may also wear this mask of pain if they have met with severely traumatic situations or have lived in homes where very little love was ever expressed. When a child does not experience love by being held or touched during the formative years of birth to eight, there can be as I explained earlier feelings of rejection even though both parents are home.

When a child is abused or molested, the victim usually puts on the mask of pain unless he is Choleric enough to push away the pain, deny reality, and forge ahead to become an achiever. The victim usually loses his own feelings and drowns in depression, guilt and shame. As adults, victims assume they have put these problems behind them and can't understand why the black cloud is always with them.

They are often negative, resentful, and complaining. No matter what people do for them, it is somehow not enough. They frequently have unexplainable physical symptoms such as headaches, body pain, asthma, and allergies. Sometimes in extreme sexual abuse cases they have blocked out the original attack and can't understand why they always feel guilty for something.

In our western society power denotes success. Everybody wants to be a somebody and those somebodies seem to be Choleric. Besides the mask of power that makes any temperament appear to be an ill-at-ease Choleric, there is the related mask of anger. Any person who represses anger over a long period of time can appear to be Cholreric when the cork blows and a temper tantrum surprises those in view.

We may be able to spot a Choleric mask when a person has Choleric weaknesses and strengths of another type, indicating valid strengths paired with controlled anger. This person may be working under extreme stress where he is helpless to do anything about it or he may have had a repressive childhood causing him to fight for survival. As he grew up the anger produced impatience, bossiness, and an argumentative nature that so overshadowed his strengths that he appeared to be Choleric. Extreme cases like this would be the person who handles his emotions at work and then one day murders his wife. Everyone is in shock as he seemed like such a nice man. Rapists and molesters are often low-key people who are carrying inside them the residue of an abusive childhood that comes out in violent acts.

The Phlegmatic mask is often the result of someone who gives up on life and becomes apathetic, deciding it's easier to mouth agreeable words than to fight for what's right. Cholerics who can't win in a given situation may put on a Phlegmatic mask of peace and pretend they don't care. Sanguines who marry mates who no longer think they're cute may turn Phlegmatic at home and save their humor for social occasions.

Personality, Birth Order & Family Roles

It is not too difficult to see how these personality biases also lend themselves to fitting into roles in a dysfunctional family. Other factors that contribute to these roles will be gender and birth order. For example, in an alcoholic family the older brother who is a Choleric can become the Hero of the family. However when he becomes an adult he is both a workaholic and an alcoholic, and is verbally abusive to his wife and neglects his children who feel unloved. He totally denies he has a problem, he is filled with hidden hostilities and repressed rage, and he believes because he keeps a job that he is not an alcoholic.

As a Phlagmatic the older sister is the "loser" of the family. She cannot function without the help of her mother who cooks for and tend to her kids. She has been married twice to "losers" and is both physically and verbally abusive to her children. She is emotionally incapable of any healthy relationships.

The Younger brother who is the Melancholy becomes the "Scapegoat." He is the black sheep of the family, a whiney sensitive little boy raised by women. He has a dependency personality and as an adult abuses drugs and sex.

Younger sister who is a Sanguine becomes the Pet. As the last, she is both spoiled and dependent. As an adult she divorces and is emotionally, verbally, and physically abusive to her children often kicking and slapping them. She seeks someone to take care of her and is pursuing a lifestyle which will lead to a destructive end.

The lies, fears, and incorrect beliefs about themselves has affected their temperaments and altered their personalities. As we consider these personalities in light of addiction we know that there are no one specific personality that will become a sex addict. What we do know is that any personality that is broken, split, wounded with feelings of shame, guilt, insecurity and insignificance and a distorted perception of what will meet their need for love are predisposed to self-medicate.

Trauma Impact

In addition to personalities and family systems, the third greatest contributor to the development of lies and distorted beliefs is traumatic experiences. I won't go into much detail because I touched on this earlier in the book, regarding wounded inner-child. For example, some experiences are burned into a child's mind. Perhaps the child was sexually abused, or the parents were divorced or there was a death in the family. Based on the age and development stage of the child, he or she might assume it was caused by something they did. Feeling it was their fault, a defense mechanism is motivated to protect the child from further harm and to get its needs met. All of these experiences are stored in our memory banks. Remember, we do not have a "clear" button in our mental computers.

World Impact

One last environmental contributor to our distorted beliefs is the fact that we are confronted daily with a world system that is not godly. Paul warned us, "Do not conform any longer to the pattern of this world" (Romans 12:2). The philosophies of the world affect our minds. That is why Paul also warned, "See to it that no one takes you captive through hollow and deceptive philosophy, which depends on human tradition and the basic principles of this world rather than on Christ" (Colossians 2:8). Because we live in this world, we will continually face the reality of temptation. For example, because alcohol is socially acceptable and sex is used to sell everything from beer to cars, we will be constantly bombarded. Our memory banks are so crammed with junk that we could fantasize for years without having to leave our own home. That is why sexual addiction is so difficult to break: because once a thought is formulated in our mind, the mental impressions are available for instant recall.

All of these factors may seem overwhelming in and of themselves, however God has provided a way of escape. He requires that we take all those shaming and condemning thoughts, all the lies and false beliefs captive to the obedience of Christ. If we allow self-defeating thoughts to ruminate in our minds, we will eventually take a path that leads to destruction. I came across a statement years ago that I have never forgotten, "Sow a thought and reap an action, sow an action and reap a habit, sow a habit and reap a character, sow a character and reap a destiny."

We have to recognize the subtle path that leads to destruction. As a sex addict consider this situation: one night a husbands wife asks him to go to the store for some milk. When he gets in his car, he briefly wrestles mentally with his selection of stores. He decides upon a local convenience store that is more likely to display pornography. He did not have to choose that particular store. He could have purchased the milk at a grocery store where the atmosphere would have been much more wholesome and less of a temptation.

The battle for his mind was already lost, however, the moment he started driving to the wrong store. Before he even left the garage, all kinds of rationalizing thoughts crossed his mind. For example, "God if you don't want me to go there, you will bring someone into my path that I know or you will cause a wreck in the intersection, etc. Because a wreck didn't happen and he didn't run into someone he knew, he tells himself it must be okay to look at the pornography. The mind has an incredible propensity to rationalize, but the rationalizations are not long lasting. Before this man leaves the store, guilt and shame overwhelm him. The choice to take the way of escape must be made before he gets into his car. It is a rare person who can turn the car around once the plan has been set in motion.

Spiritual Impact

This world is fraught with all kinds of mixed messages. Consequently, mixed emotions also abound. There are many Christians, who just like me in the past don't feel saved, don't feel like God loves them and don't feel they are worth anything. The message they have received is not true, but they believe it anyway. Scripture teaches that not all messages we receive are necessarily from the visible world. Paul wrote, "The Spirit clearly says that in later times some will abandon the faith and follow deceiving spirits and things taught by demons" (I Timothy 4:1).

If Satan can get us to believe a lie, he can destroy us emotionally and control our lives. His primary intention is to distort the perception we have of ourselves and of God. This is why Paul exhorts us to, "Finally, brothers, whatever is true, whatever is noble, whatever is right, whatever is pure, whatever is lovely, whatever is admirable-if anything is excellent or praiseworthy-think about such things" (Philippians 4:8). Our problems don't just stem from what we have believed in the past. Paul said we are to presently and continually take every "thought captive to the obedience of Christ" (2 Corinthians 10:5). The word "thought" is the Greek word "noema." Paul used that same word when he said, "I have forgiven in the sight of Christ for your sake, in order that Satan might not outwit us. For we are not unaware of his schemes" (2:10, 11).

Satan and his demons are spiritual beings. They do not have material substance, so we cannot see spiritual beings with our natural eyes, nor can we hear them with our ears. "For our struggle is not against flesh and blood, but against the rulers, against the authorities, against the powers of this dark world and against the spiritual forces of evil in the heavenly realms" (Ephesians 6:12). Losing control of our minds is a major problem with the effects of alcohol and drugs. This loss of control allows our minds to access any file in the computer. If people watched a lot horror movies or pornography, we can predict where their mind is going to go.

Satan knows how to tempt us. We consciously make a choice when we surrender to temptation. When we continue to act upon our wrong choices, we establish a habit within approximately six weeks. Habits are mental patterns of thought that have been burned into our minds over time, or by deep traumatic experiences. One writer suggests, "it is a mind-set, impregnated with hopelessness, that causes one to accept as unchangeable, something known to be contrary to the will of God."

Breaking the Patterns

So breaking these patterns we need to consider Paul's admonishment to us "to put on the armor of God" (Ephesians 6:10-18). The belt of truth defends us against the father of lies. The breastplate of righteousness is our protection against the accuser of the brethren. Then Paul summarized by saying, "In addition to all, taking up the shield of faith with which you will be able to extinguish all the flaming missiles of the evil one" (Ephesians 6:16). The "flaming missiles" are just the tempting, accusing and deceptive thoughts everybody has to deal with daily. What happens when we don't take every thought captive to the obedience of Christ? If we entertain such thoughts, we will develop these thought patterns in our minds and emotional attachments that will be difficult to break.

Don't assume all disturbing thoughts are from Satan. Where the thought came from-the television set, our memory banks, and our own creative reservoirs - doesn't matter as much as understanding that the answer is always the same. We can analyze the origin of every thought, but that won't resolve it. We will just get caught up in analysis that leads to paralysis.

One note of warning: Please do not try to cast out the demon of lust or sexual addiction. I don't believe there is a demon of lust or a demon of sexual addiction. In some of my formal and informal training that has been clearly taught. I think that kind of simplistic thinking has damaged the credibility of the Church and left the addict without an adequate answer. Trust me when I say that I have been there and it only leaves one feeling that they are too bad for God to even heal, when hours or days later they are back to using. The simplistic solution of just casting a demon out of someone doesn't take into consideration all the other factors, and I personally don't think this method of resolving spiritual conflicts is best. People have addictive problems because of the responses they have chosen in their early developmental training and the pressures of life. They have turned to the addiction as a means of coping. It's what I like to call self defeating learned behaviors. All addicts, including myself, have made choices for which we must assume personal responsibility.

No one else can become responsible "to submit therefore to God and resist the devil" (James 4:7). As a counselor I consider the role as defined by Timothy: "The Lord's servant must not quarrel; instead, he must be kind to everyone, able to teach, not resentful. Those who oppose him he must gently instruct, in the hope that God will grant them repentance leading them to a knowledge of the truth, and that they will come to their senses and escape from the trap of the devil, who has taken them captive to do his will" (2 Timothy 2:24-26). This is what I call a truth encounter verses a power encounter where people go in guns a blazing trying to cast out demons and being very presumptuous. When in fact this passage clearly shows the battle is in the mind of the individual and God can lead them into truth.

The fact of the matter is that when people don't know how to responsibly deal with their pain or resolve their conflicts, they choose other ways. Eventually they will dig some pretty deep grooves in their minds, which become the neuropaths that I spoke about earlier. They are likened to a truck that has driven on the same road for so long it has developed some deep ruts. The driver doesn't even have to steer anymore. The truck will just stay in those ruts. After awhile, any attempt to steer out of the ruts will cause the wheel to jerk in the hands of the driver. Some finally conclude it is easier to stay in the ruts and continue on down the same old path. Others break free from the ruts and commit themselves to getting on the right road to recovery.

Simply living out of the soul will keep us stuck in the same old ruts. Listen to what Paul states in Romans 7:15-19, "For that which I am doing, I do not understand; for I am not practicing what I would like to do, but I am doing the very thing I hate. But if I do the very thing I do not wish to do, I agree with the Law, confessing that it is good. So now, no longer am I the one doing it, but sin which indwells me. For I know that nothing good dwells in me, that is, in my flesh; for the wishing is present in me, but the doing of the good is not. For the good that I wish, I do not do; but I practice the very evil that I do not wish." Paul knows that the Spirit of Christ indwelt his born again spirit. Therefore, he couldn't be technically correct and say "In me…dwelleth no good thing" without the clarifying statement "that is my flesh."

Paul acknowledged his born again spirit, but declared, "there is no good thing in my flesh – my unrenewed mind and physical body, all the external parts of me functioning independent from Christ. I'm going to have to lay this flesh down and receive a new body and a new soul, which are completely renewed and think exactly like God." "For I know that in me (that is my flesh) dwells no good thing: for the wishing is present with me; but how to perform that which is good I find the principles that evil is present in me, the one who wishes to do good. For I joyfully concur with the law of God in the inner man, but I see a different law in the members of my body, waging war against the law of my mind, and making me a prisoner of the law of sin which is in my members" (Romans 7:18-23).

Sounds a lot like what he wrote in Galatians 5:17, "for the flesh sets its desire against the Spirit, and the Spirit against the flesh; for these are in opposition to one another, so that you may not do the things that you please."

Romans 7 doesn't teach that Paul was constantly trying and failing to do the right thing. He wasn't describing his present Christian life and saying that this is the way that it is. Paul wasn't confessing that after all those years, he was still struggling with lust, sexual sin, anger, and bitterness. Neither was he saying, "You have this flesh, and try as you might, but you can never beat it.

Paul was simply describing the inability of the flesh-your physical ability, natural mind, emotions, and actions all independent from Christ-to please God. You cannot overcome your flesh and addiction on your own; you have to start living from who you are in Christ. Your spirit is completely changed and infused with the life of God. You can only please Him through living by your spirit.

In your flesh you can't do what the Lord has told you to do. He's commanded you to bear it when someone insults you or falsely accuses you. I want to be honest with you, in twenty-five years of pastoring and counseling I had never been falsely accused professionally, I believe because I always did my due diligence. Yet in this particular case despite evidence to the contrary, I discovered once labelled with a criminal record you are guilty until proven innocent and an instant liability, a cancer that has to be eradicated by any organization including the church, sadly to say. Too be on the end of any such accusation and judgement is devastating at best and unfair to say the least. You all of a sudden find yourself on the outside looking in with disbelief and perplexed as to what just happened. Our flesh wants justice, it wants to make a wrong right.

For months I kept thinking how did this happen? I felt angry, hurt, betrayed not only from the organization but from God. With a deep need for vindication I would drive by my former place of employment with some kind of twisted thought and fantasizing some kind of justice for a wrong done. You know, "I will show them," scenario. The feelings of shame and rejection were so intense at times, I would think it must have been my fault, after all here I am again. All the stinking thinking had returned along with the old beliefs that stated that I am no good, a failure and deserving of rejection. My anger turned from them to me and I was now ruthless and relentless. I was faced with the choice, bitter or better and trust me when you feel like the victim it is easy to get bitter and reject better.

Compounding this was a week later I would be told that I was turned down for my pardon. When I inquired with Pardon & Wavers Canada I was told that, "it was nothing that I did, but that the Government changed the process to be five years rather than three years post your last day of your probation period and will change the name from Pardon to Suspended Sentence." I was devastated, I pleaded for understanding of what the ramifications of this meant for me. I inquired to when this ruling change occurred and could I not be grandfathered in given I was past the three year term do to their own internal delays. Unfortunately it was like talking to an answering machine, I kept getting the same response, "I know this must be difficult, but it is not our decision but the governments." Today I sit in financial crisis, applying daily anywhere and everywhere with no job prospects in sight. With moments of high anxiety I plead to the Lord for grace, for some kind of break.

Other days I am faced with great grief and depression with the prospect of having lost my two vocational ministries as a Pastor and a Therapist. Now what, at times I feel like King Saul, when the Spirit of the Lord was taken from him and out of defeat and a sense of hopelessness he falls upon his own sword. In the vernacular of the day, I feel like taking a long walk of a short peer.

Like I said, you can't overcome these things in the flesh. How do you obey God's command to just bear it, when it feels so unbearable? How do you turn the other cheek and forgive seventy times seven when every part of you wants justice and vindication for false accusations (Matthew 5:39-41). Your natural self, independent of God, just won't do things like that!

As human beings and certainly as an addict it's natural to be self-serving, self-seeking, and self-promoting! If somebody slaps you on the cheek, you want to hit both of theirs. If someone takes something from you through a lawsuit, you want to hire the best lawyer to sue them back. But the Lord tells us to do the opposite. That is why Paul declared, "It's no longer me that lives but Christ who lives through me" (Galatians 2:20).

There is tremendous amount of liberty that comes with recognizing and releasing Christ in you. You don't have to say in the flesh "Well, I will to love you" and turn the other cheek through gritted teeth. It's much better to pray, "Father, in myself, I'd like to hurt them like they hurt me; I know that is my flesh and I cannot do this," (Romans 7), "but in my spirit, I can do all things through Christ who strengthens me. I have the same spirit that Jesus had when He hung on the cross and forgave the very people who crucified Him. Father, I don't feel like it right now, but I know my spirit is the same one that enabled Jesus to extend mercy to those who mocked Him. In the flesh I can't do this; I don't have enough willpower. I can't put up with this. I just can't take it. I've come to an end in myself (soul). That is good because now the Spirit can take over. "But I can do all things through Christ who strengthens me" (spirit). So I choose to draw from your strength. I really think David got this principle. In the Psalm he would be very honest with God as to how he wanted justice to be served, but in the end would always surrender it back to God, "the King of kings and Lord of lords." It is therapeutic to be brutally honest with God, He won't strike you down. It is no surprise to Him, for He already knows your thoughts and intentions, but we need to verbalize them.

We need to say like David, Father I can't do it, but You can. This is what it means to "turn it over and let go and let God," in the 12 step program. When we humble ourselves and turn away from our own natural ability and turn to God and His divine ability, we discover God's fruit of the Spirit. I Corinthians 13:7 states, that it is an unlimited supply. Love "bears all things, believes all things, hopes all things, and endures all things." When your physical mind comes into agreement with your spiritual mind, you can literally begin to hope, endure, and believe in things you couldn't have done by your natural self! Please know that this is a work in progress, I am still having my soulish days and they are not pretty.

Remember what Paul said, "O wretched man that I am! Who shall deliver me from the body of this death?" (Romans 7:25). Deliverance from the flesh comes through living by who you are in the spirit! From here Paul launches into Romans 8. "There is therefore now no condemnation to them which are in Christ Jesus, who walk not after the flesh, but after the Spirit" (Romans 8:1).

Romans 8 is one the most victorious chapters in the whole Bible! Why? It's written from the perspective of your born again spirit. Chapter 7 speaks of a person trying to please God through their own natural effort. "O God, I am trying to do better. I want to do better, but I just can't!" Yes that pretty much sums up my first 30 years as a Christian. In Romans 7 the word, "spirit" is only used once but in Romans 8 it's used twenty one times.

Understanding the spirit, soul, and body unlocks so much for our Christian life and enables us to move on in our journey of recovery. Once we understand and believe who we are and what we have in Christ, we must begin the process and journey of rejecting the flesh and walking by the truth of who we are in the spirit. "This I say then, Walk in the Spirit, and ye shall not fulfil the lust of the flesh" (Galatians 5:16).

You overcome by being mindful of what God's Word says about you. When your Word minded, you're spiritually minded because God's words are spirit, sanctified, holy, and perfected forever. As Jesus is—so are you!

Can we break out of these ruts, or change the neuropathways? Yes we can. If we have been incorrectly trained, we can be retrained. If our brains have been incorrectly programmed, we can be reprogrammed. If we have believed a lie, we now can choose to believe the truth. This was the premise of writing this book, that despite my crash and burn, I could find out where, when and how I got derailed, body, soul and spirit and that somehow through this process I would find the right track that leads to the truth that would set me free. (See Appendix VIII: Truth Telling Exercise)

This is where studying God's Word is vital for achieving single-mindedness and releasing God's power! Your spirit mind, the mind of Christ, agrees completely with the Word of God. When a truth from God's Word takes root in your soulish realm, that same knowledge, which has already existed in your spirit mind, rises up and meshes with it. Remember, "For the Word of God is living and active and sharper than any two-edged sword, and piercing as far as the division of soul and spirit, of both joints and marrow, and able to judge the thought and intentions of the heart" (Hebrews 4:12).

Since the Father, Son, and Holy Spirit are One, they don't operate independently of each other. The Holy Spirit is the One who releases the wisdom and revelation of God. He comforts, teaches, and reminds. "But the Comforter, which is the Holy Ghost, whom the Father will send in my name, He shall teach you all things, and bring all things to your remembrance, whatsoever I have said unto you" (John 14:26). He guides into all truth, listens, speaks, shows things to come, glorifies Jesus, receives of Him, and shows it by revelation to us. "I have yet many things to say to you, but you cannot bear them now. But when He, the Spirit of truth, comes, He will guide you into all the truth; for He will not speak on His own initiative, but whatever He hears, He will speak; and He will disclose to you what is to come. He shall glorify Me (Jesus speaking); for He shall take of Mine, and shall disclose it to you. All things that the Father has are Mine; therefore I said, that He takes of Mine, and will disclose it to you" (John 16:12-15).

"As we are diligent to present ourselves approved to God as a workman who do not need to be ashamed, handling accurately the word of truth" (2 Timothy 2:15). The floodgates of our soul will open up to allow God's truth already in our spirit to manifest itself in the physical and psychological parts of our being, to become enmeshed as I stated earlier.

It may sound simple, but it's not! One of the hardest things you'll ever do is learn how to turn from your natural self-rule and let who you are in Christ dominate instead. Why is it so difficult? You must perceive your spirit by faith in God's Word because you can't see or feel it. Jesus' words are "spirit and life" (John 6:63). When you look into God's Word, you're looking into a spiritual mirror (James 1:23-25). The only way to really know what is true about who you are in the spirit is by believing God's Word. You must shift from "walking by sight to walking by faith" (2 Corinthians 5:7). All you have to do is start basing your thoughts, actions, and identity on who you are in Christ.

As long as your flesh is contrary to your spirit, you'll have conflict. "This I say then, Walk in the Spirit, and ye shall not fulfill the lust of the flesh. For the flesh lusts against the Spirit, and the Spirit against the flesh: and these are contrary the one to the other: so that you cannot do the things that you would. But if you are led by the Spirit, you are not under the law" (Galatians 5:16-18). "Contrary" means they're "opposed, enemies, adversaries." This conflict between spirit and flesh is your true spiritual warfare!

You cannot please God in your flesh. "So then they that are in the flesh cannot please God" (Romans 8:8). It's not just hard-it's impossible. This means you must identify the flesh and deal with it. As we consider step 4 and take our fearless moral inventory and identify our character defects we will see that it is characterized by the flesh - "immorality, impurity, sensuality, idolatry, sorcery, enmities, strife, jealousy, outbursts of anger, disputes, dissensions, factions, envying, drunkenness, carousing, and things like these…" (Galatians 5:19-21). These characteristics often define the characteristics of our addiction. "So let us crucify the flesh with its passions and desires" Galatians 5:24.

I know that this will take the rest of my life by renewing my thoughts and developing a new character. I used to tell my alcoholic clients that it takes a long time to get sick and it takes a long time to get better; I find myself now having to take so much of my own advice. We will never be perfect in our understanding, nor will our character be completely perfect. However, as I started by saying in the earlier chapters, I can be in the process of being restored into the likeness of Christ by faith, because we are already in His Image, perfect and complete.

However that being said, renewing your mind, also involves accountability and rigorous honesty, not only with God but with yourself and others. The *Sexaholic Big Book* states;

> "Without regular participation in the fellowship, there seems to be no recovery. The program doesn't tell us how to stop but shows us how to keep from starting up again. We pick up the phone, we ask for help, we go to a meeting. We admit that we may not fully want victory over lust. We talk about the temptation in a phone call or at the next meeting and tell all. We take the action of getting out of ourselves and making contact with another member. If we're living inside our head and the emotions we could never face overwhelm us. We have to work this as it happens each time.
>
> Lust is cunning, baffling and powerful and very patient. The Twelve Steps of Recovery won't work unless I work them. We have to get to the source of the problem ourselves. We take responsibility for our own recovery. We start working the Steps.
>
> We surrender to God and take direction from a sponsor. Asking for help and accepting suggestions are what bring results. Taking action and getting out of ourselves is what counts and feelings will follow. Every time we feel overwhelmed, our sponsor can point the way out of self-pity, resentment, or fear and onto right thinking, helping us say, 'I thank God for the good and the seemingly bad as necessary for my growth. Thy will, not mine, be done.' The program doesn't work in a vacuum; it only works in the day-to-day ebb and flow of our lives.

> Trial, tribulation, and pain are the soil in which the Steps can germinate, take root, and find fruition in our lives."

Since our condition is characterized by the relentless progression of diseased attitudes, recovery for us lies in a profound change of attitude toward ourselves, others, and God. It is for this reason that I have dedicated Appendix 4-6 to working the 12 Steps of Recovery.

Epilogue

I hope I have not come across as to preachy in this book; it was not my intention, and it has simply been a process of unpacking and trying to discover who I am in relationship to God, myself and the world. I have tried to consider all biological, physiological, psychological, sociological and spiritual factors. I know it is not exhaustive; however I have tried to use the Bible as a compass, with my core belief being that it is Man's Book from God, verses God's Book from man.

So in the end, I don't believe that we can experience complete wholeness in body, soul and spirit without a personal relationship with Christ. As I have stated throughout this book, you can go from program to program, counselor to counselor, book to book and not experience wholeness and recovery.

However, "righting our wrongs is one of the single most powerful tools for success in spiritual growth and recovery" (Sexaholics Anonymous). It is on that note that I do want to take this opportunity to apologize for the wrongs that I have done and hurt that I have caused. It is with a heavy heart that I say I am sorry and regret any and all of my actions.

We need to remember despite our amends the battle is ever before us. We battle the world, the flesh and the devil. Our flesh and neuropathways still remain long after we put our faith in Christ. We will still see things on television and computers and hear and see things at work that will trigger old thought patterns but the acid test will be who we will identify ourselves with. Who am I, an Addict or a Saint? If it is the latter then we can say as Paul, "Those who belong to Christ Jesus have crucified the sinful nature [flesh] with its passions and desires. Since we live by the Spirit, let us keep in step with the Spirit" (Galatians 5:24, 25). We can "resist the devil and he will flee" from us (James 4:7). Spiritual conflicts are the easiest to resolve, but the least understood.

"It is for freedom that Christ has set us free. Stand firm, then, and do not let yourselves be burdened again by a yoke of slavery. You, my brothers, were called to be free. But do not use you freedom to indulge the sinful nature [flesh]" (Galatians 5:1, 13). Obviously the freedom Christ purchased for us on the cross can be lost to the bondages of legalism and license. These habits can be changed if we choose to believe the truth, because the truth is what sets us free.

For most of us, including myself, winning the battle for our minds will initially be a two-steps-forward and one-step-backward process. Slowly it becomes three steps forward and one step backward; then four and five steps forward, as we learn to take every thought captive in obedience to Christ. We may despair with all the backward steps, but God is not going to give up on us. Remember, our sins are already forgiven. We need only fight for our own personal victories over our addiction. The battles are winnable because the war has already been won, hence our ability to do all things through Christ who strengthens us and with Christ all things are possible. As we learn more about our true identity as children of God and the nature of the battle going on for our minds, the process gets easier.

Pearce, points out,

> "A true break with our culture (and the flesh) involves nothing other than picking up our cross. We will drop our deadly defenses, judgements, self-justifications; we will leave behind self-pity, retribution, demands for justice, and fearful reactions that lead to war and need I say, addictions. Picking up the cross shifts us out of survival instincts and opens us to the higher frequency of love, forgiveness, and trust. We will all find, upon picking up that cross, that its burden is light."

As I stated in my opening thesis of this book, I am writing in the hope that it would help me to find my way through recovery, enlighten my family and would be a help to others in understanding their Trinitarian nature and the implication on their recovery. I have tried my best to support my position bio-psycho-social and spiritually and be open and honest about my own journey. That has been a scary part in this process as I have felt very vulnerable. I hope I have done the Word of God justice. It has not been my intention to condemn the church, 12 step groups or any physiological and psychological disciplines or modalities. I see them as all having a very important and integral part to my recovery. However, I do see the foundation and starting point of recovery to be Spirit, Soul and Body in that order. We do not change ourselves from the outside in.

Through the journey of writing this book, I have come to realize that my question, who am I? An addict or a saint, was to narrow in scope. Yes, spiritually I am a Saint, but I am much more than that. My soul, my personality, my psychology if you will is a Phlegmatic, Melancholic with all of its strengths and weaknesses and my body is Ectomorph/ Mesomorph, with all its strengths and weaknesses. Each of these parts, spirit, soul and body and there interdependent relationships make me who I am? And all three parts systemically have been impacted by the neuropathology of Sexual Compulsive Behaviors (Sex Addiction), that left me feeling unlovable, inadequate, insecure, worthless, in all parts of my being. The journey of recovery is the restoration of wholeness, which has to comprise of our Trinitarian nature. I am beginning to see myself by faith to be loved by a God that bears all, believes all, hopes all, and endure all, and that love for me never fails, and I am thankful that nothing can separate me from the love of God, body, soul or spirit.

Paul wrote, “Let the peace of Christ rule in your hearts, since as members of one body you were called to peace. And be thankful” (Colossians 3:15). He explained how we can do that in the next verse. “Let the word of Christ dwell in you richly” (verse16). We have to fill our minds with the Word of God. Merely trying to stop thinking bad thoughts won’t work. Should we rebuke all those tempting, accusing and deceiving thoughts? No! If we attempt to win the battle for our minds that way, we would be doing nothing but rebuking thoughts every waking moment for the rest of our lives.

The psalmist said it well. "How can a young man keep his way pure? By living according to your Word. I seek you with all my heart; do not let me stray from your commands. I have hidden your Word in my heart that I might not sin against you" (Psalm 119:9-11). This is why God`s Word repeatedly tells us to meditate upon His Word day and night, and let His Word be a lamp unto our feet and light unto our path. This is an area that I fail the most and understand the least, the art of meditation. To go to that place where my heart and mind are in sync with the heart of God, where all I hear is His heart beat and no longer hear all the noise in my soul.

God bless you in your journey; keep in mind there is no such thing as failure, but rather lessons and we repeat lessons until we learn them. I don't know where you are in your journey and how many times you have had to repeat lessons, if you're anything like me, probably many. I hope that what I have written will give you hope and perhaps help you to avoid one more repeat performance. If there is any form of failure, it is when we fail to get back up. Remember you're not alone; millions have gone before you and millions are currently experiencing what you're experiencing. You can do all things through Christ who strengthens you. As I began this book with a poem, I would like to end it with a song called *Unstoppable* by Rascal Flatts which I think is a fitting close as we continue in our journey.

Unstoppable

So you made a lot of mistakes
Walked down the road a little sideways
Cracked a brick when you hit the wall
Yeah, you've had a pocket full of regrets
Pull you down faster than a sunset
Hey, it happens to us all
When the cold hard rain just won't quit
And you can't see your way out of it

You find your faith has been lost and shaken
You take back what's been taken
Get on your knees and dig down deep
You can do what you think is impossible
Keep on believing, don't give in
It'll come and make you whole again
It always will, it always does
Love is unstoppable

Love, it can weather any storm
Bring you back to being born again
oh, it's a helping hand when you need it most
A lighthouse shining on the coast
That never goes dim
When your heart is full of doubt
And you think that there's no way out

You find your faith has been lost and shaken
You take back what's been taken
Get on your knees and dig down deep
You can do what you think is impossible
Keep on believing, don't give in
It'll come and make you whole again
It always will, it always does
Love is unstoppable

Like a river keeps on rolling
Like the north wind blowing
Don't it feel good knowing

Love is unstoppable
So you made a lot of mistakes
Walked down the road a little sideways
Love, love is unstoppable

Songwriter(s): *James Slater, Jay Demarcus, Hillary Lindsey, James Thomas Slater*

Appendix I
Sexual Addiction Criteria

Sex Addiction Defined

Addiction is an illness of escape. Its goal is to obliterate, medicate, or ignore reality. It is an alternative to letting oneself feel hurt, betrayal, worry, and –most painful of all-loneliness.

Sex addicts tend to come from rigid, authoritarian families. These are families in which all issues and problems are black and white. Little is negotiable and there is only one way to do things. They grow up in environments where there is the classic "elephant in the room" syndrome: everyone pretends there is no problem although there's a huge issue interfering with everyone's lives. Members of the family are "disengaged" from one another-there is little sharing or intimacy.

Common characteristics of sex addicts are:

- Compulsive behavior that completely dominates the addict's life
- Priority more important than family, friends, and work
- Organizing principle of the addict's life

- The addict is willing to sacrifice what he cherishes most in order to preserve and continue his/her unhealthy behavior
- Uses sexuality to regulate emotional life
- Sexuality is used as a pain reliever or a way to relieve anxiety
- Do things that are dangerous, exploitive, and will cause shame afterwards
- Feel lonely and non-intimate

Diagnosis of Sex Addiction

- Since this is not a widely recognized/ accepted addiction, many psychiatrists, psychologists, and therapists do not diagnose sex addiction
- *DSM IVR* identifies Sexual Compulsive Disorder

Criteria for Sex Addiction

- Recurrent failure to resist sexual impulses in order to engage in specific sexual behaviors
- Frequently engaging in those behaviors to a greater extent or over a longer period of time than intended
- Persistent desire or unsuccessful efforts to stop, reduce, or control those behaviors
- Inordinate amounts of time spent in obtaining sex, being sexual, or recovering from sexual experiences
- Preoccupation with sexual behavior or preparatory activities
- Frequent engaging in the behavior when expected to fulfill occupational, academic, domestic, or social obligations
- Continuation of the behavior despite knowledge of having a persistent or recurrent social, financial, psychological, or physical problem that is caused or exacerbated by the behavior

- The need to increase the intensity, frequency, number, or risk level of behavior in order to achieve the desired effect; or diminished effect with continued behaviors at the same level of intensity, frequency, number, or risk
- Giving up or limiting social, occupational, or recreational activities because of the behavior
- Distress, anxiety, restlessness, or irritability if unable to engage in the behavior

A minimum of three of the above ten needed are needed for sex addiction to be considered present. Most sex addicts have five signs, while over fifty percent have seven.

Material taken from research by Patrick Carnes, Ph.D.

Collateral Indicators of Sexual Addictions

In addition, there are twenty collateral indicators which assist in the assessment of sexual addiction. A minimum of ten criteria must be met.

1. Has severe consequences because of sexual behavior
2. Meets the criteria for depression and it appears related to sexually acting out
3. Meets the criteria for depression and it appears related to sexual aversion
4. Reports history of sexual abuse
5. Reports history of physical abuse
6. Reports history of emotional abuse
7. Describes sexual life in self-medicating terms (intoxicating, tension relief, pain reliever, sleep aid)
8. Reports persistent pursuit of high-risk or self-destructive behavior
9. Reports sexual arousal to high-risk or self-destructive behavior is extremely high compared to safe sexual behavior

10. Meets diagnostic criteria for other addictive disorders

11. Simultaneously uses sexual behavior in concert with other addictions (gambling, eating disorders, substance abuse, alcoholism, compulsive spending) to the extent that the desired effect is not achieved without sexual activity and/or other addiction(s) present

12. Has history of deception around sexual behavior

13. Reports other members of the family are addicts

14. Expresses extreme self-loathing because of sexual behavior

15. Has intimate relationships that are not sexual

16. Is in crisis because of sexual matters

17. Has history of crisis around sexual behavior

18. Experiences diminished pleasure for same sexual experiences

19. Comes from a "rigid" family

20. Comes from a "disengaged" family

Levels of Severity

Level One:

- Masturbation
- Affairs, chronic infidelity, romance addiction
- Sexual relationships with multiple partners
- Pornography use and collection (with or without masturbation)
- Phone sex, cybersex
- Anonymous sex

- Prostitution – strip clubs

Level Two:

- Illegal prostitution
- Public sex (bathrooms, parks, etc.)
- Voyeurism – online or live
- Exhibitionism
- Obscene phone calls
- Stalking behaviors
- Sexual harassment

Level Three:

- Rape
- Child molestation
- Obtaining and viewing child pornography
- Obtaining and viewing rape, snuff pornography
- Sexual abuse of older or dependent persons
- Incest
- Professional boundary violations (clergy, police officers, teachers, physicians, attorneys, etc.)

Pornography

- Viewing
- Downloading
- Printing
- Exchanging
- Organizing pornography images/video

- Free clips and pay sites
- Self-made porn and picture exchange
- Live viewing of sexual behaviors

Interpersonal Cybersex

- Chatting- chat rooms
- Webcam – exchange of live sexual video, pictures, group sex
- Voyeurism – exhibitionism
- E-mail – text and picture exchange
- Cell phones – picture, videos, text messaging
- Websites – hooking up, anonymous sex
- Dating sites
- Longer term cyber-affairs

Ten Types of Sex Addiction:

1. *Voyeurism* - Usually means objectifying the other person, so it is not a personal relationship.

2. *Exhibitionism* – From a relationship perspective, it is introducing oneself in an inappropriate way or seeking attention from others with no intent of going further, which is to tease.

3. *Seductive Role Sex* – Often there is a fear of abandonment so having more than one relationship is away to prevent the hurt they are sure they will receive. They are crippled in their ability to form lasting bonds and enduring relationships.

4. *Trading Sex* – If a prostitute is a sex addict, meaning that they found sex more

pleasurable with clients than in personal relationships and are "hooked on the life", it represents a significant distortion of normal courtship. The goal is to simulate flirtation, demonstration, and romance. What actually happens in most cases is about replication of childhood sexual abuse in which the child gained power in a risky game of being sexual with the caregiver.

5. *Intrusive Sex* – People who engage in intrusive sex, such as touching people in crowds or making obscene phone calls, are really perverting the touching and foreplay dimensions of courtship. Their behaviors represent both intimacy failure and individuation difficulties.

6. *Fantasy Sex* – Many sex addicts find refuge in fantasy sex because other forms of acting out are simply too complicated, too risky, or too much effort. It is about fear of rejection, fear of reality, and reduction of anxiety.

7. *Paying for Sex* - Here, sex addicts are willing participants in simulated intimacy. They are focused, however, on the touching, foreplay, and intercourse without the hassle of a relationship. Often, the failure is about the sex addict's inability to communicate feelings to his/her partner or to be willing to work on his/h*er own* attractiveness behaviors.

8. *Anonymous Sex* – Having to experience fear in order for arousal or sexual initiation. You do not have to attract, seduce, trick, or even pay for sex. It is just sex. Frequently for sex addicts, part of the high is the risk of unknown persons and situations.

9. *Pain Exchange Sex* – For a sex addict to only be aroused if someone is hurting them is a distortion of what goes into sexual and relationship health. Specifically, touching, foreplay, and intercourse become subordinated to some dramatic story line that is usually a re-enactment of a childhood abuse experience.

10. *Exploitive Sex* – Addicts in this category will use "grooming" behavior, which is to carefully build the trust of the unsuspecting victim. Attraction, flirtation, demonstration, romance, and intimacy are all used. Arousal is dependent on the vulnerability of another.

Above material excerpted from the material presented by Ellen A. Ovson, M.D., at the 21st National Conference for Lawyer Assistance Programs, WORKING TOGETHER Educating the Legal Community – four days of practical sessions on treatment, recovery, and ways to create a healthier profession, sponsored by the ABA Commission on Lawyer Assistance Programs, Little Rock, Arkansas, Oct. 21-24, 2008

Appendix II
Denial & Defense Mechanisms

Definition

Denial is the refusal to acknowledge the existence or severity of unpleasant external realities or internal thoughts and feelings. For addicts, denial is a confused kind of thinking and reasoning used to avoid the reality of behavior or the consequences of behavior. It is a way to try to manage and explain the chaos caused by addictive behavior and deflect attention and responsibility.

Theory of Denial

Defense mechanisms are indirect ways of dealing or coping with anxiety, such as explaining problems away or blaming others for problems. Denial is one of many defense mechanisms. It entails ignoring or refusing to believe an unpleasant reality. Defense mechanisms protect one's psychological wellbeing in traumatic situations, or in any situation that produces anxiety or conflict. However, they do not resolve the anxiety-producing situation and, if overused, can lead to psychological disorders.

Examples of Denial

Death is a common occasion for denial. When someone learns of the sudden, unexpected death of a loved one, at first he or she may not be able to accept the reality of this loss. The initial denial protects that person from the emotional shock and intense **grief** that often accompanies news of death.

Denial can also apply to internal thoughts and feelings. For instance, some children are taught that anger is wrong in any situation. As adults, if these individuals experience feelings of anger, they are likely to deny their feelings to others. Cultural standards and expectations can encourage denial of subjective experience. Men who belong to cultures with extreme notions of masculinity may view fear as a sign of weakness and deny internal feelings of fear.

Sexual addiction, like any other addiction involves defense mechanisms that allow the desired behavior to persist despite negative consequences. The sex addiction attributes the problems associated with his/her sexual behavior to anything but the sexual behavior. Since sexual addiction co-occurs with other addictions, the other addictions often get blamed for unintended behavior or consequences. And the combination of addictions and/or their patterns of interactions can prompt unintended behavior or consequences. Unfortunately, when there are multiple addictions along with sexual addiction, this complicates the picture enough for the addict to spend a lot of time and energy trying to solve the addiction problems independently. Michael Hurst gives a good example in an on-line article on defense mechanisms.

> "A sex addict with alcoholism or other drug addiction may attribute all the negative consequences of his addictions to the alcoholism. S/he goes to inpatient treatment, not mentioning the serial one-night stands that endangers her health, damages her self-esteem, and put her into dangerous situations. She blames those one night stands on the drinking. She was certainly drinking and getting drunk each time those events happened.

> She assumes that when she sobers up, that the sexual acting out will stop. Only it doesn't. Instead of picking men up in a bar or a club, she selects her partners at AA meetings and in other social settings. The behavior is still shaming her. It is still damaging her self-esteem. She wants to stop engaging in that behavior, but it is compulsive. She is at the beginning of recovery and has not yet learned good living skills. When she experiences hurt, anger, sadness, and even boredom, she feels compelled to engage in the sexual behavior. She may not even make the connection between her feelings and the compulsion. If she does, she probably thinks, "At least I'm not drinking". But in fact, she is engaging in mood/mind altering behavior. When sex addicts are able to connect their own sexual compulsivity to negative consequences and outcomes, they like other addicts, attempt "softer, easier ways" to get their lives back under control. These attempts usually involve trying to manage their external environment a little more closely. It could involve using an internet filter to take away their digital drug of choice, putting a parental block on the television, putting a 900 number block on the phone, or it might even involve trying to engage in a romantic relationship. Sexual addiction is also an intimacy disorder, where the addict has difficulty with being truly intimate in a relationship. The sex addict, in an attempt to get the sexual compulsivity under control, may believe that if they get married or focus all their sexual activity or energy in the relationship, that their sexual acting out will stop. They believe that their need for pornography, one-night stands, fantasy, (or whatever their sexual drug of choice is), will go away. Breaking through the denial to admit that there is a problem is a first step toward recovery.

Before we can take the first step of our recovery, we must first face and admit our denial. God tells us, "You can't heal a wound by saying it's not there!" (Jeremiah 6:14) Denial is closely related to our negative self-talk or thought distortions.

34 Types of Denial and Defense Mechanisms

Although this list is not exhaustive I have tried to make it quite extensive. Working through your denial or defense mechanism not only corresponds with Step 1 but also with Step 4, "making a searching and fearless moral inventory of yourself.

Go through the list. Mark off the ones that look like you and have your spouse, trusted friend or counselor do the same.

1.___Global Thinking: This is attempting to justify something with absolute terms like "always" or "never" or "whatsoever." It also can be something along the lines of "every guy does this."

Give your own examples:______________________________

2.___Rationalization: This is justifying unacceptable behavior saying things like "I don't have a problem, I'm just sexually liberated," or "You're crazy," or "I can go months without this, so I don't have a problem." As Rick Warren states, "Rationalizing is telling yourself Rational Lies" (Twitter).

Give your own examples:______________________________

3.___Minimizing: This is trying to make behavior or consequences seem smaller or less important than they are by saying things like "only a little," or "only once in a while," or "it's no big deal," or simply telling the story in a better light than it really should be.

Give your own examples:______________________________

4.___Comparison: This is shifting focus to someone else to justify behaviors such as "I'm not as bad as…"

Give your own examples:______________________________

5.___Uniqueness: This is thinking you are different or special and saying things like "My situation is different," or "I was hurt more," or

"That's fine for you, but I'm too busy." This one can also be considered *Entitlement*.

Give your own examples:______________________________

6.___Distraction (Carnes, *Avoiding by creating an uproar or distraction*): This is being a clown and getting everyone laughing, having angry outbursts meant to frighten or intimidate others, threats and posturing, and doing shocking behavior that may even be sexual. This can be when we simply blow up upon being confronted hoping that our explosion will draw attention rather than the actual issue.

Give your own examples:______________________________

7.___Avoiding or Lying by Omission: This is trying to change the subject, ignore the subject, or manipulate the conversation to avoid talking about something. It is also leaving out important bits of information like the fact that the lover is underage, or the person is a close friend of your spouse, or revealing enough information while keeping back the most "dangerous" information that will get you in more trouble.

Give your own examples:______________________________

8.___Blaming: This is when you shift blame and responsibility from yourself to another person, and many times this is done unconsciously since in the depth of our being we really don't want to be held responsible for something. I call this the Adam Syndrome as this is what Adam did in the Garden (Genesis 3) by wrongly blaming Eve for his rebellion. This includes, "Well, you would cruise all night, too, if you had my job," or "If my spouse weren't so cold..." or "I can't help it, the baby cries day and night and makes me nervous."

Give your own examples:______________________________

9.___ Intellectualizing: This is avoiding feelings and responsibility by thinking or by asking why. This person tries to explain everything getting lost in detail, rabbit trails, and/or storytelling. This often includes pretending superior intellect and using intelligence as a weapon.

Give your own examples:______________________________

10.___Victim Mentality (Carnes, ***Hopelessness/Helplessness***): This is where a person says, "I'm a victim," or "I can't help it," or "There is nothing I can do to get better," or "I'm the worst."

Give your own examples:___________________________________

11.___Manipulative Behavior: This usually involves some distortion of reality including the use of power, lies, secrets, or guilt to exploit others.

Give your own examples:___________________________________

12.___Compartmentalizing: Separating your life into compartments in which you do things that you keep separate from other parts of your life. This is like a Jackal and Hyde or a separation of Public and Private Life to the point where it is unhealthy driven by thoughts of "If they only knew, then…"

Give your own examples:___________________________________

13.___Crazymaking: This occurs when we are confronted by others who DO have a correct perception… we simply tell them that they are totally wrong. We act indignantly toward them attempting to make them feel crazy by simply positing that they cannot trust their own perceptions.

Give your own examples:___________________________________

14.___Seduction: This is the use of charm, humor, good looks, or helpfulness to gain sexual access and cover up insincerity.

Give your own examples:___________________________________

15.___Denial: Is probably the most common weapon in our arsenal. Everyone around us sees what is happening to us, but we're blind to it. The real purpose of denial is to keep ourselves from facing the truth. Denial protects us from the truth.

Give your own examples: ___________________________________

16.___Isolation: If we tell ourselves that we almost have everything under control, we will gradually withdraw from anyone who presses the truth upon us.

Give your own examples: ___________________________________

17. ___ Attacking: Becoming angry and irritable when reference is made to the existing condition, thus avoiding the issue.

18. ___Willpower: "I should be able to handle this on my own," we tell ourselves. In fact, I can handle this all by myself!" We convince ourselves we don't need a program or anyone else to help us. To prove the strength of our willpower, we may succeed in breaking the pattern of our problems or our dependency for a period of time-sometimes for six months or more. "The problem has gone away," we tell ourselves. But then, invariably, because our enemy is stronger than we are, we once again experience defeat and humiliation-left to face the reality of our powerlessness. No matter how hard we try we always end up back in the same place.

Give your own examples: ______________________________

19.___ Ignoring the Positive: A belief that we should pay attention only to problems, shortcomings, or areas needing improvement. Disregard for positives in our personalities, skills, relationships, and accomplishments ensures a dreary outlook on all of life.

Give your own examples: ______________________________

20.___Arbitrary Inference: Jumping to illogical conclusions that create fear and anxiety. Question peoples motives and build a case against them. If someone doesn't say "hello" you begin to build a case, to assume they want something. If they don't say "hello" you begin to assume they don't like you and you have done something wrong.

Give your own examples: ______________________________

21.___Magnification/ Catastrophizing: Caricatured detectives go through life holding a magnifying glass before their eyes. Make something small into a big deal. They convince themselves that circumstances they don't like are major disasters. An example may be obsessing over something you said to someone, and playing it over and over again in your head, or simply making a mountain out of a mow hill.

Give your own examples: ______________________________

22.___Reification of Feelings: Convinced that feelings are the infallible barometer of a given incident or set of circumstances. Believe the feelings represent reality. They rely on their feelings as a guide and compass through life because they are so real to them. When they are having a down or difficult day, reification of feelings can be a self-perpetuating spiral of negative feelings and self-defeating self-talk.

Give your own examples: ________________________________

23.___Labeling: It is the childhood form of name calling. Instead of objectively describing behavior or actions (our own or someone else's), we attach a derogatory label to the person. For example, idiot, stupid, hypocrite, irresponsible or any other self-depreciating label.

Give your own examples: ________________________________

24.___Fortune-Telling: Tell yourself you know what the outcome will be. By fortune-telling you in effect, play it safe, avoid taking risks, and miss opportunities for reconciliation and personal growth because you habitually predict dismal outcomes.

Give your own examples: ________________________________

25.___Projection: Dumping feelings of self-hate on others. Any negatives in others that we don't like in ourselves. We cannot like or dislike something in someone else that we don't first like or dislike within ourselves.

Give your own examples: ________________________________

26.___Repression: Unconscious blocking of events that are too difficult to deal with. This is often associated with trauma and grief.

Give your own examples: ________________________________

27.___Lying by Commission: A lie is a false statement to a person or group made by another person or group who knows it is not the whole truth, intentionally. It can be deemed a barefaced (or bald-faced) lie is one that is obviously a lie to those hearing it. For example being asked if you were doing something or where somewhere and you simply state "no" knowing that it is not true, you where there or where doing something.

Give your own examples:________________________________

28.___Worrier: The Worrier creates anxiety by imagining the worst-case scenario. They promote your fears that what is happening is dangerous or embarrassing. ("What if I have a heart attack?" "What will they think if they see me?")

Give your own examples:______________________________

29.___Shoulds (Musts/Oughts): Shoulds are demands we make of ourselves. For example: "I should have known better"; or "I should be happy and never depressed or tired." We think we motivate ourselves with such statements. Usually, however, we just feel worse. I then feel inadequate, frustrated, ashamed, and hopeless.

Give your own examples: ______________________________

30.___Personalizing: Is seeing yourself as more involved in negative events that you really are. For example, a student drops out of college and the mother concludes, that it is all my fault.

Give your own examples: ______________________________

31.___Ingratiating (Kissing up): Being pleasing and agreeable, calculated to please and win favor.

Give your own examples: ______________________________

32.___Personality Masks: Is a process in which an individual changes or "masks" his or her natural personality to conform to social pressures. There is an inconsistency in behavior. Some examples of masking are a single overly dominant temperament, or humor, two incongruent temperaments, or displaying three of the four main temperaments within the same individual. You may not even know your wearing a mask because it is a behavior that can take many forms. (See Appendix 12)

Give your own examples:______________________________

33.___Awfulizing: Imagine something to be as bad as it can possibly be. It is a method people use to try to head off potential disappointment, or try to start preparing ourselves for the negative situation we're sure is on the horizon. It is just a negative thought habit.

Give your own examples: ______________________________

34.___Pride (Closed Minded): A high or inordinate opinion of one's own dignity, importance, merit, or superiority, whether as cherished in the mind or as displayed in conduct. Pride will often lead the individual to not listen to others and being closed minded.

Give your own examples: ______________________________

Read your examples out loud to your therapist, sponsor or trusted friend. We are only "as sick as our secrets," and usually sex addicts have a significant number of secrets. So take a moment and list your secrets and who you kept the truth from. Consider your lies of omission as well?

Look realistically at the consequences of your behavior in each category below. Put a check in the box by each of the ones that you have experienced:

Emotional Consequences

____Thoughts or feelings about committing suicide

____Attempted suicide

____Homicidal thoughts or feelings

____Feelings of hopelessness and despair

____Failed efforts to control your sexual behavior

____Feeling like you had two different lives-one public and one secret

____Depression, paranoia, or fear of going insane

____Loss of touch with reality

____Loss of self-esteem

____Loss of life goals

____Acting against your own values and beliefs

____Strong feelings of guilt and shame

____Strong feelings of isolation and loneliness

____Strong fears about the future

____Emotional exhaustion

____Other emotional consequences

Physical Consequences

____Continuation of addictive behavior, despite the risk to health

____Extreme weight loss or gain

____Physical problems (ulcers, high blood pressure, etc.)

____Physical injury or abuse by others

____Involvement in potentially abusive or dangerous situations

____Vehicle accidents

____Injury to yourself from your sexual behavior

____Sleep disturbances (not enough sleep or too much sleep)

____Physical exhaustion

____Other physical consequences related to your sexual behavior such as venereal diseases.

Spiritual Consequences

____Feelings of spiritual emptiness

____Feeling disconnected from yourself and the world

____Feeling abandoned by God or your Higher Power

____Loss of faith in anything spiritual

____Other spiritual consequences

Consequences Related to Family

___Risking the loss of partner or spouse

___Loss of partner or spouse

___Increase in marital or relationship problems

___Jeopardizing the well-being of your family

___Loss of family's or partner's respect

___Increase in problems with your children

___Estrangement from your family of origin

___Other family or partnership consequences

Career and Educational Consequences

___Decrease in work productivity

___Demotion at work

___Loss of co-workers' respect

___Loss of the opportunity to work in the career of your choice

___Failing grades in school

___Loss of educational opportunities

___Loss of business

___Forced to change careers

___Not working to your level of capability

___Termination of job

___Other career or educational consequences

Other Consequences

____Loss of important friendships

____Loss of interest in hobbies or activities

____Few or no friends who don't participate in or condone your sexual behavior

____Financial problems

____Illegal activities (arrests or near-arrests)

____Court or legal involvement

____Lawsuits

____Provincial or Federal Incarceration

____Stealing or embezzling to support behavior

____Other consequences

(Consequences by Patrick Carnes)

Give several examples for each consequence you identified. Talk to your therapist, sponsor or trusted friend regarding the consequences.

Often addicts like me will feel that consequences are unfair, that the punishment doesn't match the crime. Remember that no one promised justice and fairness. You have to deal with what is real and face the truth. You may have lived with the illusion that others will respond with sympathy, because of all the good you have done or how hard you have worked. None of that will help you now.

The people who gave you the consequences are not your enemies although it is very hard not to think or feel that way. If you see them in that light then you will keep yourself stuck in justifying your behavior. The real problem is your denial and your capacity for self-delusion. You are responsible for making yourself vulnerable to them. It is your addiction that got you there in the first place. When you chose your behavior, you opened the door to consequences. You have to ask whether the risk was worth it.

At this point see your consequences as teachers. We are enrolled in a full time school called life and we will receive lessons, but we will repeat lessons until we learn them.

Appendix III
Your Addictive Cycle

Each phase of the cycle has a place for you to record examples of your cycle. Provide as many examples as you can:

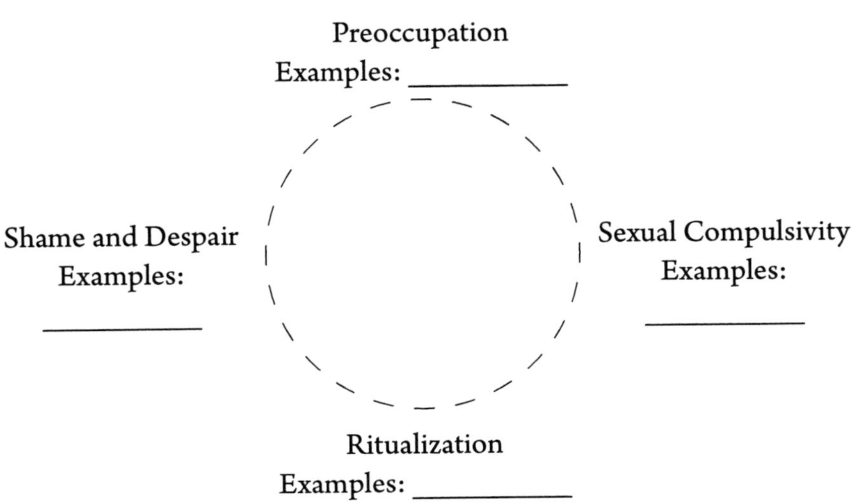

Some people have found it helpful to take a large piece of newsprint and diagram their one addictive system. Take each component-beliefs, thinking, addiction cycle, and unmanageability-and map out what happens in your addiction. Talk to your therapist, sponsor or trusted friend to enable them to get the big picture.

Appendix IV
Spiritual Focus Steps 1-3

The 12 Steps can be broken down into four parts, Spiritual, Mental and Physical and Social. (Body, Soul & Spirit) I would suggest that the goal of the first three steps is spiritual as we make peace with God. The goal of steps 4-7 is making peace with us as it relates to our Mind (soul). The goal of step 8-9 is making peace with others as it relates to our social and physical world (body) and the goal of the last three steps, 10-12 is keeping the peace (Social). Please note that I am only attempting to summarize the concepts of the steps as they relate to Spirit, Soul and Body as I consider a holistic (Trinitarian) approach to recovery. The exercises are a brief introduction to the steps but are by no means exhaustive. I believe the most comprehensive guide to working the Steps are found in the Alcoholics Anonymous Big Book. A second choice would be Sexaholics Anonymous Study Guide of the Steps. You will note that I have referred to John Baker in his book *Celebrate Recovery* who gives us very practical acronyms for understanding the process of working through each of the steps. I hope you find this practical and helpful as it has been for me.

Steps 1 and 3 offers the chance to embrace our shame and vulnerability. Only by embracing the shame can we come out of hiding and give up trying to control shame. It is important not only to recognize but to admit that shame has been a huge catalyst to our addiction. Because of shame we have learned to trust no one and yet the steps ask us to trust someone or something greater than ourselves.

Step One

We admitted we were powerless over our compulsive sexual behaviors - that our lives had become unmanageable.

Principle 1: Realize I'm not God. I admit that I am powerless to control my tendency to do the wrong thing and that my life is unmanageable.

Key Scripture: "I know that nothing good lives in me, that is, in my sinful nature. For I have the desire to do what is good, but I cannot carry it out" (Romans 7:18).

Be Attitude: "Happy are those who know they are spiritually poor" (Matthew. 5:3).

Key 1: Realization: "I realized that I was powerless and that my life was unmanageable.

Subject: Conviction: I accept that I have reached the point that my life is out of control and I am totally helpless. This sense of helplessness is the beginning of God working in my life by His Spirit.

The Condition: Consists of the utter inability to initiate and sustain a desired from of behavior.

The Result: Unmanageability-the inability to control life situations, due primarily to condition of powerlessness.

Reality: We did not contain the necessary power to return our lives to manageability.

Components of Powerlessness:
The knowledge that you need help
The necessity of seeking help
The difficulty in asking for help
The necessary attitudes for obtaining help (humility)

Concepts:
Admission-to sincerely and honestly ADMIT
Powerlessness-recognition of denial of the problem
Unmanageable- In all areas of my life, not just the presenting problem

Scripture Support:
Luke 15: 11-24 Prodigal Son
Deuteronomy 30: 19, 20 Choose life
John 15: 5-8 "God is the vine;" Cor. 12:9-10; Romans 7:18-20;
2 Matthew 5:3; Psalms 6:6-7; I Corinthians 8:2; Mark 4:35-40
2 Corinthians 12:9 "my grace is sufficient;" Jeremiah 6:14;
Ecclesiastes 11:4; Job 30:27; Romans 7:15-17; Proverbs
14:12; Job17:11; Psalm 6:6- 7; 2 Corinthians 1:9

Step Summary:

The ideas presented in Step One are overwhelming to most of us until we begin to see our lives as they really are. It is threatening to us at times to imagine we are powerless. Thinking of us as being unable to manage our own lives is frightening. In our daily experience we are reminded regularly that our behavior and attitudes do not always produce peace and serenity. The recognition of this truth is necessary for growth.

We would, however, rather feel that we have power and are in control of our lives. Surrendering is not an easy thing to do. We want answers. As we accept the reality of our condition, we wonder why the quality of life we desire is escaping us. Basically, this is what life is all about. Working through Step One can be applied to any problem in life. In our daily life we must continually surrender our problems to God rather than attempt to take total control of our own lives.

The Twelve Steps for Christians states,

> "We may have been taught to believe that we only have to accept Christ as our Lord and Savior for our lives to be complete and satisfying. We may have relied upon this to prepare us for the hereafter. Our proclamation that "I am born anew; the past is washed clean; I am a new creature; Christ has totally changed me" is true. Our Spirits are born anew, but since our soul and spirit are separate entities, we need to realize that we have a

> lifetime of habits and wounds in our soul and we need more than salvation. We need transformation-the hard work of change. To over-spiritualize the initial work of salvation may be to deny the actual condition of our lives.

The fact that we still feel pain from our past is not a sign of a failed relationship with God. The presence of pain does not lessen the impact of salvation in our lives. This is simply a signal we need to begin the process of healing by daily working the steps with God's help. In time, God will bring the healing and make the necessary changes in our lives. To admit the pains and problems may seem a contradiction of our strong claim to salvation, but it is not.

John Baker in his book *Celebrate Recovery* gives us an acrostic of **POWERLESS**

P- Pride:

Proverbs 29:23 "Pride ends in a fall, while humility brings honor."

O- Only ifs:

Our "if only's" in life keep us trapped in the fantasyland of rationalization!

"Whatever is covered up will be uncovered, and every secret will be made known. So then, whatever you have said in the dark will be heard in broad daylight" (Luke 12:2-3).

W- Worry:

Worrying is a form of not trusting God enough!

"So don't be anxious about tomorrow, God will take care of your tomorrow too. Live one day at a time" (Matthew 6:34).

E- Escape:

By living in denial we may have escaped into a world of fantasy and unrealistic expectations of ourselves and others.

"For light is capable of showing up everything for what it really is. It is even possible for light to turn the thing it shines upon into light" (Ephesians 5:13-14).

R- Resentments:

Resentments act like an emotional cancer if they are allowed to fester and grow.

"In your anger do not sin': Do not let the sun go down while you are still angry, and do not give the devil a foothold" (Ephesians 4:26-27).

L- Loneliness:

Loneliness is a choice. In recovery and in Christ, you never have to walk alone.

"Continue to love each other with true brotherly love. Don't forget to be kind to strangers, for some who have done this have entertained angels without realizing it" (Hebrews 13:1-2).

E- Emptiness:

You know that empty feeling deep inside. The cold wind of hopelessness blows right through it. Jesus said, "My purpose is to give life in all its fullness" (John 10:10).

S- Selfishness:

We often pray: "Our Father which art in heaven: give me, give me, give me."

Whoever clings to his life shall lose it, and whoever loses his life shall save it" (Luke 17:33).

S- Separation:

Some people talk about finding God – as if He could ever get lost!

"For I am convinced that nothing can ever separate us from His love. Death can't and life can't. The angels won't, and all the powers of hell itself cannot keep God's love way... Nothing will ever be able to separate us from the love God demonstrated by our Lord Jesus Christ when He died for us"(Romans 8:38-39).

Process:

Stop denying the pain:

"Pity me, O Lord, for I am weak. Heal me, for my body is sick, and I am upset and disturbed. My mind is filled with apprehension and with gloom" (Psalm 6:2-3).

Stop playing God

"No one can be a slave to two masters; he will hate one and love the other; he will be loyal to one and despise the other" (Matthew 6:24).

Start admitting your powerless

"Jesus ... said, "With man this is impossible, but with God all things are possible" (Matthew 19:26).

Start admitting that your life has become unmanageable

"Problems far too big for me to solve are piled higher than my head. Meanwhile my sins, too many to count, have all caught up with me and I am ashamed to look up" (Psalm 40:12).

Sexaholics Anonymous Step Study Guide states:

> "In the written review of our past we face ourselves as we really are. The words, "I am a sexaholic" come out of this insight. Bringing what we are to the light keeps us from hiding what we are and becomes the act of putting it all behind us and sending it away.
>
> The idea is to look fearlessly at the whole of our lust, fantasy, sex and relationship history from the very beginning to face who and what we really are, detect the destructive patterns of thinking and behavior, and see the powerlessness and unmanageability of our lives."

Exercise:

What are your fears concerning the pain and suffering you may experience as a result of self-examination?

Sexual History (Answer the following questions by giving the approximate age and the specific event that was part of your sexual development.)

Your Age_____

Key childhood sexual experiences up to age 10 (strong memories, traumatic events; events that evoke strong feelings; child abuse by parents or other persons).

Your Age_____

Key adolescent sexual experiences up to age 18 (sexual experimentation; masturbation; onset of menstruation; sexual abuse; fantasy life; sexual partners; dating; other).

Your Age_____

Key adult experiences up to age 25 then 26 to present age (dating; marriage; divorce; sexual partners; other).

List as many examples as you can that show how powerless you have been to stop your behavior. Remember, "Powerless" means being unable to stop the behavior despite obvious consequences. Be very explicit about types of behavior and frequency. Start with your earliest examples. Remember you do not need to complete this inventory in one sitting. When you have completed it share it with your therapist, sponsor or trusted friend.

List as many examples as you can that show how your life has become totally unmanageable because of your dependency. Remember, "Unmanageability" means that your addiction created chaos and damage in your life. Go back and review your list of consequences under the denial appendix. Use the acronym **BECHRISTLIKE** as a guide to exploring different areas of your life. Again when you finish this inventory, stop and talk to your therapist, sponsor or trusted friend. You will need the support.

B- Behavior:

Addictive behavior and behavior strengths and deficits for example; perfectionism, controlling, physical, emotional and sexual abuse, intimidating and argumentative, people pleasing, irresponsible, lazy and a procrastinator, over driven and achiever, seductive, workaholic, withdrawal, avoidant and silent treatment, compulsive and impulsive, arrogant and bossy, critical, deceitful and defensive, exaggerate, indecisive, passive, passive-aggressive, aggressive and hostile, self-reliant and self-serving, vain, arrogant, rebellious and greedy, etc. (Review your denial and self-defense mechanism Inventory; Appendix II)

E- Emotions:

What are your common emotional patterns? What are your emotional themes? Controlled by what emotions? Deny feelings? Describe what emotions you experience and give several examples, depression, envy, fear and anxiety, fear of failure, fear of rejection, hateful, irritable, moody, negative, angry, resentful, sadness, self-pity, self-righteous, stubborn, suspicious, worry, lonely and easily intimidated, inadequate, unwanted, worthless and unacceptable, helpless, insignificant, insure, unloved, unimportant, rejected, hopeless, a nobody and worthless, inferior, bad and evil, guilty, shameful, abandoned, stupid, dumb and no good, etc.

C- Cognitions:

What is your self talk for example, self-condemning, sexual fantasy and lust, suicidal thoughts, self-depreciation, revengeful and covetous, self-hatred, self-justification, etc. (Review Self-Talk Inventory; Appendix IX)

H- Health:

Medical issues, eating, sleeping and exercise habits, weight loss or gain. Are you currently on any prescription medication?

R- Religion:

What have been some of your religious affiliations in the past or present? Have you had any changes over the years for example an increase or decrease in attendance, and why? Have you ever been involved in Cult or Occult practices? What is your general attitude and belief towards God, Jesus, prayer and spirituality?

I- Idols and incorrect beliefs:

What desires and values compete with God? What do you believe is going to meet your emotional needs for significance and security, your sense of worth?

S- Substances:

Are you currently using any illicit drugs or abusing alcohol or any other substance? What is your pattern of use and age of onset? Do you have any kind of eating disorder, diagnosed or self-diagnosed?

T- Teachability:

Are you motivated or resistant to change? Do you believe you can change? Are there people in your life that you are willing to be open and honest with and let them speak into your life and be truth tellers?

L- Law and ethics:

Is there a risk to yourself or another human being? Any suicide attempts in the past, how many and how? Any current legal problems and charges, past or present and include money spent, time in jail? Do you currently have a criminal record?

I- Interpersonal relationships:

Describe current issues and history with family and friends. What are the best and worst traits in each of your parents? How did they make you feel? Did they have a favorite child? How was there relationship? Was your family rigid and authoritarian, with no allowance for emotional expression? What did you learn about men and women from your parents? How did your parents handle stress and hardship? Is there a history of addictions in your family? How old where you when you first saw pornography of any kind and what was the context? Who was the disciplinarian and how? Where you ever emotionally, physically or sexually hurt? If you have siblings how would you describe your relationship with them? Describe spousal relationship, divorce history, etc. Specify any ongoing support of those for whom you have felt guilt or have been legally required to support? Describe sexual behaviors and problems in your relationship. What are your secrets and overt and covert lies? If you have children how would you describe your parenting style?

K-Knowledge:

What is your current education level and any learning disabilities? What do you know about sexual addiction and addictions in general? Do you believe you know more or less than most people or average?

E-Environment:

What are your external obstacles and triggers? What strength and resources are available to you? What is your current living arrangements and financial status? Include money spent on your addiction, from pornography, prostitution to cosmetic surgery.

How has family attitudes and religious experiences, ethnic or cultural heritage affected and impacted your sexual development?

What difficulties are you experiencing in recognizing your powerlessness and your inability to manage your life?

How do you feel, when, after looking carefully at yourself, you recognize an area of your life that needs change or improvement?

Read 2 Corinthians 12:9, 10: How does God comfort you and help you accept the powerlessness and unmanageability of your life?

Step Two

Came to believe that a Power greater than ourselves could restore us to sanity.

Principle 2: Earnestly believe that God exists, that I matter to Him, and that He has the power to help me recover.

Key 2: Recognition: I recognized that I needed help beyond myself.

Be Attitude: "Happy are those who mourn, for they shall be comforted." (Matthew. 5:4)

Key Scripture: "For it is God who works in you to will and to act according to His purpose."

Scripture Support: Ephesians 2:12-13; 2 Corinthians 4:7-8; Colossians 1:27; Romans 12:2; Isaiah 42:3: Matthew14:22-34; Matthew 17:20; Mark 9:23-24; Psalm 34:18-22; 2 Corinthians 1:9; Philippians 2:13; 2 Corinthians 3:5; Isaiah 40:28-31; Isaiah 41:10; John 3:16-17

Components:

"**Came**" – the first word means a slow process

"**To believe**" – This brings up the question of faith in God. Keep an open mind – get out of the debating society and be willing to listen – stop fighting to preserve your point of view.

"**Sanity**" – means in this step "soundness of mind." Dictionary defines insanity as inability to manage one's own affairs and perform one's social duties and without recognition of one's own illness." Insanity has often been described as doing the same thing over and over and expecting different results. Sanity has been defined as "wholeness of mind; making decisions based on the truth."

Step Summary:

Step two is about faith – trust and believing. As I discussed in chapter 8, faith is the hinge to our recovery and it is our faulty belief system that became the foundation in which our addiction rests.

With the help of Step One we came to grips with the fact that we are powerless and our lives are unmanageable. So this step is about acknowledging the existence of a power greater than ourselves. Believing in God does not always mean that we accept His power.

For many of us, this step presents major obstacles. As I stated early in the book, addicts have a hard time with trusting others and even God and out of our loneliness we have tended to rely on our own resources. Belief in our self-will and our ability to manage our own lives is all we have. We may even doubt that God can heal us or even be interested in doing so. Unless we let go of our distrust and begin to lean on God, we will continue to operate in an insane manner. The chaos and confusion of our lives will only increase.

The 12 Steps Spiritual Journey states,

> "Depending on our religious background, some of us may have been taught that God is an authority to be feared. We never saw him as a loving God. Our fear of displeasing God magnified our growing sense of guilt and shame. Or we may be harboring childhood anger at God because he often disappointed us. Some of us have even rejected God because He did not relieve our pain.

For some of us like my good friend in the recovery program who started out as an Atheist believing there is no God in response to his legalistic religious upbringing. However, in His recovery program he has come to believe in a personal God and addressed his early childhood rejection of Him.

On the other hand I had a colleague who is a licensed psychologist that I worked closely with as co-facilitator of psycho-educational groups for abused men and for children of domestic violance. About 4 months ago out of desperation she pulled me aside and began to share some of her childhood trauma and her current sexual exploits. She disclosed that her sex life was beginning to unravel and she felt overwhelmed with the prospect of losing her second husband and their child. I explored her belief system and her willingness to explore a higher power. She responded in no uncertain terms and with a level of hostility that there is no God and she would not need a spiritual program to recover. I had since left that place of employment and just heard today that she had taken her own life and was found dead in her office, leaving behind her second husband and three children. My heart is broken over this news yet I am only reminded that without God the chaos, confusion and feelings of powerlessness and unmanageability only increases.

Others of us are Agnostics and say, "There may be a God but I cannot know for certain." Others are Polytheistic and believe that there are many gods" and yet others are Pantheist and see that God is simply the forces and laws of the universe, God in nature. It is clear that people approach this step from many and varied perspectives. I strongly propose Monotheism, the belief that there is only one God.

It does raise the question, if there is a God, can He be known? Rather how does one come to know God? To a degree God can be known through His creation, Psalm 19:1-4; Romans 1:18-20. There are other ways in which God has revealed Himself, through history as we worked on behalf of His people. He most explicitly revealed Himself in Jesus, His incarnate Son, John 14:8-11. The Bible which is a collection of 66 books, written over a period of at least 1600 years by approximately 40 human writers is also a way in which God is revealed. The crucial issue is to what degree are you willing to acknowledge the authority of the Word of God. Does the Bible contain the word of God and is it, in all parts, reliable and trustworthy? 2 Timothy 3:15; Psalm 19:7-11; Psalm 119:89. Personally I have come to believe the Bible as the Word of God in its entirety, in part due to the fact that it is eighty percent prophecy and its inerrancy in this regard over all these millennia. For this reason I believe the Bible serves as a plum-line to inform us of what is truth or error, Amos 7:7-9.

In the process of coming to believe we begin to see God's true nature and a weight is lifted from our shoulders. We begin to view life from a different perspective. In the Bible we are shown that through him all things are possible. This brings new hope as we begin to see that help is available to us. We must simply reach out and accept what our Higher Power has to offer. "Anyone who comes to God must believe that He exists and that He rewards those who earnestly seek Him." (Hebrews 11:6)

John Baker in *Celebrate Recovery* gives us an acronym for **HOPE**:

H-Higher Power:

Our Higher Power has a name: Jesus Christ! Jesus desires a hands-on, day-to-day, moment by moment relationship with us. He can do for us what we have never been able to do for ourselves.

"Everything comes from God alone. Everything lives by His power" (Romans 11:36; 2).

"My grace is enough for you; for where there is weakness, my power is shown the more completely" (II Corinthians 12:9).

O- Openness to change:

Throughout our lives, we will continue to encounter hurts and trials that we are powerless to change. With God's help, we need to be open to allow those trials to change us. To make us better not bitter.

"Now your attitudes and thoughts must all be constantly changing for the better. Yes, you must be a new and different person" (Ephesians 4:23).

P- Power to change:

In the past, we have wanted to change and were unable to do so. We could not free ourselves from our hurts or habits.

"For I can do everything God asks me to with the help of Christ who gives me the strength and the power" (Philippians 4:13).

"Lead me; teach me; for you are the God who gives me salvation. I have no hope except in you" (Psalms 25:5).

E-Expect to change:

Remember you are only at the second step, remember it takes a long time to get sick, it takes a long time to get better, one step at a time,

"I am sure that God who began the good work within you will keep right on helping you grow in His grace until His task within you is finally finished on that day when Jesus Christ returns" (Philippians 1:6).

"Now faith is being sure of what we hope for and certain of what we do not see" (Hebrews 11:1).

So no matter what you have done in the past, God wants to forgive it! "While we were still sinners, Christ died for us" (Romans 5:8). No matter what shape your life is in today, together God and you can handle it! "And God is faithful" He will not let you be tempted beyond what you can bear. But when you are tempted, He will also provide a way out" (I Corinthians 10:13).

A simple prayer to begin this new relationship with God is simply stating, dear God, I have tried to "fix" and "control" my life's hurts, and habits all by myself. I am powerless to change. I need to begin to believe and receive your power to help me recover. You loved me enough to send Your Son to the cross to die for my sins. Help me be open to the hope that I can only find in you. Please help me to start living my life one day at a time. In Jesus' name I pray, Amen.

The purpose of writing this Step is to help us become aware of the acquired destructive thinking and character defects that has wrecked our lives.

Exercise:

Read Romans 1:18-20 Paul says we "have no excuse for not knowing God." What excuses have you used in the past and present for not knowing God's power?

Read Romans 1:21-23 if in the past and present you have created your own understanding of God how has that led to your disappointment with God?

Our recovery begins "when we come to believe." Describe any new insights you have discovered about God.

Describe your first few steps in coming to believe.

Read Luke 15:11-32 what has your insanity looked like to you? To others who cared about you? How did you come to your senses? And in which ways have you been humbled?

The son received grace rather than judgment, what are some of pleasant surprises of grace that you have received since starting recovery?

Read Hebrews 11:1-3 what would sanity look and feel like to you?

Read Hebrews 12:1-2 the text talks about our running with endurance. What resources are you gathering to help you do this? Who is your cloud of witnesses?

Step Three

Made a decision to turn our will and our lives over to the care of God as we understood God.

Principle 3: Consciously choose to commit all my life and will to Christ's care and control

Key 3: Responsibility: "I made firm commitments concerning my sobriety, my program, and my future."

Key Scripture: "Therefore, I urge you, brothers, in view of God's mercy, to offer your bodies as living sacrifices, holy and pleasing to God – this is your spiritual act of worship" (Romans 12:1).

Be Attitude: "Happy are the meek" (Matt. 5:5).

Scriptures Support: Romans 10:9; Matthew 17:20; Matthew 11:28-30; Psalm 37:5; Psalm 25:5; 2 Corinthians 1:9; Psalm 143:10; Proverbs 3:5-6; James 4:1-10

Components:

- **Turn it over**; Give God control, surrender is the key idea.

-**Self-will**: Which is a determination in us all to control our own lives. Our choices have brought about pain, hardships, addictions, compulsions, and self-defeating behaviors. God's will for our lives bring us hope, healing, and peace.

Step Summary:

Step One and Two have laid the groundwork for our recovery, but Step Three calls us to act. We must make a decision! It is one thing to admit that our lives are out of control, and that we need someone more powerful than we are to restore us to sanity. But all too often, on the inside, we're still thinking there are some parts of our recovery we need to do on our own. Recovery involves truly surrendering; it is a leap of faith.

Sexaholics Anonymous Step Study Guide states:

> We become convinced that any life run on self-will can hardly be a success. Obviously, the first two steps show, in no uncertain terms, the confusion caused by using self-will (self-will is a part of the acquired false self). Self-will includes selfishness and self-centeredness. This self-centeredness is the root of our troubles. We found that we could not reduce the self-centeredness much by wishing or relying on our own power. Thus, we had to quit playing God. It did not work.

Step Three is an affirmative step. It is time to make a decision. In the first two Steps, we became aware of our condition and accepted the idea of a power greater than ourselves. Although we began to know and trust Him, we may find it difficult to think of allowing God to be totally in charge of our lives.

As we surrender our lives and stop carrying the burdens of our past, we will begin to feel better about ourselves. The more we learn to trust in God, the more we will trust ourselves.

John Baker in *Celebrate Recovery* gives us an acronym for how to **TURN** our life over to the one and only Higher Power, Jesus Christ

T- Trust:

Deciding to turn your life and your will over to God requires only trust. Trust is putting the faith you found in Principle into action.

"If you declare with your lips, 'Jesus is Lord,' and believe in your heart that God raised him from the dead, you will saved" (Romans 10:9).

U- Understand:

Relying solely on our own understanding got you into recovery in the first place! After you make the decision to ask Jesus into your life, you need to begin to seek His will for your life in all your decisions.

"Trust in the Lord with all our heart and lean not on your own understanding; in all your ways acknowledge Him, and He will make your paths straight" (Proverbs 3:5-6).

R- Repent:

To truly repent, you must not only turn away from your sins, but turn toward God. Repentance allows you to enjoy the freedom of your loving relationship with God.

"Turn from your sins and act on this glorious news!" (Mark 1:15)

N- New Life:

After you ask Jesus into your heart, you will have a new life! You will no longer be bound to your old sin nature. God has declared us 'not guilty' if we trust Jesus Christ to take away our sins.

"Now God says he will accept and acquit us-declares us 'not guilty'- if we trust Jesus Christ to take away our sins" (Romans 3:22).

The second component: **"As we understood him"** as shared in Step two and our understanding of God may be based on past frustrations with Him. We've developed an image of God based on his seeming failure to help us in the past. We need to understand that God desires to be our refuge, our place of safety. Over and over throughout the Psalms, David affirms that God is his safe place, he writes, "Those who live in the shelter of the Most High will find rest in the shadow of the Almighty. This I declare about the Lord: He alone is my refuge, my place of safety; He is my God, and I trust him" (Psalm 91: 1-4).

Next we need to understand that God is a God who loves. When we live in the shame of our problems and dependencies, our perception of God may center on His judgment. God's very nature is love and He doesn't judge us-He accepts us and receives us. I John 4:8-10 states, "Anyone who does not love does not know God, for God is love. God showed how much He loved us by sending His one and only Son into the world so that we might have eternal life through Him. This is real love- not that we loved God, but that He loved us and sent His Son as a sacrifice to take away our sins."

Lastly, we must understand that we can depend on God. When we surrender our wills and our lives to Him, we can trust Him to be faithful. This is an act of our wills. Rick Warren implies that faith requires action. He gives us the acronym for **ACTION**.

A-Accept Jesus Christ as your Higher Power and Savior!

Make a decision to ask Jesus into your heart. Now is the time to commit your life, to establish that personal relationship with Jesus that He so desires.

"If you confess with your mouth, 'Jesus is Lord,' and believe in your heart that God raised him from the dead, you will be saved" (Romans 10:9).

C-Commit to seek and follow HIS will!

We need to change our definition of willpower: Willpower is the willingness to accept God's power. We see that there is no room, for God if we are full of ourselves. I once heard it said that EGO means, Edging God Out.

"Teach me to do your will, for you are my God; may your good Spirit lead me on level ground" (Psalm 143:9-10).

T-Turn it over:

"Let go; let God!" There is nothing to big or too small that God can't handle.

"Come to me I will give you rest- all of you who work so hard beneath a heavy yoke. Wear my yoke-for it fits perfectly- and let me teach you; for I am gentle and humble, and you shall find rest for your souls"(Matthew 11:28-30).

I-It's only the beginning:

Our walk with our Higher Power, Jesus Christ, begins with this decision and is followed by a lifelong process of growing and maturing.

"God who began the good work within you will keep right on helping you grow in His grace until his task within is finally finished" (Philippians 1:6).

O- One day at a time:

My mother always told me, if you have one day in yesterday and one day in tomorrow, then you're shitting all over today. Okay my mom's language wasn't completely refined but her point was well taken. Recovery happens one day at a time.

"So don't be anxious about tomorrow. God will take care of your tomorrow too. Live one day at a time" (Matthew 6:34).

N- Next:

How do I ask Christ into my life?

Believe Jesus Christ died on the cross for me and showed He was God by coming back to life (I Corinthians 15:2-4)
Accept God's free forgiveness for my sins (Romans 3:22)
Switch to God's plan for my life (Romans 12:2)
Express my desire to Christ to be the director of my life (Romans 10:9)

A Prayer of Surrender: Dear God, I have tried to do it all by myself, on my own power and I have failed. Today, I want to turn my life over too You. I believe you sent Your Son, Jesus, to die for my sins so I can be forgiven. I am sorry for my sins and I ask You to be my Lord and my Savior. You are the One and only Higher Power! I ask that You help me start to think less about my will. I want to daily turn my will over to You, to daily seek Your direction and wisdom for my life. Please continue to help me overcome my hurts and habits and may that victory over them help others as they see Your power at work in changing my life. Please put Your Spirit in my life to direct me. Help me to do your will always. In Jesus' name I pray, Amen.

Exercise:

If you have said this prayer for the first time, from the depth of your heart, God tells us that we must "confess it with our mouth." Tell someone, friend, sponsor, pastor, etc. of your decision.

What do you fear turning over to His Care?

How do your childhood memories continue to frighten you?

What is keeping you from turning them over?

Read 118: 8-9; where has trusting in man failed you?

Read Isaiah 54:7-8; describe a time when you felt abandoned by God?

Read 2 Peter 1:2; where in your recovery journey do you still need to experience God's grace and peace?

Read Matthew 11:28-30; how will coming to the Lord for guidance lighten your burden?

How do you plan to practice Step Three in your daily routine of living?

Read John 14: 12-13; how do you see your life improving because of your decision to surrender to God's will?

Appendix V
Soul Focus: Steps 4-7

The goal of steps 4-7 is making peace with us as it relates to our Mind (soul). We move from shame to guilt. We become aware of how our character defects were strategies we used to transfer our shame to others and live out of our false self. The admission to self, others and God in step 5 is a way to come out of hiding. Shame loves secrecy and darkness. To come out into the light is a way to overcome it. Steps 6 and 7 focus on becoming willing to ask for help, something no shame based person would do. Shame believes that is doesn't have any right to depend on others and therefore ask for help.

Step Four

Made a searching and fearless moral inventory of ourselves.

Principle 4: Openly examine and confess my faults to myself, to God, and to someone I trust.

Key 4: Reason: "I came to understand that my three dimensional problem requires a three dimensional solution."

Key Scripture: "Let us examine our ways and test them, and let us return to the Lord." (Lamentations 3:40)

Be Attitude: "Happy are the pure in heart" (Matt. 5:8).

Scriptures Support: Lamentations 3:40; Galatians 6:3-5; Psalm 139:23-24; James 1:19-21; 2 Corinthians 13:5-6; Ephesians 4:31; Colossians 3:5-8; I John 14:26; Philippians 3:7-12; I Peter 4:1-6

Components: "Moral Inventory"

Step Summary:

The purpose of "taking inventory" of our lives is to help us face the truth about ourselves. Truth is the opposite of denial. By putting the truth in writing, we demonstrate that we are ready to break free from the patterns and behaviors of denial.

Facing the truth is painful because we must face the reality of our behavior and expand our understanding of ourselves. I heard it once said that our true character is not determined by what we do in the light but in the darkness. This inventory is an attempt to shine light in the darkness and come clean with ourselves and others.

As our self-discovery unfolds, we begin to recognize the role that denial has played in our lives. This realization is the basis for our acceptance of the truth of our personal history.

12 Steps – Spiritual Journey states,

> "Resentment and fear are two issues that need to be dealt with before we begin the process of preparing our inventory. Our resentment toward people, places and things that have injured us keeps us preoccupied and limits our ability to live in the present moment. Resentment results from hiding the bitter hurts and evokes anger, frustration and depression. Fear limits our ability to be rational. When fear is present, it is difficult to see situations in their true perspective. Fear is the root of other repressive and painful feelings. It prevents us from expressing ourselves honestly and stops us from responding in appropriate ways to threatening situations. In order to change our behaviors, we must first face and accept our fears.

Sexaholics Anonymous states:

> The Fourth Step allows us to uncover and discover the acquired character defects that are a part of the false self. These defects are not a part of the real you. Only when you detach yourself from these acquired character defects can you start to uncover and discover, in a fearless manner, these acquired character defects that have controlled you in the past. These acquired character defects have been the primary cause of our lusting and our failure at life; we must now be willing to work hard at the elimination of the worst of these defects.

John Baker in *Celebrate Recovery* gives us an acronym, **MORAL** to show us how to begin the inventory.

M – Make time:

Set aside a special time to begin your inventory. Schedule an appointment with yourself. Set aside a day or a weekend to get alone with God! Clear your mind of the present hassles of daily life.

"Then listen to me. Keep silence and I will teach you wisdom!" (Job 33:33)

O – Open your heart and your mind to allow the feelings that the pain of the past has blocked or caused you to deny:

Try to "wake up" your feelings! Ask yourself, "What do I feel guilty about? What do I resent? What do I fear? Am I trapped in self-pity, alibis, and dishonest thinking?"

"Let me express my anguish. Let me be free to speak out of the bitterness of my soul" (Job 7:11).

R – Rely on Jesus, your Higher Power, to give you the courage and strength this exercise requires.

"Love the Lord, all of you who are his people; for the lord protects those who are loyal to Him...So cheer up! Take courage if you are depending on the Lord" (Psalm 31:23-24).

A – Analyze your past honestly:

To do a "searching and fearless moral inventory," you must step out of your denial! That's all that the word "moral" means – honest! This step requires looking through your denial of the past into the truth!

"The Lord gave us mind and conscience; we cannot hide from ourselves" (Proverbs 20:27).

L –List both the good and the bad:

Keep your inventory balanced! If you just look at all the bad things of your past, you will distort your inventory and open yourself to unnecessary pain.

"Let us examine our ways and test them" (Lamentations 3:40).

Exercise:

Under each subject heading list that behavior, the reason you do it, the effects and what it activates. For example under resentments you may say I resent my boss because he doesn't care to hear my explanation of why I am depressed. This affects my self-esteem. This activates unexpressed anger. Also give examples how you're improving in this area.

Inventory List: (Examples taken from 12-Step Journal Workbook)

Fear: (In anxious states of mind, people typically can't see the forest for the trees. The process of worrying takes a greater toll on a person than the negative consequences of what they worried about) Indicators of recovery is that you let go and let God and you seek to clarify your problems and put them into proper perspective.

Repressed Anger (May show as self-pity, jealousy, anxiety, depression, sadness stress, bitterness, resentments and or physical discomfort) Indicators of recovery is that you express anger, identify hurt feelings, make reasonable requests, set limits for yourself, enjoy inner peace, reduce stress and anxiety.

Approval Seeking (we may people please, fear criticism, fear failure, feel unworthy, ignore our own needs, lack confidence) Indicators of recovery are that you recognize your own needs, tell the truth about how you feel, be loyal to yourself, building confidence.

Caretaking (we may make ourselves indispensable, rescue people, ignore our own needs, lose our identity, feel super-responsible, become co-dependent) Indicators of recovery is that you stop rescuing others, take care of yourself, set limits, develop your own identity, recognize dependent relationships

Control (we may overreact to change, lack trust, fear failure, be judgmental and rigid, be intolerant, manipulate others) Indicators of recovery is that you accept change, trust in yourself, empower others, reduce your stress load, find ways to have fun, accept others as they are.

Fear Abandonment (we may feel insecure, be caretakers, avoid being alone, worry excessively, feel guilty when standing up for ourselves, become co-dependent) Indicators of recovery are being honest about your feelings, feel comfortable being alone, express confidence, consider your own needs in a relationship, reduce your caretaking and co-dependency traits.

Fear of Authority Figures (may cause us to fear rejection, take things personally, be arrogant to cover up, compare ourselves to others, react rather than act, feel inadequate) Indicators of recovery is that you act with increased self-esteem, stand up for yourself, accept constructive criticism, interact easily with people in authority.

Frozen Feelings (we may be unaware of our feelings, have distorted feelings, suppress our feelings, experience depression, developed physical illness) Indicators of recovery is you feel free to cry, openly express feelings, experience our true self, express your needs to others.

Isolation (we may fear rejection, experience loneliness, procrastinate, feel defeated, non-assertive, see ourselves as different from others) Indicators of recovery is you accept yourself, freely express your emotions, cultivate supportive relationships, complete projects, actively participate with others.

Low Self-Esteem (we may be non-assertive, fear failure, appear inadequate, fear rejection, isolate from others, need to be perfect). Indicators of recovery is that you become more confident, act more assertively, easily interact with others, love yourself, openly express feelings, take risks.

Overdeveloped sense of responsibility (we may take life too seriously, appear rigid, be a perfectionist, be a high achiever, have false pride, and manipulate others). Indicators of recovery is that you take care of yourself, enjoy leisure time, accept your limitations, delegate responsibility.

Repressed Sexuality (we may feel guilt and shame, lose our sense of morality, be confused about our sexual identity, be lustful, be incest victim, experience being frigid or impotent, manipulate others by seductive behavior) Indicators of recovery is that you communicate openly about sex, accept your sexual self, consider your own sexual needs, share intimate feelings.

Step Five

Admit to God, to ourselves, and to another human being the exact nature of our wrongs.

Principle 5: Openly examine and confess my faults to myself, to God and to someone I trust.

Key 5: Redirection: "I came to believe that only God could restore me to sanity and wholeness."

Key Scripture: "Therefore confess your sins to each other and pray for each other so that you may be healed." (James 5:16)

Be Attitude: "Happy are the pure in heart" (Matt. 5:8).

Subject: Reconciliation: I will share the sins of my past with God and someone else so that by the act of sharing I will find God's forgiveness.

Scripture Support: Proverbs 28:1-3; I John 1:9; James 4:7-8; Jeremiah 14:20; Romans 14:12; Luke 15: 17-19; James 5:16; Proverbs 30:32; Romans 3;23-26

Components:

-Shadow: We discovered what has been in the shadows causing us problems and we confess it openly.

-Confession: We speak the truth about ourselves; we tell our story. We end the silence, the isolation and secrets.

Step Summary:

Completing our Step Four inventory has made us aware of many truths about ourselves. If we have been open, honest and thorough, it identified the unresolved feelings, unhealed memories and personal defects that have produced resentment, depression and loss of self-worth. Now that we have identified all of our character defects and our false self, it is possible to relieve ourselves of the burden of guilt and shame associated with our wrong-doings. This step requires that we put our pride aside, face our fear of rejection and step out of isolation and admit our faults to ourselves, others and God.

As I heard it once said, "we are only as sick as our secrets." Our natural instinct at this point is to keep our inventory a secret. If we have been open and honest in our inventory then it is a major embarrassment to us. I remember thinking to myself, isn't there an easier way? Please! Jeremiah 6:14 puts it succinctly by stating, "You can't heal a wound by saying it's not there! They offer superficial treatments for people's mortal wounds. They give assurance of peace when there is no peace."

What happens when we admit to ourselves, others and God? James 5:16 tells us that, if we confess our sins to each other and pray for each other we will be healed. The word "admit" and "confess" mean the same thing. It means "to speak the same thing." We admit that we agree with what happened. Remember David when Nathan came to him and told him that he was guilty of murder and adultery and David's response was, "I have sinned." He was in agreement with Nathan as to what had happened.

If we confess the exact nature of our wrongs to ourselves, to God and to another human being, we become more able to accept the bad parts along with the good parts of who we really are. We move out of isolation and a distorted perception of reality and it takes us to a new level of willingness and humility. And last but not least we find forgiveness, which allows us to experience real intimacy with God and others. Our soul and our spirit can be in agreement and peace with each other.

So how do we do this? Again John Baker in *Celebrate Recovery* gives us an acronym for **CONFESS** which sets out the guidelines for the process.

C – Confess your shortcomings, resentments and sins:

God wants us to come clean. We need to admit that "what is wrong is wrong. We're guilty as charged." We need to own up to the sins we discovered in our inventory.

"He who conceals his sins does not prosper, but whoever confesses and renounces them finds mercy" (Proverbs 28:13).

O – Obey God's directions:

We confess our sins to God.

"As surely as I am the living God, says the Lord, everyone will kneel before me, and everyone will confess that I am God, 'Every one of us, then, will have to give an account of himself to God" (Romans 14:11-12).

"Therefore confess your sins to each other and pray for each other so that you may be healed" (James 5:16).

N – No more guilt:

This step begins to restore our confidence and our relationships, knowing that there is now no more condemnation for those who are in Christ Jesus. (Romans 8:1).

"All have sinned...yet now God declares us 'not guilty... if we trust in Jesus Christ, who...freely takes away our sins" (Romans 3:23-24).

F – Face the truth:

Recovery requires honesty! After we complete this principle we can allow the light of God's truth to heal our hurts, hang-ups, and habits. We stop denying our true feelings.

"Jesus... said, 'I am the light of the world. Whoever follows me will never walk in darkness, but will have the light of life" (John 8:12).

E – Ease the pain:

As I stated already "We are only as sick as our secrets!" When we share our deepest secrets we divide the pain and shame. We begin to see a healthy self-worth develop, one that is no longer based on the world's standards, but on those of Jesus Christ.

"There was a time when I wouldn't admit what a sinner I was. But my dishonesty made me miserable and filled my days with frustration... My strength evaporated like water on a sunny day until I finally admitted all my sins to you and stopped trying to hide them. I said to myself, 'I will confess them to the Lord.' And you forgave me! All my guilt is gone" (Psalm 32:3-5).

S – Stop the blame:

We cannot find peace and serenity if we continue to blame ourselves or others. Our secrets have isolated us from each other. They have prevented intimacy in all our relationships.

"Why do you look at the speck of sawdust in your brother's eye and fail to notice the plank in your own? How can you say to your brother, 'Let me get the speck out of your eye,' when there is a plank in your own? ...Take the plank out of your own eye first, and then you can see clearly enough to remove your brother's speck of dust" (Matthew 7:3).

S- Start accepting God's forgiveness:

Once we accept God's forgiveness we can look others in the eye. We understand ourselves and our past actions in a "new light." We are ready to find the humility to exchange our shortcomings.

"For God was in Christ, restoring the world to Himself, no longer counting men's sins against them but blotting them out" (2 Corinthians 5:19).

"But if we confess our sins, he will forgive our sins, because we can trust God to do what is right. He will cleanse us from all the wrongs we have done" (I John 1:9).

Exercise:

What are your expectations and fears surrounding Step Five?

Read Jeremiah 14:20, which of your faults is the most difficult to acknowledge? Why?

How does denial prevent you from being honest with yourself?

Read I John 1:8-9, how will completing Step Five stop you from deceiving yourself?

What is your resistance to sharing your story with another person?

What qualities do you look for when choosing a person with whom to share your Fifth Step?

Read Psalms 32:3-5, how has carrying the burden of your wrongs caused you to groan and have no strength?

Read Proverbs 28:13, as you complete Step Five, how will confessing your sins help you find mercy?

Step Six

Were entirely ready to have God remove all these defects of character.

Principle 6: Voluntarily submit to every change God wants to make in my life and humbly ask Him to remove my character defects.

Key 6: Regeneration: "I came to know that Jesus Christ is God's only provision for man's powerlessness."

Key Scripture: "Humble yourselves before the Lord, and he will lift you up." (James 4:10)

Be Attitude: "Happy are those whose greatest desire is to do what God requires" (Matthew. 5:6).

Subject: Sanctification: I will allow the Holy Spirit to show me the defects of character and areas of problem which He wants to change in my life. I will also allow Him to produce within me the "Fruit of the Spirit." I will allow Him to become "Lord of my life.

Scripture Support: I Thessalonians 5:23,24; Ephesians 4:20-24; Romans 6:11-14; Galatians 5:22,23; I Peter 1:3; Psalm 37:4-5; Philippians 3: 12-14; Romans 12:2; James 1:5-6; 2 Thessalonians 3:3

Components:

-Readiness: Is a time to overcome fear. We need readiness and willingness for God to change us. We now know the truth about ourselves, now fear must be removed.

-Defects of character: They are called many things, weaknesses, faults, shortcomings, harmful behaviors, survival skills, negative traits, etc. They must be removed and replaced with godly character. They began in childhood as a means of survival. We learned to manipulate in order to have our needs met, to lie to protect ourselves, and to hide our emotions in defense against overwhelming pain. They were a way to manage our environment, minimize our threats, and take care of ourselves.

-Willingness: We may have the best intentions, but until we are willing to act, we won't. With God's help we are entirely ready and willing to change.

Step Summary:

Step One through Five helped to steer us in the right direction as we built a foundation for ultimate surrender. In Step Six, we confront the need to change our attitudes and behaviors. We prepare to make these changes and totally alter the course of our lives.

Step Six is similar to Step Two. Both steps deal with our willingness to allow God to work through us to change our lives. Both steps acknowledge the existence of problems and require that we seek God's help in being freed from them. The fact that we "came to believe" will strengthen our capacity to be "entirely ready."

Our past has been dominated by our self-will, through which we sought to control our environment. We victimized ourselves by our self-will, rarely calling on God for help. Our life condition shows us that self-will (the soul) has never been enough to help us.

Recognizing the need for change and being willing to change are two different matters. The space between recognition and willingness to change can be filled with fear. Fear arises when we feel as though everything is our responsibility. This is often where we believe the lie that God helps those who help themselves. Remember what I shared earlier in the book, that God helps those who can't help themselves. Our ability to talk to God is an important part of Step Six. We need to communicate with him in a way that shows our humility and invites his intervention.

Sexaholics Anonymous Study Guide reminds us that:

> Step Six does not mean that we should expect all the defects to be removed as was the obsession of lust. A few of the acquired character defects may be, but with most of them we shall have to be content with patient improvement. Once we are aware of the acquired character defects (being part of our false self), then we must exercise self-discipline. This will deepen our awareness that we must ask for God's help in eliminating them.

So how do we do this John Baker in *Celebrate Recovery* gives us an acronym for **READY** which sets out the guidelines for the process.

R – Release Control:

A willingness to let God into every area of your life. He won't come in where He is not welcomed.

"Help me to do Your will, for You are my God. Lead me in good paths, for your Spirit is good" (Psalm 143:10).

E – Easy does it:

It is not a quick fix, you need to allow time for God to work in your life. This principle goes further than helping you to stop doing wrong. It goes after the very defect that causes you to sin!

"Commit everything you do to the Lord, trust Him to help you do it and He will" (Psalm 37:5).

A – Accept the change:

Seeing the need for change and allowing the change to occur are two different things. Self-will is your enemy, you need to be ready to accept God's help throughout the transition.

"So then, have your minds ready for action. Keep alert and set your hope completely on the blessing which will be given you when Jesus Christ is revealed. Be obedient to God, and do not allow your lives to be shaped by those desires you had when you were still ignorant" (I Peter 1:13-14).

D – Do replace your character defects:

You spent a lot of time with your old hang-ups, compulsions, obsessions, and habits. When God removes one, you need to replace it with something positive, such a recovery meetings, church, volunteering! If you don't, you open yourself for a negative character effect to return.

"When an evil spirit goes out of a person it travels over dry country looking for a place to rest. If it can't find one, it says to itself "I will go back to my house." So it goes back and finds the house empty... then it goes out and brings along seven other spirits even worse than itself, and they come to live there" (Matthew 12:43-45).

Y – Yield to the growth:

Your old self-doubt and low self-esteem may tell you that you are not worthy of the growth and progress that you are making in the program. Yield to the growth—it is the Holy Spirit work within you.

"The person who has been born into God's family does not make a practice of sinning, because God's life is in him; so he can't keep on sinning, for this new life has been born into him and controls him—he has been born again"(Spirit) (I John 3:9).

Exercise:

Read Philippians 3:12-14; what areas do you have to work the hardest to give up your defects?

What anxieties do you feel when considering having your character defects removed?

Identify any character defects you are not entirely ready to have removed. Explain why you are attached to them.

Read Romans 6:11-12; What character defects have caused the most pain and need to be removed first?

What inappropriate sexual behavior will you be giving up?

How will removing your lustful tendencies change your current social behavior?

What anxiety do you feel when you realize the need to tell the truth?

How will honesty improve the quality of your life?

What difficulty are you having in letting go of your preoccupation with self?

What steps have you taken to eliminate your habit of procrastination?

Step Seven

Humbly asked God to remove our shortcomings

Principle 7: Voluntarily submit to every change God wants to make in my life and humbly asked Him to remove my character defects.

Key 7: Repentance: "I made a conscious decision to turn my entire life over to the care and keeping of God."

Key Scripture: "If we confess our sins, He is faithful and just and will forgive us our sins and purify us from all unrighteousness." (I John 1:9)

Be Attitude: "Happy are those whose greatest desire is to do what God requires" (Matthew 5:6).

Scripture Support: Psalm 25:8-11; Philippians 4:6; Matthew 23:12; James. 4:6-8. Psalm 51:10-12; I Peter 5:6-7; Acts 3:19

Components: -Humility: True biblical humility implies that we see ourselves as God sees us. We can be Christ like in our humility as we place ourselves under God's control and submit to his will and plan for our lives. It is putting ourselves into proper perspective in light of his plan.

Step Summary:

Sexaholics Anonymous Study Guide states:

> The whole emphasis of Step Seven is on humility. The Step allows us to change our attitude, which permits us with humility to be instrumental in destroying the acquired false self. Humility is part of the True Inner Self (God's image in us), which allows us to move from being self-centered to being self-less. This then produces harmony with God and with other people.

So Step Seven requires surrendering our will to God so that we may receive the serenity necessary to achieve the happiness we seek. Asking God to remove our faults is a true measure of our willingness to surrender control. For those of us who have spent our lives thinking we were self-sufficient, the surrender of control can be an extremely difficult task. If we are sincerely ready to abandon these deceptions we can ask God to help us let go of your past and nurture the new life within us. Use your Step Four inventory as your Step Seven guide to prayer. This is truly the process of living out of your spirit and not your soul.

Letting go of negative behaviors, however destructive they are, may create a sense of loss and require that we allow ourselves to grieve.

This is an opportunity to rely on our love and trust in God to heal our memories, repair the damage, and restore us to wholeness.

So how do we do this John Baker in *Celebrate Recovery* gives us an acronym for **VICTORY** which sets out the guidelines for the process.

V – Voluntarily submit:

Submit to every change God wants me to make in my life and humbly ask Him to remove my shortcomings.

"Offer yourselves as a living sacrifice to God, dedicated to His service and pleasing to Him ... Let God transform you inwardly by a complete change of your mind" (Romans 12:1-2).

I – Identify character defects:

The ones you want to work on first. Go back to the wrongs, shortcomings, and sins you discovered in your inventory. Ask God to first remove those that are causing the most pain.

"In his heart a man plans his course, but the Lord determines his steps" (Proverbs 16:9).

C – Change your mind:

When you become a Christian you are a new creation—a brand new person inside; the old nature is gone (Spirit). But you have to let God (change) transform you by renewing your mind (Soul). Your responsibility is to take the action to follow God's directions for change.

"Do not conform any longer to the pattern of this world, but be transformed by the renewing of your mind. Then you will be able to test and approve what God's will is—His good, pleasing and perfect will" (Romans 12:2).

T – Turn over character defects:

You have tried to change your hurts, hang-ups, and habits by yourself and were unsuccessful. "Let go; let God."

"Humble yourselves before the Lord, and He will lift you up" (James 4:10).

O – One day at a time:

It took a long to get sick, it takes a long time to get better. Life by the yard is hard; life by the inch is a cinch." One day at a time, one moment at a time.

"So don't be anxious about tomorrow. God will take care of your tomorrow too. Live one day at a time" (Matthew 6:34).

R – Recovery is a process:

Don't look for perfection; instead rejoice in steady progress.

"And I am sure that God who began a good work within you will keep right on helping you grow in His grace until His task within you is finally finished on that day when Jesus Christ returns" (Philippians 1:6).

Y – You must choose change:

To ask for help to change your hurts, hang-ups, and habits requires humility. We need to stop trying to make the changes on our power. We need to rely on His power to change us!

"God gives strength to the humble… so give yourself humbly to God. Resist the devil and he will flee from you. And when you draw close to God, God will draw close to you" (James 4:6-8).

Exercise:

List areas in which you are discouraged about your level of progress in having your defects removes.

Read Philippians 4:6 In what ways does prayer relieve your feelings of anxiety?

List examples that indicate you are practicing humility.

What do you fear by not knowing what is ahead?

Cite examples that indicate you are focusing more on God and less on yourself?

What affirmations do you use as a part of your ongoing commitment to recovery?

Read the Serenity Prayer

God, grant me the serenity
To accept the things I cannot change,
The courage to change the things I can,
And the wisdom to know the difference.
Living one day at a time,
Enjoying one moment at a time;
Accepting hardship as a pathway to peace'

Taking, as Jesus did,
This sinful world as it is,
Not as I would have it;
Trusting that You will make all things right
If I surrender to your will;
So that I may be reasonably happy in this life
And supremely happy with You forever in the next.
Amen

By Reinhold Niebuhr

List examples of your behavior that indicate you have the courage to change the things you can.

Appendix VI
Physical/Social Focus: Steps 8-9

The goal of steps 8-9 is to make peace with us as it relates to our Physical (social). These two steps are action steps and take us into guilt, conscience and reparation. As shame is externalized it becomes a feeling again. I can feel shame over some things I've done without concluding that I'm defective as a person. Shame as an emotion moves us to do something about what we have done. Shame triggers our guilt which triggers our conscience. I can then take action to repair the damage that I have done. With guilt I made a mistake and I can correct it wherever possible. These steps restore us to respectability. I become a self-responsible person with a conscience.

Step Eight

Made a list of all persons we had harmed and became willing to make amends to them all.

Principle 8: Evaluate all my relationships. Offer forgiveness to those who have hurt me and make amends for harm I've done to others, except when to do so would harm them or others.

Key 8: Review, Restore, Receive: "I got honest with God and others and experienced freedom.

Key Scripture: "Do to others as you would have them do to you." (Luke 6:31)

Be Attitude: "Happy are the peacemakers" (Matthew 5:9).

Scripture Support: Colossians 3:13; Romans 2:1; Luke 6:37; Matthew 6:12; Romans 8:31; Luke 19:8; Ephesians 4:32; Romans 15:1-3; Matthew 7:3-4; Mark 11:25

Components: -Amends is defined as repairing damages of the past. It can be a simple apology or as complex as restitution for physical or financial liability.

-Forgiveness: It is not an emotion. It is a decision. God alone can give us the grace, desire, and ability to release those who have hurt us.

Step Summary:

In Step Eight, we begin the process of releasing the need to blame others for our misfortune and accepting full responsibility for our own lives. Reviewing our Fourth Step inventory will help us determine who belongs on our list. This step will help to improve our relationships, both with ourselves and others. It invites us to leave behind our isolation and loneliness. We will develop a new openness with others.

Forgiving ourselves and others helps us overcome our resentments. God has already forgiven us for the harmful actions that separated us from him. The amends that we make are primarily for our own benefit.

Sexaholics Anonymouse Step Study Guide suggests that:

> "We do Step Eight to deepen our awareness of the acquired personality traits that led to defective relations with other human beings. This awareness should then spur us on to become willing to make amends to all persons that we had harmed."

The three areas of making amends are material wrongs, moral wrongs and spiritual wrongs.

Again John Baker in *Celebrate Recovery* gives us an acronym for **AMENDS** which sets out the guidelines for the process.

A – Admit the hurt and the harm:

You need to once again face the hurts, resentments, and wrongs others have caused you, or wrongs that you have caused others. Holding on to resentments not only blocks your recovery but blocks God's forgiveness in your life.

"Do not judge others, and God will not judge you; do not condemn others, and God will not condemn you; forgive others, and God will forgive you" (Luke 6:37).

We need to forgive others so Satan cannot take advantage of us (2 Corinthians 2:10, 11). We are commanded to get rid of all bitterness in our lives and forgive others as we have been forgiven (Ephesians 4:31, 32). In winning our spiritual battles we need to understand that this is foundational.

One of the best explanations I have come across is from Neil Anderson in his third step to "Freedom in Christ," entitled "Bitterness vs. Forgiveness."

> "He states that forgiveness is not merely forgetting. People who want to forget all that was done to them will find they cannot do it. Don't put off forgiving those who have hurt you, hoping the pain will one day go away. Once you choose to forgive then healing will begin to come into your lives.
>
> Forgiveness is a choice, a decision of your will. Since God requires you to forgive, it is something we can do. Sometimes it is very hard to forgive someone because we naturally want revenge for the things we have suffered. Forgiveness seems to go against our sense of what is right and fair. So we hold on to our anger, punishing people over and over again in our minds for the pain they've caused us.
>
> But we are told by God never to take our own revenge (Romans 12:19). Let God deal with the person. Let

him or her off your hook, because as long as you refuse to forgive someone, you are still hooked to that person. You are still chained to your past, bound up in your bitterness. By forgiving, you let the other person off your hook; but he or she is not off God's hook. You must trust that God will deal with the person justly and fairly, something you simply cannot do. "But you don't know how much this person hurt me!" you say. You're right. We don't, but Jesus does, and He tells you to forgive others for your sake. Until you let go of your anger and hatred, the person is still hurting you. You can't turn back the clock and change the past, but you can be free from it. You can stop the pain; but there is only one way to do it—forgive from your heart. Forgive others for your sake so you can be free from your past."

Forgiveness is agreeing to live with the consequences of another's sin. You are going to live with those consequences whether you like it or not, so the only choice you have is whether you will do so in the bondage of bitterness or in the freedom of forgiveness. This can seem unfair, and you may wonder, "where is the justice?" The Cross makes forgiveness legally and morally right.

Consider Jesus took the eternal consequences of sin upon Himself. God "made Him who know no sin to be sin on our behalf, that we might become the righteousness of God in Him" (2 Corinthians 5:21). We, however, often suffer the temporary consequences of other people's sins. That is simply a harsh reality of life all of us have to face. Do not wait for the person to ask for your forgiveness. Remember what Jesus said, "Father, forgive them, for they do not know what they are doing" (Luke 23:34)

Forgiveness comes from the heart. Allow God to bring the painful memories to the surface, and then acknowledge how you feel toward those who've hurt you. If your forgiveness doesn't touch the emotional core of your life, it will be incomplete. Too often we're afraid of the pain, so we bury our emotions deep down inside of us. Let God bring them to the surface so He can begin to heal those damaged emotions.

Forgiveness is choosing not to hold someone's sin against him or her anymore. It is common for bitter people to bring up past issues with those who have hurt them. They want the other people to feel as badly as they do! But we must let go of the past and choose to reject any thought of revenge. This doesn't mean you continue to put up with the future sin of others. God doesn't tolerate sin and neither should you. Don't allow yourself to be abused by others. Take a stand against sin while continuing to exercise grace and forgiveness toward those who hurt you.

Forgiveness cannot wait until you feel like forgiving. You will never get there. Once you make the choice to forgive, Satan will lose his power over you in that area, and God will heal your damaged emotions.

Now you are ready to forgive. Don't say, Lord, please help me to forgive." Or that "I want to forgive..." but rather say "Lord, I choose to forgive..."

M – Make a list:
Go back to your fourth step inventory and you see the list of people you need to forgive and a list of people you need to make amends to.
"Treat others as you want them to treat you" (Luke 6:31).

E – Encourage one another:
Speak to sponsor, friend or spouse to get an objective opinion, which will ensure that you stay on track.
"And let us consider how we may spur one another on toward love and good deeds" (Hebrews 10:24).

N – Not for them:

You need to approach these people humbly, sincerely, and willingly. Do not offer excuses or attempt to justify your actions. Focus only on your part. Don't expect anything back.

"Love your enemies and do good to them, lend and expect nothing back" (Luke 6:35).

D – Do it at the right time:

It is key at this time to prayerfully ask Jesus for His guidance and direction. It requires sound judgment.

"Each of you should look not only to your own interests, but also to the interests of others" (Philippians 2:4).

S – Start living the promises of recovery:

We will become ready to embrace God's purpose for our lives.

"If it is possible, as far as it depends on you, live at peace with everyone" (Romans 12:18).

Exercise:

Write an Amends list: (Romans 12:17-18)

Harm that I have done:

Person (Effects on Me)	**Relationship**	**My wrong doing** (Action)	**Effects on Others** (Feelings& damage)

Harm done to me:

Person (Effects on Me)	**Relationship**	**Their wrong doing** (Action)	**Effect on me** (Feelings& damage)

Have you accepted God's forgiveness? (Romans 3:22-25)

Have you forgiven yourself ? (Romans 8:1; Isaiah 1:18-19)

What hurt from the past are you still holding on to?

Do you owe God an amends? When will you give it?

Step Nine

Made a direct amends to such people where ever possible, except when to do so would injure them or others.

Principle 9: Evaluate all my relationships. Offer forgiveness to those who have hurt me and make amends for harm I've done to others, except when to do so would harm them or others.

Key 9: Revelation: I made a firm commitment to increase my knowledge of God through daily Bible Study

Key Scripture: "Therefore, if you are offering your gift at the alter and there remember that your brother has something against you, leave your gift there in front of the altar. First go and be reconciled to your brother; then come and offer your gift." (Matthew 5:23-24)

Be Attitude: "Happy are the merciful" (Matthew 5:7).

Scripture Support: Matthew 5:23-24; I John 4:20; Luke 6:35; Matthew 5:43-44; Romans 12:17-18; Romans 13:8

Components:

-Indirect Amends: Non personal may include those who are deceased, location unknown, etc.

-Amends to self by writing a letter to yourself and then read it out loud to yourself in front of a mirror.

Step Summary:

Step Nine is similar to the repairs and rebuilding that take place after a disaster. Through the process of making amends, we begin to mend the damage of our past. In Step Eight we surveyed the damage and made a plan. Now, in step Nine we go into action.

We are ready to face our faults, to admit the degree of our wrongs, and to ask for and extend forgiveness. Accepting responsibility for the harm done can be a humbling experience because it forces us to admit the effect we have had on others.

The *Sexaholics Anonymous Study Guide* states that:

> This step requires good judgment, a careful sense of timing, courage and prudence. It goes on to say that we must be sure to remember that WE CANNOT BUY

OUR PEACE OF MIND AT THE EXPENSE OF OTHERS. We must be aware when the time is right.

Some people in our lives feel bitter toward us. Others feel threatened by us and resent our changed behavior. We can pray about these people and ask that Christ's wisdom be made known to them. God gives us the discernment to consider the appropriateness of facing these people directly.

So how do we do this? John Baker in *Celebrate Recovery* gives us an acronym for **GRACE** which sets out the guidelines for the process.

G – God's gift:

Grace cannot be bought. It is a freely given gift by God to you and me.

"All need to be made right with God by his grace, which is a free gift. They need to be made free from sin through Jesus Christ" (Romans 3:24).

R – Received by our faith:

We cannot work our way into heaven. Only by professing our faith in Christ as our Savior can we experience his grace and have eternal life. It is only through our faith in Christ that we can find the strength and courage needed for us to make our amends and offer our forgiveness.

"For it is by grace you have been saved, through faith and this is not from yourself, it is the gift of God, not of works so that no one can boast" (Ephesians 2:8-9).

A – Accept by God's love:

We can love others because God first loved us, and we can also forgive others because God first forgave us.

"Let us then feel very sure that we can come before God's throne where there is grace. There we can receive mercy and grace to help us when we need it" (Hebrews 4:16).

C – Christ paid the price:

Jesus loves us so much that He died on the cross so that all our sins, all our wrongs, are forgiven. We also need to sacrifice our pride and our selfishness. We must speak the truth in love and focus on our part in making amends or offering forgiveness.

"In Christ we are set free by the blood of his death, and so we have forgiveness of sins. How rich is God's grace" (Ephesians 1:7).

E – Everlasting gift:

Once you have accepted Jesus Christ as you Lord and Savior, God's gift of grace is forever.

"And I am sure that God who began the good work within you will keep right on helping you grow in his grace until his task within you is finally finished on that day when Jesus Christ returns" (Philippians 1:6).

Exercise:

Forgiving harm I have done to Others:

I was____________(scared, overwhelmed, feeling…) when___________ happened between us. I ask your forgiveness for _____________(harm done) and for anything else I may have done in the past through my thoughts, words, or actions to cause you pain. I ask your forgiveness and assure you of my intention to change and to extend goodwill to you.

Forgiving others for harm done to me:

Lord, I choose to forgive__________________________(name the person) for_____________________ (what they did or failed to do), and I felt___________________ (share the painful feelings).

Pray, Lord,

I choose not to hold on to my resentment. I thank You for setting me free from the bondage of my bitterness. I relinquish my right to seek revenge and ask You to heal my damaged emotions. I now ask You to bless those who have hurt me. In Jesus' name, amen.

Forgiving myself:

I was ________ (scared, overwhelmed, feeling….) when_______ (harm done) and anything else I may have done in the past through my thoughts, words, or actions to cause myself harm.

Appendix VII
Steps 10-12

Step Ten

These last steps are a maintenance step. It asks us to continue to be in touch with the healthy feeling of shame. Such a feeling tells us we are limited, finite and human. It tells us that we will make mistakes and that it is healthy to acknowledge them. It reminds us that we have accepted our humanness and our limitations. We can stop playing God. Our wills are restored.

Continued to take personal inventory and when we were wrong promptly admitted it.

Principle 10: Reserve a daily time with God for self-examination, Bible reading, and prayer in order to know God and His will for my life and to gain the power to follow His will.

Key 10: Relationship: I made a firm commitment to increase my knowledge of God through daily Bible Study.

Key Scripture: "So if you think you are standing firm, be careful that you don't fall!" (I Corinthians 10:12)

Scripture Support: Romans 12:3; I Timothy 1:19; Psalm 26:2; Proverbs 27:12; I Timothy 4:16; I Corinthians 10:12; Matthew 5:25; Proverbs 14:30

Components:

-Personal Inventory: It is much more like a moral inventory, and personally reminds us that it is about us and not others.

-Spot check Inventory: We monitor throughout the day.

Step Summary:

In Step Ten, we begin the maintenance part of the steps. This journey requires that we continue to rely on God's Holy Spirit and the inspiration of His Word. Our success can be maintained only if we are willing to depend upon God and practice the principles of the steps daily for the rest of our lives.

In Step Ten, we consciously examine our daily conduct and confess our wrongs where necessary. We look at ourselves, see our errors, promptly admit them, and seek God's guidance in correcting them. We must be careful not to judge ourselves too harshly. It examines our strengths and weaknesses, motives and behaviors. It should not be time consuming and should be around 15 minutes. We are looking for signs that we are returning to our old ways and slipping into stinking thinking. Maintaining our honesty and humility allows us to continue to develop. Our personal inventory helps us to discover who we are, what we are, and where we are going. It helps us to become more focused and better prepared to live the Christian life we desire.

The *Sexaholics Study Guide* states:

> This practice will become easier as we become aware that all people, including ourselves, are to some extent emotionally ill as well as frequently wrong. The false self will resist admitting its wrongs. The only way to decrease the control of the false self and ego (what I call Edging God Out) is by continually admitting the wrongs done.

So how do we do this? Again John Baker in *Celebrate Recovery* gives us some simple guidelines for the process.

O – Ongoing: Do it periodically through the day.

D – Daily: At the end of the day write in a journal and the next day promptly admit mistakes and make amends.

P – Periodic: Every 90 days go on a little retreat and read and pray through your journal.

Exercise:

What do the following steps mean to you? Proverbs 16:23; Ephesians 4:29: Proverbs 16:21; 12:25; I Corinthians 13:1; Mark 14:38

What are the recurring events or issues that you are constantly needing to make amends for?

Step Eleven

Sought through prayer and meditation to improve our conscious contact with God, as we understood God, praying only for knowledge of God's will for us and the power to carry that out

Principle 11: Reserve a daily time with God for self-examination, Bible Reading, and prayer in order to know God and His will for my life and to gain the power to follow His will.

Key 11: Renewal: "As a result of these commitments I have begun a new adventure in victorious living, walking by faith, not by sight."

Key Scripture: "Let the word of Christ dwell in you richly. (Colossians 3:16)

Scripture Support: 2 Timothy 3:16; Ephesians 4:23; Job 37:14; Isaiah 30:21; Psalm 1:1-2; I Peter 1:13-14; Proverbs 4:26-27; Mark 14:38; Romans 12:2; Colossians 3:10; James 1:5

Components:

-Prayer: Conversation with someone who loves us very much

-Meditation: Increases insight into scriptures, it is a way to listen to God

-Conscious Contact: Practicing the presence of God

-God's Will: Pray for the knowledge of God's will and the power to carry that out.

Step Summary:

Step 11 is a tool that helps us trust God more fully and sustain the progress we have made in the earlier steps. It helps us to become more sensitive and responsive to God's guidance. When properly done, this process will calm us emotionally and relax us physically. We will release the energy we normally expend keeping our emotions in high gear and our bodies tense with anxiety.

Praying only for knowledge of God's will for us and the power to carry it out helps us set aside our self-serving motives and interact well with others. If we are progressing satisfactorily with Step Eleven we will see signs along the way. We will feel more at peace in our daily affairs. We will experience deep gratitude for our ongoing healing. We will feel as though we have finally achieved a rightful place in the world. Feelings of self-worth will replace feelings of shame.

So how do we do this? John Baker in *Celebrate Recovery* gives us his version of the "B" attitudes.

"B" Attitudes which sets out the guidelines for the process.

Be thankful to God

"Let us give thanks to the Lord for His unfailing love and wonderful deeds for men" (Psalms 107:15).

Be thankful for others

"Let the peace of Christ keep you in tune with each other, in step with each other. None of this going off and doing your own thing. And cultivate thankfulness. Let the word of Christ have the run of the house" (Colossians 3:15-16).

Be thankful for your recovery

"As for us, we have this large crowd of witnesses around us. So then, let us rid ourselves of everything that gets in the way, and the sin which holds on to us tightly, and let us run with determination the race that lies before us" (Hebrews 12:1).

Exercise:

Why do you think it is important for you to maintain an "attitude of gratitude" in your recovery?

How does meditating improve your conscious contact with God?

Cite a recent situation in which you were under pressure and took control away from God.

How does your communication with God reduce your anxiety?

Step Twelve

Having had a spiritual awakening as the result of these Steps, we tried to carry this message to other sex addicts and to practice these principles in all of our activities.

Principle 12: Yield myself to God to be used to bring this Good News to others, both by my example and my words.

Key 12: Resolution: "Having had a Spiritual Awakening I am strengthened by the fellowship of others who have, and am challenged to share my strength with those who have not."

Key Scripture: "Brothers, if someone is caught in a sin, you who are spiritual should restore him gently. But watch yourself, or you also may be tempted" (Galatians 6:1).

Be Attitude: "Happy are those who are persecuted because they do what God requires" (Matt. 5:10).

Scripture Support: 2 Corinthians 1:3-4; Deuteronomy 4:9; James 2:17; 2 Corinthians 3:18; Hebrews 10:24; Romans 12:13,9; Galatians 6:1; Ecclesiastes 4:9-12

Components:

-Spiritual Awakening: is a gradual change in the control of our lives. We eventually realize that we sincerely trust God and can depend on him.

-Carrying the Message: The message that we carry is that God can save us from our sin, from our self-defeating behavior, from addiction and despair and our torment. That God is able to control our lives and heal us.

Step Summary:

Our spiritual awakening is a gift that instills in us a new perspective. It is usually accompanied by a positive and significant change in our value system. Our pursuit of worldly goals has been subdued and redirected.

Carrying the message gives us an opportunity to describe the ways in which God's Spirit works through the Twelve Steps to transform our lives. Each day our life experiences remind us how we are renewed in our relationship with God. Through our sharing, we convey the message of our experience, strength, and hope.

So how do we do this John Baker in *Celebrate Recovery* gives us the Acronym **GIVE** which sets out the guidelines for the process.

G – God first:

You will realize that everything you have is a gift from Him. You realize that your recovery is not dependent on material things. It is built upon your faith and your desire to follow Christ.

"He did not even keep back His own Son, but offered him for us all! He gave us His Son—will he not also freely give us all things?" (Romans 6:24)

I – I becomes we:

The first word in Step 1 is "we." The road to recovery is not meant to be traveled alone.

"Two are better than one, because together they can work more effectively. If one of them falls down, the other can help him up. But if someone is alone… there is no one there to help him… Two men can resist an attack that would defeat one man alone" (Ecclesiastes 4:9-12).

V – Victories shared:

God never wastes a hurt! He will give us the opportunities to share our experience and victories.

"Let us give thanks to the God and Father of our Lord Jesus Christ, the merciful Father, the God from whom all help comes! He helps us in all our troubles, so that we are able to help those who have troubles, using the same help that we ourselves have received from God" (2 Corinthians 1:3).

E – Example of your actions:

In James 1:22 it says we are to be "doers of the word." But to be of help to another, we are to "carry the message in all our affairs."

"My children, our love should not be just words and talk; it must be true love, which shows itself in action" (I John 3:18).

"No one lights a lamp and then covers it with a wash tub or shoves it under the bed. No, you set it up on a lamp stand so those who enter the room can see their way...We're not hiding things; we're bringing everything out into the open. So be careful that you don't become misers...Generosity begets generosity. Stinginess impoverishes" (Luke 8: 16-18).

John Baker gives us a second Acronym **YES** which further sets out the guidelines for the process and brings a conclusion to the 12 Steps.

Y – Yield myself to God:

To bring this good news to others, both by example and by word.

"If a Christian is overcome by some sin, humbly help him back onto the right path, remembering that the next time it might be one of you who is in the wrong. Share each other's troubles and problems, and so obey our Lord's command" (Galatians 6:1-2).

E – Your walk needs to match your talk because your lifestyle reflects what you believe. Does it reflect selfishness, pride, and lust—or does it reflect the love, humility, and service of Christ?

"Let us not love with words or tongue but with actions and in truth" (I John 3:18).

S- Serve others as Jesus Christ did:

You are ready to pick up the "Lord's towel."

"And since I, the Lord and Teacher, have washed your feet, you ought to wash each other's feet. I have given you an example to follow: do as I have done to you" (John 13:14-15).

Exercise:

What does Matthew 10:8 "Freely you have received, freely give" mean to you?

Ecclesiastes 4:9 tells us that "two are better than one." List specific instances in your own recovery that you have seen this verse in action.

What are some of recent victories that you could share with others.

In James 1:22 we are told to be "doers of the Word." How can you be a doer of the Word?

What are some ways you can pick up the Lord's towel (John 13:14-15) today and start serving others?

In the words of Step 12, how will you "practice these principles in all your affairs"?

Describe what the phrase "You can't keep it unless you give it away" means in your recovery.

Sexaholics Anonymous Study Guide concludes that:

> If we find ourselves still challenged by the lesser and more continuous problems of life, our answer is still more spiritual development. As we grow spiritually, we find that the old ideas and negative thinking associated with the False Self slowly disappear. So in order to grow, we must continue to practice the SA Principles in all our affairs.

Appendix VIII
Spiritual Work: Spiritual Battle

There is a battle:

I believe the Bible is quite clear in describing to us, not only that we are in a battle, but also what type and who is all involved in this battle. We are in a battle and we should not be "ignorant of the Enemy's devices" "in order that no advantage be taken of us by Satan; for we are not ignorant of his schemes (2 Corinthians 2:11).

Be of sober spirit, be on the alert your adversary, the devil, prowls about like a roaring lion, seeking someone to devour. But resist him, firm in your faith, knowing that the same experiences of suffering are being accomplished by your brethren who are in the world" (I Peter 5:8, 9).

"Put on the full armor of God, that you may be able to stand firm against the schemes of the devil. For our struggle is not against flesh and blood, but against the rulers, against the powers, against the world forces of this darkness, against the spiritual forces of wickedness in the heavenly places" (Ephesians 6:11, 12).

"For though we walk in the flesh, we do not war according to the flesh, for the weapons of our warfare are not of the flesh, but divinely powerful for the destruction of fortresses. We are destroying speculations and every lofty thing raised up against the knowledge of God, and we are taking every thought captive to the obedience of Christ" (2 Corinthians 10:3-5).

We must understand our enemy, his tactics, his weapons, the battle ground, and the weapons that God has given to us to fight this battle and emerge victorious through Him. "For the weapons of our warfare are not carnal, but mighty through God to the pulling down of strong holds."

Where is the battle taking place?

According to the previous passage, it occurs in our thoughts and imaginations, "bringing into captivity every thought to the obedience of Christ" (2 Corinthians 10:5), literally subjecting our thoughts to scrutiny and seeing whether they stand before God as truth.

A warning is given to us in 2 Corinthians 2:11 "in order that no advantage is taken of us by Satan; for we are not ignorant of his schemes."

Our Enemy, the devil, studies and knows us. He knows exactly where our weaknesses are and how we react to situations, and, therefore, he often defeats us and puts us in bondage. We must be proactive to defend ourselves against his schemes.

Ephesians 6:11, 12 states: "Put on the full armor of God, that you may be able to stand firm against the schemes of the devil. For our struggle is not against flesh and blood, but against the rulers, against the powers, against the world forces of this darkness, against the spiritual forces of wickedness in the heavenly places."

We can see that the Enemy is deceptive by the fact that in most cases, we aren't even aware that we are operating against the Enemy. We think that it is our own problem:

"In addition to all, taking up the shield of faith with which you will be able to extinguish all the flaming missiles of the evil one."

Satan infuses thoughts into our mind, imposes feelings into our emotions, and invokes plans for actions. Example:

David: I Chronicles 21:1

"And Satan stood up against Israel, and provoked David to number Israel." David did not know that Satan was behind him, prodding. He took for granted that this was his own idea and plan. In verse 7 of this same chapter, it says, "And God was displeased with this thing; therefore he smote Israel." The reason God was displeased was that David chose to depend upon the size of his army rather than upon God. What was the result? Verse 14 tells us, "So the Lord sent pestilence upon Israel: and there fell of Israel seventy thousand men." What a price to pay – when duped by Satan by evaluating problems through our natural understanding!

Job:

The devil destroyed everything Job had, inflicted sickness upon him, accused him of sinning and tried to discourage him through his wife.

Peter: Mark 8:31-33

"And he began to teach them, that the Son of man must suffer many things, and be rejected of the elders, and of the chief priests, and scribes, and be killed, and after three days rise again. And He was stating the matter plainly. And Peter took Him aside and began to rebuke Him. But turning around and seeing His disciples, He rebuked Peter, and said, "Get behind Me, Satan: for you are not setting your mind on God's interests, but man's."

As I shared in the book, Satan spoke through Peter to rebuke Jesus. Peter was unaware that it was Satan speaking through him; he thought this was his own thought, yet Jesus recognized where it came from and therefore said. "*Get behind me, Satan.*"

Jesus: Luke 4:1-13

Satan attempted to dissuade Jesus from fulfilling God's purpose. He pretended to be sympathetic toward Jesus' physically weakened condition. He challenged Jesus to use God's power for His own purpose, to worship Satan or the things he stood for, and to tempt God to protect Him from harm, even though He would not be in God's will.

Paul: 2 Corinthians 12:7-10

"And because of the surpassing greatness of the revelations, for this reason, to keep me from exalting myself, there was given me a thorn in the flesh, a messenger of Satan to buffet me—to keep me from exalting myself!"

It was a messenger of Satan that buffeted Paul.

Stealing the Word: Mark 4:15

"And these are the ones who are beside the road where the Word is sown; and when they hear, immediately Satan comes and takes away the word which has been sown in them."

Judas: Luke 22:3-6

"And Satan entered into Judas..."

Saul: I Sam 18:9-11

"An evil spirit came upon Saul"

These examples from Scripture clearly indicate that the devil is out to kill, steal, and destroy. He uses the same tactics today.

Paul is making us aware that the enemy is a real foe today, as he was in the time of Jesus.

Jesus first sermon according to Luke 4:18-19 was purposed to heal the broken hearted, set the captives free, and to set at liberty those who were bruised.

"The Spirit of the Lord is upon me, because He anointed me to preach the gospel to the poor. He has sent me to proclaim release to the captives, and recovery of sight to the blind, to set free those who are downtrodden, to proclaim the favorable year of the Lord."

Jesus wants people to be free. "If therefore the Son shall make you free, you shall be free indeed" (John 8:36).

If you believe

"And when they came back to the disciples, they saw a large crowd around them, and some scribes arguing with them. And immediately, when the entire crowd saw Him, they were amazed, and began running up to greet Him. And He asked them, "What are you discussing with them?" And one of the crowds answered Him, "Teacher, I brought You my son, possessed with a spirit which makes him mute; and whenever it seizes him, it dashes him to the ground and he foams at the mouth, and grinds his teeth, and stiffens out, and they could not do it." And He answered them and said, "O unbelieving generation, how long shall I be with you?" How long shall I put up with you? Bring him to Me!" And they brought the boy to Him, and when he saw Him, immediately the spirit threw him into a convulsion, and falling to the ground, he began rolling about and foaming at the mouth. And He asked his father, "How long has this been happening to him?" And he said, "From childhood. And it has often thrown him both into the fire and into the water to destroy him. But if you can do anything take pity on us and help us!" And Jesus said to him, "If you can!" All things are possible to him who believes." Immediately the boy's father cried out and began saying, "I do believe; help my unbelief." And when Jesus saw that a crowd was rapidly gathering, He rebuked the unclean spirit, saying to it, "You deaf and dumb spirit, I command you, come out of him and do not enter him again." And after crying out and throwing him into terrible convulsions, it came out; and the boy became so much like a corpse that most of them said, "He is dead!" But Jesus took him by the hand and raised him; and he got up. And when He had come into the house, His disciples began questioning Him privately, "Why could we not cast it out?" And He said to them, "This kind cannot come out by anything but prayer" (Mark 9:14-29).

Jesus expects us to believe not only in the reality of demons, but also that God wants to set us free from them. He does not want us to co-exist with them or be fooled into believing that they are part of us. All things are possible to him who believes" (vs. 23). The fathers response was, "I believe but help my unbelief." If we have a hard time believing the reality of demons in everyday life, or if we struggle in believing that we can walk in victory and be more than conquerors, then we need to say as this father did. "Lord, I choose to believe, give me the faith that I lack!"

We are told to search the Scriptures to find the truth.

"Be diligent to present yourself approved to God as a workman who does not need to be ashamed, handling accurately the word of truth" (2 Timothy 2:15).

What does the Bible say when you are in need of:

Courage: Psalm 27:14; 30:5; 118:17; Isaiah 43:2; I Peter 4:12, 13; Romans 8: 25, 38, 39; Isaiah 41:10; 51:11; Philippians 4: 6, 8, 13; Psalm 31:24

Patience: Galatians 5:22; Isaiah 40:31; Psalm 27:14; Lamentations3:26; Romans 8:25; Hebrews 6:12; 10 35-37; 12:1; Ecclesiastes 7:8,9; Romans 15:4, 5; Psalm 37: 7-9; Psalm 40:1; Romans 5:3-5; James 1: 3,4; 5:7, 8

Peace: Isaiah 26: 3, 12; 55:12; 57:2; John 14:27; Philippians 4: 6, 7; Romans 5:1; Psalm 37:37; 119:165; 37:11; Romans 8:6; 14: 17-19; 15:13

In Doubt of God: Mark 11: 22-24; Luke 12: 29-31; Romans 4: 20,21; Isaiah 46: 10b, 11b; I Thessalonians 5:24; 2 Peter 3:9; Psalm 18: 30; Isaiah 59:1; I Peter 4: 12, 13; Romans 10: 17; Isaiah 55: 10, 11

Need Confidence: Philippians 4:13; Hebrews 13:6; 10: 35, 36; Philippians 1: 6; Habakkuk 3: 19; Romans 8:37; I John 5: 14, 15; John 14: 12; Zechariah 4: 6; Isaiah 43: 2; Proverbs 3: 26; 2 Corinthians 7:16; Ephesians 3: 12; I John 3: 21; Isaiah 40: 31

When Troubles Hit Your Life: Nahum 1:7; 2 Corinthians 4: 8,9; Psalm 138: 7; John 14: 1; Isaiah 43: 2; Romans 8: 28; Psalm 31: 7; 121:1, 2; Hebrews 4: 15, 16; I Peter 5:7; Matthew 6: 34; 2 Corinthians 1: 3, 4; Philippians 4: 6, 7; Isaiah 51:11

Financial Trouble: Psalm 34: 10; 23:1; Deuteronomy 28: 2-8; 11-13; Luke 6: 38; Matthew 10:8; 2 Corinthians 9: 6-8; Matthew 19:29; Joshua 1:8; Ecclesiastes 2: 26; Matthew 6: 31-33; Philippians 4:19

Marital Problems: Ephesians 4: 31, 32; Genesis 2:24; Ephesians 5: 21-33; I Peter 3: 1-7; Joshua 24: 15; Psalm 101: 2; I Peter 3: 8-11; Proverbs 3: 5,6; Proverbs 10:12; I Peter 1: 22

Deserted by Loved Ones: Psalm 9:10; Psalm 94: 14; 27: 10; 91: 14, 15; 37: 25; Matthew 28:20; Isaiah 62:4 41: 17; 2 Corinthians 4:9; I Peter 5: 7; Deuteronomy 4: 31; Isaiah 49: 15, 16; Deuteronomy 3: 16; I Samuel 12: 22

You Do Not Understand God's Ways: Isaiah 55: 8, 9; 41: 10; Jeremiah 33:3; 32:40; Romans 8:28, 31, 35-37; Psalm 34:19; 18:30; 138:8; Hosea 6:3; Hebrews 10:23; I Peter 4:12, 13

Waiting On God: Psalm 27:14; 33:20; 130:4; 62: 5; 145:15, 16; Isaiah 40:31; 25:9; Habakkuk 2:3; Hebrews 10:23; 3:14

Guidance for your Life: Psalm 119:105; Proverbs 6:22, 23; Psalm 119:11, 24; 37:23; 23:3; John 8:31, 32; Isaiah 30:21; Luke 1:70, 79; Joshua 1:8; 2 Timothy 3:16, 17

Strength: Daniel 10:19; Isaiah 30:15; Ephesians 3:16, 17; Colossians 1:10-12; Isaiah 40:31; Nehemiah 8:10; Philippians 4:13; Isaiah 41:10, 29; Proverbs 8:14; Psalm 18:2; 27:1; Ephesians 6:10

Sufficiency: 2 Corinthians 9:8; Philippians 4:19; Mark 11:24; 2 Corinthians 3:5; Philippians 4:13; Ephesians 1:19; 2 Corinthians 12:9; Romans 8:37; Ephesians 1:3; John 15:7; John 15:7; John14:13; John 16:23, 24; Matthew 21:22; 2 Peter 1:3, 4 Psalm 103:2-4

What the Bible has to say about:

Love: I John 4:7, 8; I Corinthians 13:1-8a, 13; I John 4:10-12; John 15:9, 10; 14:21; 15:12-14, 17; 3:16; 13: 34, 35; Mark 12:30, 31, 33; I John 4:16, 21; Jeremiah 31:3; Romans 5:8; 8:38, 39

Obedience: Deuteronomy 5:1, 32, 33; 11:26-28; I Samuel 15:22; Isaiah 48:18; Jeremiah 7:23; John 14: 15, 21; Acts 5:29; I John 2:3-6; I Kings 3:14; Psalm 143:10; Colossians 3: 22-24; I Peter 2: 13-20; Ephesians 6:1; Colossians 3:20-24

The Carnal Mind: Romans 8:6-8; Galatians 6:8; James 4:4; Proverbs 14:12; Philippians 3:18, 19; I Timothy 5:6; 2 Timothy 2:4, 22; 3:2-7; I Peter 2:11; I John 2:15-17; Romans 12:1, 2; Philippians 2:5; 4:8; Isaiah 26:3; Colossians 3:2, 5

The Holy Spirit: I Corinthians 6:19; Romans 5:5; John 14:16, 17; 16:7, 13; 7:38, 39; Matthew 3:11; Luke 11:13; Joes 2:28; Acts 1:4, 5, 8; 2:4; 2:38; 4:31; 8:14-17; 10:44-46a; 19:2-6

God's Faithfulness: Psalm 119:65; 36:5; 89:1, 2, 33, 34; I Thessalonians 5:24; Genesis 9:16; 28:15; Deuteronomy 7:8, 9; Joshua 23:14; I Kings 8:56; I Corinthians 1:9; 10:13; 2 Peter 3:9; 2 Timothy 2:13, 19

The Bible, Infallible Authority: 2 Timothy 3:16; 2 Peter 1:20, 21; Hebrews 4:12; Isaiah 55:10, 11; John 5:39; I Peter 1:23; Psalm 33:9; 119:89; 33:6; Proverbs 30:5; 2 Corinthians 1:20; I Peter 1:24, 25; Mark 13:31

Forgiving Others: Matthew 6:14, 15; 18:21, 22; Luke 17:3; Mark 11:25; Colossians 3:13; Philippians 3: 13, 14; Isaiah 43:18, 19; I Peter 2:19-23; Matthew 5: 10-12; Hebrews 10:30; I Peter 4:12-14; Romans 12:21; I Peter 3:9, 10; Ephesians 4:31, 32

Appendix IX
Soul Work: Truth Telling

As I started out by saying in Chapter 11 under the subject of the soul, our brains like a computer have recorded every experience we have ever had. These impressions have a lasting impact on our physical and psychological being. Because of the trauma, lies, fears, and false belief about ourselves it has affected how we see God, and has affected our temperaments and altered our personalities. It takes time to renew our minds, and to replace the lies we have believed with the truth of God's Word. Until we identify our lies and replace them with the truth, emotional well-being is impossible. One of the ways that we are able to do that is by what is formally called cognitive restructuring; God's Word would call it "renewing your mind."

What we tell ourselves can be either truth or a lie. Proverbs reads, "As a man thinks in his heart, so is he." What we too often fail to recognize is the connection between our feelings, or thoughts, and the ongoing internal monologue we carry on with ourselves at all times. This internal monologue –our self-talk—is the way we interpret events, emotions, and circumstances.

The words and images running through our minds begin at an early age and determine our feelings and actions, our moods and habits. For many of us our self-talk can be largely misinformed and distorted, causing emotional turmoil, maladaptive behavior, relational difficulties, or may I say a sin sick soul. By never addressing the "false beliefs" that inform our self-talk, we become victims of circumstances, events, and painful emotions. This is what Backus calls the "false belief trinity;" devaluing yourself, your life and your future.

The fact is you feel the way you think; you think the way you believe. Learning to control your emotions begins when you learn to listen to your self-talk. It is not events either past or present which make us feel the way we feel, but our interpretation of those events. If you believe something, you'll act as though you believe it. That is why your beliefs are the most important factors of your mental and emotional health (Soul Health).

False beliefs generally appear as truth to the person repeating them to themselves. They might even seem to be true to an untrained counselor. That is partly because they often do contain some shred of truth, and partly because the sufferer has never examined or questioned these erroneous assumptions.

Before I go on any further, perhaps I need to define these two pivotal terms, lies and truth. I now have made reference to this several times in the book, but I want to punctuate the point because it is paramount that we understand it. Simply put, lies are beliefs, attitudes, or expectations that don't fit reality. And we don't have to go out looking for them. They come to us. We learn our lies from a variety of sources—our parents, our friends, the culture we live in, even the church we attend—and they can make life emotionally miserable, even at times unbearable.

Some of the lies we tell ourselves we know to be lies. But some we believe have actually become the "truth" because we have practiced them for so long. These are the most dangerous lies of all because we rarely, if ever, dispute them. We don't dispute what we believe to be true.

Which leads me to the next question, what is truth? I know I have stated that "God is the Way the Truth and the Life..." and "if we know the truth it will set us free." That is objective and positional in nature, but there is also truth that is more subjective in nature but I don't want to open up a big philosophical can of worms because truth can be such a difficult thing to uncover. Facts can be twisted, even innocently, to back whatever belief or lie we want them to. Remember, not too many centuries ago, the facts known at the time suggested that the world was flat.

So what is truth? Dr. Thurman states,

> "Truth is reality as it is, not as it seems to be. Can we know the whole truth of a situation? Yes, but seeing and understanding the truth are skills that have to be learned, and as with most skills, learning them can be quite difficult and painful at times. But the more you practice, the better you get. The better you get, the healthier you become. The more you're able to see truth about yourself and life, the more you'll be able to see past your lies.
>
> He adds one important caveat about truth. He believes that certain truths, "ultimate truths" that give focus and meaning and substance to life, can only be learned through spiritual means. Truth is like an iceberg. What we can learn from day-to-day experiences is just the tip of the truth that we can learn on our own. Knowing the deeper, spiritual truths of life that lie below life's surface requires that we depend on a greater power than ourselves.

Thomas Aquinas put it like this: "Human salvation demands the divine disclosure of truths that surpass reason." If we accept the Bible as God's Word, we have a guide. We can learn why and how to explore the Bible for truth: "All Scripture is given by inspiration of God, and is profitable for doctrine, for reproof, for correction, for instruction in righteousness, that the man of God may be complete, thoroughly equipped for every good work" (2 Timothy 3:16-17). Timothy goes on to say that if we are "diligent workman…we can accurately divide (teach) the Word of truth."(2 Timothy 2:15).

So as we consider the way we interpret events, emotions, and circumstances in our lives it is important that we become cognisant of our internal dialogue known as self-talk. Those words we tell ourselves in our thoughts. The words we tell ourselves about people, self, experiences, life in general, God, the future, the past, the present; it is specifically, all of the words you say to yourself all the time. By never addressing the lies we have come to believe, those distorted perceptions of truth "false beliefs" that inform our self-talk, we become victims of circumstances, events, and painful emotions.

As addicts, identifying our old self-talk and clearing away long-held false beliefs may be difficult initially; you have to "unlearn" attitudes and ways of thinking that are deeply entrenched. William Backus in his book *Telling Yourself the Truth* calls it "emotional remodeling." He states that it involves five steps.

> "Firstly, identify what needs to be changed. Secondly, use a blueprint or design for the remodeling. Thirdly, assemble tools and materials necessary for the project. Fourthly, clear out the old to make way for the new and lastly, be willing to live with the inconvenience, discomfort, and adjustments of a "work in progress" while trusting that the results will be worth the effort.

The fact is the truth hurts, it is painful. Most of us don't like to hear the real truth about ourselves and will sometimes react with hurt, even anger, when we do. Also truth is sometimes painful because it forces us to give up lies that we have grown accustomed to and/or ones with which we feel secure. Giving up what makes us feel secure—even if it is miserable security—is hard.

Dr. Chris Thurman in his book *The Lies We Believe* quotes Psychiatrist Scott Peck in stating that truth is the prerequisite for health. Peck shares that,

> "Truth is reality. That which is false is unreal. The more clearly we see the reality of the world, the better equipped we are to deal with the world. The less clearly we see the reality of the world—the more our minds are befuddled by falsehood, misperceptions, and illusions—the less able we will be to determine a correct course of action and make wise decisions. Our view of reality is like a map... If the map is true and accurate, we will generally know where we are, and if we have decided where we want to go, we will generally know

> how to get there. If the map is false and inaccurate, we generally will be lost."

The following inventory is a self-analysis questionnaire to discover some of the lies that you may be living by and telling yourself.

1	2	3	4	5	6	7
Strongly Disagree			Neutral			Strongly Agree

Do not spend too much time on any one statement, but give the answer which describes how you really feel. Try to avoid using the neutral (4) response.

1.______I must be perfect.

2.______I must have everyone's love and approval

3.______It is easier to avoid problems than to face them.

4.______Things have to go my way for me to be happy.

5.______My unhappiness is externally caused.

6.______You can have it all.

7.______You are only as good as what you do.

8.______Life should be easy.

9.______Life should be fair.

10._____You shouldn't have to wait for what you want.

11._____People are basically good.

12._____My marriage problems are my spouse's fault.

13._____If my marriage takes hard work, my spouse and I must not be right for each other.

14._____My spouse should meet all my needs.

15._____My spouse owes me for what I have done for him/her.

16._____I shouldn't have to change who I am in order to make my marriage better.

17._____My spouse should be like me.

18._____I often make mountains out of molehills.

19._____I often take things personally.

20._____Things are black and white to me.

21._____I often miss the forest for the trees.

22._____The past predicts the future.

23._____I often reason things out with my feelings rather than the facts.

24._____God's love can be earned.

25._____God hates the sin and the sinner.

26._____Because I'm a Christian, God will protect me from pain and suffering.

27._____All of my problems are caused by my sins.

28._____It is my Christian duty to meet all the needs of others.

29._____Painful emotions such as anger, depression, and anxiety are signs that my faith in God is weak.

30._____God can't use me unless I am spiritually strong.

Each of the statements listed above is a lie or a way that we lie to ourselves. Go back through your responses and put a check mark by any statement that you gave a (5) (6) or (7) to. These are the lies that you tend to believe the most and want to pay the most attention to.

Taken from *The Lies We Believe* by Dr. Chris Thurman

Identifying your old self-talk and clearing away long-held false beliefs may be difficult initially; you are having to "unclean" attitudes and ways of thinking that are deeply entrenched.

The following corresponds with your Fourth Step, as they relate to your defects of character. The following inventory is taken from *Learning to tell Myself the Truth* by William Backus.

Here is a list of self-talk statements based on common false beliefs. Read them over and check those you can relate to, those which express how you think or feel. These statements may not necessarily reflect how you think and/or feel currently; if you recognize your own thoughts, past or present, in these statements, go ahead and check the statement.

Depression

1.____Things will never get better.

2.____My life isn't worth living.

3.____I have nothing to look forward to.

4.____Why bother? I'll never amount to anything anyway.

5.____I just don't have anything to live for.

6.____Nothing I do turns out right.

7.____No matter what I do, my past controls my life.

8.____The way I was raised will always determine how I feel and what I do.

9.____If I do something bad, it means I am a bad person.

10.____I can't do anything right.

11.____I feel worthless.

12.____No matter how hard I try, I feel like a failure.

13.____If my life doesn't go the way it should, I know it's my fault.

14.____When anyone else screws up, things seem to work out; anytime I screw up, it's a major disaster.

15.____When one thing goes wrong for me, everything goes wrong.

16.____If I do something wrong, it's because I am a bad Christian.

17.____I am a failure at everything that really matters.

18.____God despises people who have not lived up to His law.

19.____ I am tired of hurting, tired of trying. I don't even want to get out of bed in the morning.

20.____I can't change or control the way I feel.

Total_____

Very high score is between 16-20; Experiencing significant emotional turmoil or relational difficulty. These statements represent some of the self-talk that governs your attitudes and actions, based on your false beliefs.

High 10-15; Many of your reactions, emotions and attitudes are still grounded in false beliefs.

Moderate 5-9; Determines where you need to devote your efforts first.

Low 0-4; Indicates that this is not a pressing area of concern for you.

Sit down and write out the negative thoughts most frequently or consistently running through your internal monologue. You know them well because, when you are depressed, they stay with you almost always. You might use the examples in the checklist to help you see what you're looking for. What do you tell yourself about yourself? About your life? About your future? ____

____

____

____

Check your painful automatic thoughts to find any of these words like, always, never, must, have to , need, should, ought, at all and replace them with more truthful words like, sometimes, seldom, preferred.

____

____

____

____

Write the truth statement instead of the lie. ____________________

____

____

____

____

Anxiety

1.____I can't stand it if anyone is upset with me.

2.____I worry about everything that could possibly go wrong.

3.____Whatever I do, I want to do it perfectly.

4.____If something bad happens, I should be able to handle it better than I do.

5.____When someone disapproves of me, I feel like something is wrong with me.

6.____I can hardly stand it if someone doesn't like me.

7.____I can't let myself make a mistake.

8.___When things are going OK for me, I always feel like something terrible is going to happen to me.

9.___I'd rather avoid confrontation or conflict; putting off dealing with difficulties is easier than facing them.

10.___I should avoid things that frighten me.

11.___When I see a potentially dangerous situation, I worry constantly about what might have happened.

12.___I should "let go and let God" do things instead of trying to do something myself.

13.___I'd rather avoid taking any risks.

14.___Trying to be self-disciplined is too hard for me.

15.___I shouldn't take chances.

16.___I shouldn't worry so much about my problems.

17.___God will love me as long as I do the things I should.

18.___Jesus was gentle and meek, always thinking of the welfare of others; therefore, I should let others do what they wish and not be assertive about what I want or need.

19.___If I don't perform perfectly, I'm a failure.

20.___Anytime I screw up, it's a major disaster.

Total_____

High score is between 16-20 Experiencing significant emotional turmoil or relational difficulty. These statements, represent some of the self-talk that governs your attitudes and actions, based on your false beliefs.

High 10-15 Many of your reactions , emotions and attitudes are still grounded in false beliefs.

Moderate 5-9 Determine where you need to devote your efforts first.

Low 0-4 Indication that this is not a pressing area of concern for you.

What is causing you the greatest anxiety right now? ____________________

____

____

____

Is my anxiety caused primarily by a person, place, object, difficult task, inner fear? ____

____

____

____

Try to imagine you are in the anxiety-arousing situation and ask yourself what your thoughts are in that situation. Write out your thoughts about it. Don't write the thoughts you have about your anxiety itself, but about the situation that elicits the anxiety. Look for negative, threatening thoughts you find in your self-talk. ____________________

____

____

____

What do you think you might say to yourself instead? What would be more truthful? ____

____

____

____

In what ways do I avoid dealing with my inner fear? ______________

____

____

____

Anger

1.____I think I should get what I want most of the time.

2.____My family should respect and appreciate me more than they do.

3.____My spouse and children (or co-workers, relatives, etc.) should do what I want because I only have their best interests at heart.

4.____When things don't go the way I planned, I get very frustrated.

5.____Getting angry is a sin.

6.___If my husband/wife would just listen to me, things would be better.

7.___I shouldn't have to go through these unpleasant experiences.

8.___ I need to keep my anger to myself until I'm over it; a good Christian doesn't express anger, especially to family or church members.

9.___I never learned how to control my temper when I was a kid and it's too late now.

10.___I get mad because other people upset me.

Total_____

High score is between 8-10; Experiencing significant emotional turmoil or relational difficulty. These statements, represent some of the self-talk that governs your attitudes and actions, based on your false beliefs.

High 5-7; Many of your reactions , emotions and attitudes are still grounded in false beliefs.

Moderate 3-4; Determine where you need to devote your efforts first.

Low 0-2; Indication that this is not a pressing area of concern for you.

Can you identify the situations in which you get most angry? ________

____

____

____

What are the predisposing conditions that create this? ____________

____

____

____

What precautionary steps can I take to change the situation in the future? ________________________________

____

____

Perfectionism

1.____When something goes wrong, my first thought is, "Whose fault is this?"

2.____If I wasn't so successful, I don't think people would be interested in being with me.

3.____I don't think relationships should be this hard.

4.____I can hardly stand it if someone doesn't like me.

5.____There's a right way and a wrong way to do things, and I am inpatient with others when they don't do things right.

6.____I shouldn't have to go through unpleasant experiences.

7.____I can change whatever is wrong with me if I just try harder.

8.____When I feel bad it's usually because of the way other people have acted.

9.____I shouldn't have to suffer like this.

10.____If I don't live up to my own expectations, I'm a failure.

11.____I am the way I am and I can't change.

12.____I don't expect any more of others than I expect of myself.

13.____I can't stand the way some people treat others.

14.____I am usually right.

15.____If my family would treat me differently, I would be happier.

16.____I can just sit back and let things happen, since everything comes to the person who waits.

17.____I frequently put off doing something, because I know how it should be done and doing it "right" feels overwhelming.

18.____When I accepted Jesus as my Savior, I thought God would make all my difficulties better.

19.____No matter how much I get done, it's not enough.

20.____Things should be easier than this.

Total_____

Very high score is between 16-20 Experiencing significant emotional turmoil or relational difficulty. These statements, represent some of the self-talk that governs your attitudes and actions, based on your false beliefs.

High 10-15; Many of your reactions , emotions and attitudes are still grounded in false beliefs.

Moderate 5-9; Determine where you need to devote your efforts first.

Low 0-4; Indication that this is not a pressing area of concern for you.

Think about some of your past decisions or choices that turned out all right, and briefly describe the results :_________________________

____

____

____

____

Now, can you think of a few of your past choices that did not turn out as well as you had hoped, and briefly describe the results? ______________

____

____

____

____

Is it possible that even many of your past, less-than-perfect choices, ultimately had positive outcomes? If so, in what way? _____________

____

____

____

There are no norms for this inventory. You may find your self-talk tends to cluster into one or more areas of concentration, such as anxiety or depression. This survey is simply a helpful tool to clarify what areas of emotional health you will want to focus on.

Yet none of our painful emotions, erroneous self-talk, and damaging false beliefs could exist without an underlying spiritual disease. Human behavior, whether caused by inherited biochemistry, dysfunctional family systems, traumatic experiences, or economic disadvantages, has fundamental spiritual dimension. Sick or inappropriate behavior has its roots in spiritual sickness—and this is where secular psychotherapy fails.

According to the Christian faith, there is an age-old reason for human problems. The sinfulness of human nature, man's deepest spiritual disorder, involves a quarrel with God. Springing from this rift are underlying false beliefs about God and His attitude toward us which in turn lead to untruthful thoughts, thoughts that affect our feelings and behavior and create difficulties in our relationships with others. Influenced by our spiritual false beliefs, we may become convinced that God isn't there at all, and that if He is there, He doesn't care about us, or that God intends bad things for us and our troubles are His fault.

These spiritual false beliefs, and countless others, handicap our efforts to improve our mental and emotional health. Truth therapy is simply learning to incorporate the truth of God into the deepest part of your spirit and soul. I want you to understand that this is much more than just Cognitive Therapy. I believe it is based on the Word of God and the best of modern psychology. I had a client say to me that she has tried Cognitive Therapy in the past and it didn't work, but this is different because it is helping her to understand her relationship with Christ. It is key that we don't simply see it as soul work, but embracing the fundamental truths of who we are in spirit and in truth.

Read through this list and check any statement that reflects thoughts you've had:

Spiritual

1.____If God really love me, I wouldn't suffer so much hurt and pain.

2.____When I pray, nothing ever changes, so I really doubt that God cares, hears, or answers.

3.____I must be so wicked and sinful that God won't help me.

4.____Because I feel so guilty and unworthy, it must be true that God hates me.

5.____No matter how much I pray or how hard I try, it's never enough to satisfy God (or me).

6.____God has no right to tell me what to do and what not to do.

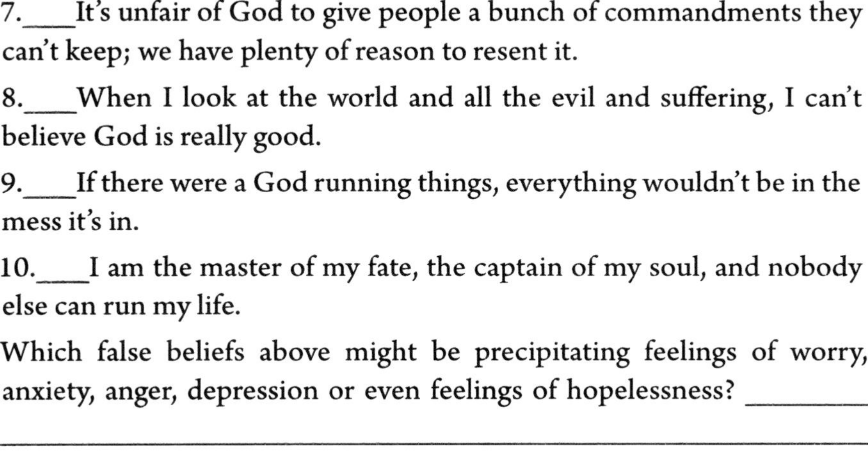

7.____It's unfair of God to give people a bunch of commandments they can't keep; we have plenty of reason to resent it.

8.____When I look at the world and all the evil and suffering, I can't believe God is really good.

9.____If there were a God running things, everything wouldn't be in the mess it's in.

10.____I am the master of my fate, the captain of my soul, and nobody else can run my life.

Which false beliefs above might be precipitating feelings of worry, anxiety, anger, depression or even feelings of hopelessness? ________

____

____

Identifying the false beliefs that prompt your self-talk is the first step to freeing yourselves from their control. Remember what Paul said, "I am confident of this, that he who began a good work in you will carry it on to completion...for it is God who works in you to will and at act according to his good purpose" (Philippians 1:6;2:13).

Now begins the practicum. When I was working on my Masters of Theology degree I remember the professor stating from the onset that he wanted this educational experience to be more than just informational but to be formational. That is my hope for you. How do we take all this information that I have written about and make it formational in your life, "so we are no longer conformed to this world (by way of attitudes and self defeating behaviors) but transformed by the renewing of our minds so we can prove what is the good, and acceptable and perfect will of God" (Romans 12:1,2).

We seldom stop to realize how our emotions affect our bodies and how integrated all of our bodily systems are with our thoughts and feelings. That has been part of my objective in writing about the Trinitarian nature of man so that we don't see our problems from a one dimensional perspective but rather understanding how our belief system affects our emotions which in turn affects our bodies.

It is paramount to our recovery and spiritual formation that we understand our emotions, internal self-talk and false beliefs. So learning to sort through our thoughts and feelings is essential in getting at our core false beliefs.

We can always find four elements in an episode of anger, anxiety, frustration, depression or other intense emotions.

Provocation: Is the event that triggers the bad feelings.
Cognitions: Which is your self-talk about the meaning of the event.
Physical reactions: The bodily changes that you experience.
Response: What you do about the situation—your
decisions, choices, actions and reactions.

Remember that this happens all very quickly and often below our conscience awareness. Our automatic thoughts spring from underlying beliefs, or more to the point, false beliefs. If examined in the light of the truth, are irrational, false and misinformed. Backus states that all too frequently we fall into the trap of "post hoc ergo propter hoc thinking, assuming that our feelings and reactions are caused by external factors—frustrating encounters, difficult relationships, past experiences, etc." In reality the cause of our emotional ups and downs comes from within us—not what happens to us, but what we tell ourselves as we interpret what's happening to us.

The exercise that you will be starting will be to integrate truthful beliefs into your self-talk, turning your self-talk into living faith. We can only do this by becoming very cognisant or consciously aware of our self-talk.

I want to use the very simple acronym that Thurman uses, TRUTH as a very practical tool to aid in the monitoring of yourself monologue. I have taken some liberty to the content of each letter. As a form of journaling take some time throughout the day or at the end of the day to record events that were emotionally defining moments in your day.

T – Trigger event:

Describe the event that "made you" feel… …. (consider biologically, physically, emotionally, spiritually)

R – Reckless or wrong thinking:

Your automatic thoughts and interpretation of the event (event being a person, place, thing, situation, or circumstance). What do you see as the past cause to this thinking and belief? Your predominant feelings and self-talk may correspond to the inventories that you did earlier in this section (i.e. Depression, Anger, Anxiety or Perfectionism, etc.) also label the distortion by using the Denial/Self-Defense Inventory. (Appendix II)

U – Unhealthy response:
Self-defeating learned behaviors, compulsive activities, sexual acting out.

T – Truthful Response:
Talk back! Indentify the lie (we directly or indirectly denied God's truth) therefore, confess the self lie, the denial, the self-defense strategies (I John 1:9), ask God to forgive you for believing the lie, thank God for the forgiveness, take authority over the enemy who is the father of lies (Luke 10:9), confess the truth in this area (John 8:32) and change to new truth-filled self-talk (Ephesians 6:10-18). Positive counterstatements and ask God to fill the released area with the Holy Spirit (Luke 11:24-26).

H – Healthy Response:
Trusting in the Lord with all your heart and leaning not on your own understanding….Thinking on those things that are true, and honorable, right, lovely and pure, anything excellent and anything worthy of praise. Bearing the fruit of the Spirit which is love, joy, peace, patience, kindness, goodness, faithfulness, gentleness and self-control.

I have made a list of Truth counterstatements to oppose the lies and false beliefs. The more we meditate on these passages the more we will be able to refute the lie. I wrote in the book, that the best way to identify the counterfeit, is not to know every counterfeit that exists but rather to know the original so well that when you see any counterfeit you will recognize it right away.

We need to know the truth in all areas of our lives, body, soul and spirit. I have made a list of truth statements that we need to meditate and reflect on and ultimately believe in if we hope for any sustained change and recovery in our lives. I will start with a list of positional truths of who we are in Christ by Neil Anderson in his workbook *Ministering the Steps to Freedom in Christ* titled statement of faith:

1. I recognize that there is only one true and living God who exists as the Father, Son and Holy Spirit. He is worthy of all honor, praise and glory as the One who made all things and holds all things together. (Exodus 20:2,3; Colossians 1:16,17).

2. I recognize that Jesus Christ is the Messiah, the Word who became flesh and dwelt among us. I believe that He came to destroy the works of the devil, and that He disarmed the rulers and authorities and made a public display of them, having triumphed over them (John 1:1,14; Colossians 2:15; I John 3:8).

3. I believe that God demonstrated His own love for me in that while I was still a sinner, Christ died for me. I believe that He has delivered me from the domain of darkness and transferred me to His kingdom, and in Him I have redemption and the forgiveness of sins (Romans 5:8; Colossians 1:1314).

4. I believe that I am now a child of God and that I am seated with Christ in the heavenlies. I believe that I was saved by the grace of God through faith, and that it was a gift and not a result of any works on my part (Ephesians 2:6,8,9; I John 3:1-3).

5. I choose to be strong in the Lord and in the strength of His might. I put no confidence in the flesh, for the weapons of warfare are not of the flesh but are divinely powerful for the destruction of strongholds. I put on the full armor of God. I resolve to stand firm in my faith and resist the evil one (2 Corinthians 10:4; Ephesians 6:10-20; Philippians 3:3).

6. I believe that apart from Christ I can do nothing, so I declare my complete dependence on Him. I choose to abide in Christ in order to bear much fruit and glorify my Father. I announce to Satan that Jesus is my Lord. I reject any and all counterfeit gifts or words of Satan in my life (John 15:5, 8; I Corinthians 12:3).

7. I believe that the truth will set me free and that Jesus is the truth. If He sets me free, I will be free indeed. I recognize that walking in the light is the only path to true fellowship with God and man. Therefore, I stand against all of Satan's deception by taking every thought captive in obedience to Christ. I declare that the Bible is the only authoritative standard for truth and life (John 8:32, 36; 14:6; 2 Corinthians 5:17; Colossians 3:9, 10).

8. I choose to present my body to God as a living and holy sacrifice, and the members of my body as instruments of righteousness. I choose to renew my mind by the living Word of God that I may prove that the will

of God is good, acceptable, and perfect. I put off the old self with its evil practices and put on the new self. I declare myself to be a new creation in Christ (Romans 6:13; 12:1, 2; 2 Corinthians 5:17; Colossians 3:9, 10).

9. By faith, I choose to be filled with the Spirit so that I can be guided into all truth. I choose to walk by the Spirit so that I will not carry out the desires of the flesh (John 16:13; Galatians 5:16; Ephesians 5:18).

10. I renounce all selfish goals and choose the ultimate goal of love. I choose to obey the two greatest commandments: to love the Lord my God with all my heart, soul, mind and strength, and to love my neighbor as myself (Deuteronomy 6:5; Matthew 22: 37-39; I Timothy 1:5).

11. I believe that the Lord Jesus has all authority in heaven and on earth, and He is the head over all rule and authority. I am complete in Him. I believe that Satan and his demons are subject to me in Christ since I am a member of Christ's body. Therefore, I obey the command to submit to God and resist the devil, and I command Satan in the name of Jesus Christ to leave my presence (Matthew 28:18; Ephesians 1:19-23; Colossians 2:10; James 4:7).

He also goes on to capture the implications of what it means to be "In Christ," as it relates to our basic need for significance and security which in essence forms our sense of self-worth.

I Am Accepted: I renounce the lie that I am rejected, unloved, dirty or shameful because in Christ I am completely accepted. God says that

John 1:12	I am God's child
John 15:15	I am Christ's friend
Romans 5:1	I have been justified
I Corinthians 6:17	I am united with the Lord, and I am one spirit with Him.
I Corinthians 6:20	I have been bought with a price. I belong to God.
Ephesians 1:1	I am a saint
Ephesians 1:5	I have been adopted as God's child.
Ephesians 2:18	I have direct access to God through the Holy Spirit
Colossians 1:14	I have been redeemed and forgiven of all my sins

Colossians 2:10	I am complete in Christ

I Am Secure: I renounce the lie that I am guilty, unprotected, alone or abandoned because in Christ I am totally secure. God says;

Romans 8:1, 2	I am free from condemnation
Romans 8:28	I am assured that all things work together for good
Romans 8:31-34	I am free from any condemning charges against me.
Romans 8:35-39	I cannot be separated from the love of God
2 Corinthians 1:2, 22	I have been established, anointed and sealed by God.
Colossians 3:3	I am hidden with Christ in God
Philippians 3:20	I am a citizen of heaven.
2 Timothy 1:7	I have not been given a spirit of fear, but of power, love, and a sound mind.
Hebrews 4:16	I can find grace and mercy to help in time of need
I John 5:18	I am born of God and the evil one cannot touch me.

I am Significant: I renounce the lie that I am worthless, inadequate, helpless or hopeless because in Christ I am deeply significant. God says;

Matthew 5:13, 14	I am the salt and light of the earth.
John 15:1, 5	I am a branch of the true vine, a channel of His life
John 15: 16	I have been chosen and appointed to bear fruit
Acts 1:8	I am a personal witness of Christ
I Corinthians 3:16	I am God's temple
2 Corinthians 5:17-21	I am a minister of reconciliation for God
2 Corinthians 6:1	I am God's co-worker

Ephesians 2:6	I am seated with Christ in the heavenly realm
Ephesians 2:10	I am God's workmanship
Ephesians 3:12	I may approach God with freedom and confidence
Philippians 4:13	I can do all things through Christ who strengthens me

I am not the great "I AM," but by the grace of God I am what I am (Exodus 3:14; John 8:24, 58; I Corinthians 15:10).

I renounce the lie that I will never be free.
I announce the truth that Christ has set me free (John 8:32).

I renounce the lie that I am a product of my past
I announce the truth that I am a product of the Cross

I renounce the lie that I can do it myself. All I have to do is try harder, get stronger and learn how to cope or deal with my addiction.
I announce that apart from Christ I can do nothing, but in Christ all things are possible (Philippians 4:13).

I renounce the lie that I need to rely on my own understanding.
I announce the truth that I need to acknowedge God (Proverbs 3:5, 6).

I renounce the lie that my Heavenly Father is distant and disinterested, insensitive and uncaring, stern or demanding, passive and cold, absent, dissatisfied with me, harsh, a killjoy, controlling and manipulating, condemning or unforgiving.

I announce the truth that my Heavenly Father is intimate and involved, kind and compassionate, accepting and loving, warm and affectionate, always with me, approving and affirming, gentle and protective of me, came to give me abundant life, full of grace and mercy and tender hearted and forgiving (I John 4:16).

I renounce the lie that what I do and have done determines who I am, a sinner and an addict.

I announce the truth that what Christ has done determines who I am and what I do. I am a saint who sins and a child of God who struggles with a sexual addiction (I John 3:1-3)

I renounce the lie that if I am the problem, I need to change who I am as a person. Or that I need to find the right program and work it.

I announce the truth that I believe the truth of who I am in Christ, my behavior will change. Knowing the truth will bring freedom but I need to acknowledge the battle is in my mind.

Twenty "cans" of success

Why should I say, "I can't" when the Bible says, "I can do all things through Christ who strengthens me" (Philippians 4:13)?

Why should my needs not be met knowing that "my God shall supply all my needs according to His riches in glory in Christ Jesus" (Philippians 4:19)?

Why should I fear when the Bible says that "God has not given me a spirit of fear, but of power and of love and of a sound mind" (2 Timothy 1:7)?

Why should I doubt or lack faith knowing that "God has allotted to each a measure of faith" (Romans 12:3)?

Why am I weak when the Bible says, "the Lord is the strength of my life" (Psalms 27:1) and "people who know their God will display strength" (Daniel 11:32)?

Why should I allow Satan to have supremacy over my life, for "greater is He who is in me than he who is in the world" (I John 4:4)?

Why should I accept defeat when the Bible says, thanks be to God, who always leads us in His triumph in Christ" (2 Corinthians 2:14)?

Why should I lack wisdom when Christ "became to us wisdom from God" (I Corinthians 1:30) and God gives wisdom to all men generously and without reproach who ask Him for it (James 1:5)?

Why should I be depressed when I can recall to my mind and therefore have hope that “the Lord’s loving kindnesses indeed never cease, for His compassions never fail. They are new every morning; great is Thy faithfulness” (Lamentations 3:22, 23)?

Why should I worry and fret when I can cast all my anxiety upon Christ, because He cares for me” (I Peter 5:7)?

Why should I ever be in bondage, for “where the Spirit of the Lord is, there is liberty” (2 Corinthians 3:17” and “it was for freedom that Christ set me free” (Galatians 5:1)?

Why should I feel condemned when the Bible says, “There is...no condemnation for those who are in Christ Jesus” (Romans 8:1)?

Why should I ever feel alone when Jesus said, “I am with you always, even to the end of the age” (Matthew 28:20) and “I will never desert you, nor will I ever forsake you” (Hebrews 13:5)?

Overcoming Emotional Traps

Select what emotional trap you are most prone too. Read the passages that correspond to the emotional traps that you selected. Write down how this truth can be applied to your life and recovery.

___Discouraged: Isaiah 51:11; I Peter 1:6-9; Philippians 4:6-8; John 14:1; John 14:27; 2 Corinthians 4:8,9; Hebrews 10:35,36; Philippians 1:6; Galatians 6:9; Psalm 31:24; Psalm 27:1-4

___Worried: I Peter 5:7; John 14:1; Philippians 4:6, 7; Colossians 3:15; Isaiah 26:3; Psalm 4:8; Philippians 4:19; Matthew 6:25-34; Romans 8:6; Proverbs 3:24; Hebrews 4:3, 9; Psalm 119:165; Psalm 91:1, 2; John 14:27

___Lonely: Hebrews 13:5; Matthew 28:20; I Samuel 12:22; Isaiah 41:10; John 14:18; John 14:1; Deuteronomy 33:27; Psalm 147:3; Romans 8:35-39; Deuteronomy 4:31 and 31:6; Psalm 27:10; Isaiah 54:10; I Peter 5:7; Psalm 46:1

___Depressed: Psalm 34:17; Isaiah 43:2; Psalm 30:5; I Peter 4:12, 13; Isaiah 61:3 and 40:31; 2 Corinthians 1:3, 4; Romans 8:38, 39; Philippians 4:8; Psalm 147:3; Isaiah 41:10; I Peter 5:6, 7; Luke 18:1; Nehemiah 8:10; Isaiah 51:11

____Dissatisfied: Psalm 34:10, 37:3, 63:1-5, 103: 1-5, 107:9; Isaiah 44:3, 12:2,3, 55:1; Philippians 4:12, 13; Jeremiah 31:14b; Joel 2:26; 2 Corinthians 9:8; Matthew 5:6

____Condemned: Romans 8:1; Psalm 103:10; 12: 2 Corinthians 5:17; John 3:17,18; John 5:24; Hebrews 8:12; Isaiah 43:25; 55:7; Psalm 32:1, 5; I John 1:9; Revelation 12:10, 11; John 8:10, 11; Jeremiah 31:34; Hebrews 10:22; 2 Chronicles 30:9

____Confused: I Corinthians 14:33; 2 Timothy 1:7; James 3:16-18; Isaiah 50:7; I Peter 4: 12, 13; James 1:5; Proverbs 3:5, 6; Psalm 32:8; Psalm 119:165; 55:22; Isaiah 43:2; 40:29; 30:21; Philippians 4:6, 7

____Tempted: I Corinthians 10:12, 13; Hebrews 4: 14-16; 2:18; 2 Peter 2:9a; Romans 6:14; Psalm 119:11; James 1:13,14; Proverbs 28:13; I John 1:9; I Peter 5:8,9; Ephesians 6: 10, 11, 16; James 4:7; I John 4:4; James 1:2,3,12; Jude 24,25a; I Peter 1:6, 7

____Anger: James 1:19, 20: Ephesians 4:26; Proverbs 15:1; Matthew 6:14; Proverbs 14:29; 16:32; Ecclesiastes 7:9; Romans 12:19-24; Proverbs 25:21, 22; Hebrews 10:30; Ephesians 4:31, 32; Matthew 5:22-24; Proverbs 14:16, 17; Colossians 3:8; Psalm 37 8

____Rebellious: Hebrews 13:17; Proverbs 14:16, 17; I Samuel 15:22, 23; I Peter 1:13, 14; Isaiah 1:19, 20; I Peter 2:13-15; Philippians 2:5-8; Hebrews 5:8; I Peter 5:5, 6; Ephesians 5:21; Proverbs 12:21; Romans 6:12, 13; Ephesians 4: 17, 18; Ephesians 5:8; James 4:7

____Fear/Anxiety: 2 Timothy 1:7; Romans 8:15; I john 4:18; Psalm 91:1, 4-7, 10, 11; Proverbs 3:25,26; Isaiah 54:14; Psalm 56:11; 23:4,5; 31:24; 27:1,3; Romans 8:29, 31, 35-39; John 14:27; Hebrews 13:6; Isaiah 41:10; 50:7; Psalm 55:22; Philippians 4: 6,7,8; Isaiah 43:2; 2 Corinthians 1:3,4; Psalm 57:1-3; Ephesians 2:8, 10, 14; 2 Thessalonians 3:5, 6; Psalm 46:1-3, 7; Psalm 13: 1-2; 121: 1-2, 7-8; 125: 1-2; Jeremiah 29"11-13;

These are all incredible spiritual truths related to our position in Christ and it is foundational to our recovery. However as I have written throughout this book, I do not want to be guilty of a one dimensional approach, but rather consider our Trinitarian nature even as we consider cognitive restructuring and renewing our minds.

The following exercises are a list of affirmations related to your character, personalities, bodies, minds and accomplishments. This is not the power of positive thinking, but rather the truth of who you are. It is not an easy exercise because your mind will want to "ya but" these statements, but stick to it. Remember practice makes better, not perfect. It can also be helpful to ask a trusted friend to offer some objectivity to some of these statements and give you some concrete examples. One rule you need to follow is, "no ya butting" when they are talking to you. The following exercises are taken from *The Anxiety & Phobia Workbook* by Edmund J. Bourne and *The Self-Esteem Workbook* from Glenn R. Schiraldi., note I have taken some liberty with the content.

What I Am

I am lovable and capable.
I fully accept and believe in myself just the way that I am, and the way God made me.
I am a unique and special person. There is no one else quite like me in the entire world.
I accept all the different parts of myself.
My feelings and needs are important.
It's O.K. to think about what I need.
It's good for me to take time for myself.
I have many good qualities.
I believe in my capabilities and value the unique talents I can offer the world.
I am a person of high integrity and sincere purpose.
I trust in my ability to succeed at my goals.
I am a valuable and important person, worthy of the respect of others.
Others perceive me as a good and likable person.
When other people really get to know me, they like me.
Other people like to be around me. They like to hear what I have to say and know what I think.
Others recognize that I have a lot of offer.
I deserve to be supported by those people who care for me.
I deserve the respect of others.
I trust and respect myself and am worthy of the respect of others.

I now receive assistance and cooperation from others
I'm optimistic about life. I look forward to and enjoy new challenges.
I know what my values are and am confident of the decisions I make.
I easily accept compliments and praise from others.
I take pride in what I've accomplished and look forward to what I intend to achieve.
I love myself just the way I am.
I don't have to be perfect to be loved
The more I love myself, the more I am able to love others.

Positive Qualities (Check off if sometimes are, or have been, reasonably)

____Clean

____Handy

____Literate

____Punctual

____Assured or self-confident

____Enthusiastic, spirited

____Humorous, or amusing

____Friendly

____Gentle

____Loyal, Committed

____Trustworthy

____Trusting, seeing the best in others

____Loving

____Strong, powerful

____Determined, Resolute, Firm,

____Patient

____Rational, Reasonable, Logical

____Intuitive or Trusting of own instincts

____Creative or Imaginative

____Compassionate, Kind, or Caring

____Disciplined

____Persuasive

____Talented Cheerful

____Sensitive, or Considerate

____Generous

____Appreciative

____Respectful, or Polite

____Responsive to beauty or nature

____Principled, Ethical

____Industrious

____Responsible, Reliable

____Organized, Orderly, or Neat

____Sharing

____Encouraging, Complimentary

____Attractive

____Well-groomed

____Physically fit

____Intelligent, perceptive

____Cooperative

____Forgiving, or able to look beyond mistakes or shortcomings

____Conciliatory

____Tranquil or Serene

____Successful

____Open-minded

____Tactful

____Spontaneous

____Flexible or Adaptable

____Energetic

____Expressive

____Affectionate

____Graceful, Dignified

____Adventurous

Good At (Words that describe you are sometimes reasonably good at)

____Socialized

____Listener

____Cook

____Athlete

____Worker, Doer

____Friend

____Musician or Singer

____Learner

____Leader or Coach

____Organizer

____Decision Maker

____Counselor

____Helper

____"Cheerleader," supporter

____Planner

____Follower

____Mistake corrector

____Pleasant Demeanor

____Debater

____Mediator

____Story Teller

____Letter Writer

____Thinker

____Administrator

____Mate

____Taker of Criticism

____Risk Taker

____Cleaner

____Entrepreneur

____Enjoy Hobbies

____Volunteer

____Giver

____Financial manager, or Budgeter

____Family Member

____Other______________________________

What I Am Learning:

____To love myself more every day

____To believe in my unique worth and capabilities

____To trust myself and others

____To recognize and take care of my needs

____That my feelings and needs are just as important as anyone else's

____To ask others for what I need

____That it is okay to say "no" to others when I need to

____To take life one day at a time

____To approach my goals one day at a time

____To take better care of myself

____To take more time for myself each day

____To let go of worry

____To let go of guilt and shame

____That others respect and like me

____To be more comfortable around others

____I am learning to take every thought captive in obedience to Christ (who He states I am)

____To be open and honest with my feelings, and trusting others

____I am learning to take risks, especially with intimacy

____I am learning to feel more confident________________(name the situation)

____I am learning to be more assertive__________________(give examples)

____I am learning to have healthy boundaries_________________(give examples)

____That it's okay to make mistakes. (no failures, just lessons)

____I am learning that I don't have to be perfect to be loved

____I am learning that I am not inadequate or inferior

____I am learning that there is hope and that I am not hopeless

____I am learning that there is help, and that I am not helpless

____I am learning that I can't change myself solely with self-help materials

____I am learning that I am not a victim of circumstance

____I am learning to accept myself just the way that I am

____I am learning that I am significant and secure

____I am learning that I am not a bad person and unworthy of love but that I am worthy person and I am loved

____I am loved just as I am

____That my needs are going to be met as I depend on God and others

____That I can live without sex

____That I can recover and be the person that God purposed me to be

____I am learning to manage stress

____I am learning to eat healthy

____I am learning the importance of regular exercise

____I am learning that depression, anxiety, anger and perfectionism are a choice

____I am learning that real power in my life is Christ in me

____I am learning to say "thanks" in all things and have an "attitude of gratitude"

____I am learning to "accept" every person, place, thing, situation and circumstance to be exactly the way it is suppose to be and what needs to change is me and my attitude.

____I am learning to walk by faith and not by sight

____I am learning to not let my feelings dictate my life but rather God's Word.

____I am learning not to lean on my own understanding, but to simply acknowledge God.

____I am learning how to meditate

____I am learning how to surrender my will and "let go and let God"

____Other things that I am learning______________________________

Now comes the tough part. Select one or two affirmations each week from each of the lists (Statement of Faith, I Am Significant, I Am Secure, I Am Accepted, I Can, What I Am, , Positive Qualities, What I Am good at, What I Am Learning) and write them down individually on 3X5 cards. Then read through the stack slowly and with feeling once or twice a day. Doing this while alternately looking at yourself in a mirror is an excellent idea. They say that your eyes are the window to your soul, however, I would suggest that it is the window to your spirit. Look at yourself in your eyes and speak these truths, you can alternate between "I am" statements and "you are" statements. You will know when it connects with your spirit, because it will connect with the emotional core of your being. You will want to turn away or feel like this is silly and stupid and believe it won't work; stick with it, you're worth it. When you use the TRUTH acronym you will want to use these positive affirmations of truth under the second letter "T" for truthful response to counter the lies under the "R."

Appendix X Soul Ties: Dysfunctional Family Systems

Profile

When we think of a DYSFUNCTIONAL FAMILY it's like a machine which is run by gears with weak or cracked cogs. As one cog breaks it puts more stress on the other cogs of that gear and then on other cogs of other gears. Eventually the whole machine shuts down. *DYSFUNCTION* means just that: unable to FUNCTION properly. Each individual in a family is like a gear and each perceived responsibility is like the cog. The main or original DYSFUNCTIONAL person may show their DYSFUNCTION in many ways: they may have difficulty coping, may yell, rage, isolate, verbally abuse, physically abuse, chemically abuse, gamble, cheat on their partner, threaten to leave, threaten suicide, give the silent treatment etc. This causes everyone to walk on eggshells and lots of CRAZY MAKING goes on.

So what constitutes dysfunctional family? I touched on it in the book, but using the acronym DYSFUNCTIONAL complete the profile. Place an "X" beside letters that would describe your family of origin. (*The Family*, Bradshaw)

D.____ Denial and Delusion—Your family denied that there was any problems. So the problems never got solved. The five freedoms were denied in your family were feelings, perceptions, thoughts, wants and imaginings, especially the negative ones like fear, loneliness, sadness, hurt, rejection and dependency needs.

Y.____ Yin/Yang Disorder—There was no intimacy in the family which has caused a vacuum.

S.____ Shame-based—Your parents internalized their shame and acted shameless towards the kids by shutting down feelings. You felt ashamed of the family.

F.____ Fixed, Frozen and Rigid Roles—Roles were created by the needs of the family as a system. If we consider an adaptability scale, low would be inflexible or Rigid is high and overly flexible which is enmeshed with no boundaries. The middle would be flexible and most adaptable.

The grown-ups or parent figures assume two roles: Dysfunctional person and the other plays the enabler. You decide which applies to your situation. In some cases the mother may be the dysfunctional person and father the enabler and vise versa in other cases. Both roles play off each other. The dysfunctional person is trapped in self delusion. They actually believe that they are justified in what they do and how they act. They have very distorted thinking. They seem to find ways to strengthen their own credibility and weaken everyone else's in the family. Therefore, if anyone were to tell someone outside the family who the dysfunctional person really was, many people would not really believe them because of the way they present themselves to the public.

The enabler also has distorted thinking and believes that they are basically responsible for the other person's dysfunction. And they are therefore very fixated on the other person and often times appear to be uncaring or neglectful toward their children. But this person has only so much energy to go around and most of it goes toward the "squeakiest wheel," the dysfunctional person.

The children in the family may play more than one role at a time or only one. Each role gives the child their basic identity and shapes their script and future. The role also gives them their sense of worth and value. So they too get trapped in their roles and also develop distorted thought patterning. This is how the tapes, to be carried through life, about who we are and who we will become, begin to develop. Each role carries some aspect about the DYSFUNCTION of the whole family.

The following are roles of the typical behaviors of children from dysfunctional families. Put an "X" beside the one that would best describe you in your family of origin.

_____The Dysfunctional Person/Addict

- other family members revolve around this person
- likely to be experiencing quite a bit of pain and shame even though they may not see it as the result of addiction
- as things get worse, the addict is faced with increasing feelings of shame, guilt, inadequacy, fear, and loneliness
- develop a number of defenses to hide their shame and guilt - may include irrational anger, charm, rigidity, grandiosity, perfectionism, social withdrawal, hostility, and depression
- project blame or responsibility for their problems onto others including family members who take on unhealthy roles in order to survive.

_____Codependent/Enabler/Caretaker

-Phlegmatics are prone to this role
- steps up and takes control if the addict loses power
- enabling is anything that protects the dependent person from the consequences of their actions
- spouse often takes on the role, but children and siblings can also be enablers
- tends to everyone's needs in the family
- loses sense of self in tasks of a domestic nature
- never takes the time to assess his/her own needs and feelings
- person never gains what they need most in order to get better: insight
- as long as the enabler and the dependent family members play their

game of mutual self-deception, things never get better - they get worse

- others cannot bond with the caretaker due to the bustle of activity

Caretaker's purpose: to maintain appropriate appearances to the outside world.

_____Hero

-Melancholics and Choleric personality would be prone to this role
- high achiever; takes focus off the addict because of his/her success; perfectionist; feels inadequate; compulsive; can become a workaholic
- addict bestows this role onto the individual whose accomplishments compensate for the addictive behavior
- often the oldest child who may see more of the family's situation and feels responsible for fixing the family pain
- child excels in academics, athletics, music or theatre
- gets self worth from being "special"
- rest of family also gets self worth ("we can't be that bad if one of us is successful")
- hero does not receive attention for anything besides an achievement; therefore, inner needs are not met
- he/she loses the ability to feel satisfied by whatever feat he/she has manifested
- as things get worse, the hero is driven to higher and higher levels of achievement. No level of super responsible, perfectionist, over achievement can remove the hero's internalized feelings of inadequacy, pain, and confusion
- many others grow up to become workaholics and live under constant stress as they work in the service of others seeking approval for their extraordinary effort
- they often end up distancing themselves from their family of origin
- interestingly, many family heroes grow to marry addicts and become enablers

Hero's purpose: to raise the esteem of the family.

_____Scrapegoat

-Choleric personality would be prone to this role.
- goes against rules; acts out to take the focus off the addict; feels hurt & guilt; because of behavior, can bring help to family
- lightening rod for family pain and stress
- direct message is that they are responsible for the family's chaos
- family assigns all ills to the person who harbors this role, e.g. "Mom would not drink so much if (Scapegoat's name) were not always in trouble."
- in reality the misbehavior of the Scapegoat serves to distract and provide some relief from the stress of the dependency
- child has issues with authority figures as well as negative consequences with the law, school and home
- on the inside the child is a mass of frozen feelings of anger and pain
- may show self-pity, strong identification with peer values, defiance, and hostility or even suicidal gestures
- this role may seem strange in purpose. However, if there were no scapegoat, all other roles would dismantle. He/she allows others a pretense of control
- The scapegoat is identified as 'The Problem.'
Scrapegoat's purpose: puts the focus away from addict thereby allowing the addict to continue to use.

_____Mascot/Cheerleader/Clown

-Sanguine would be prone to this role
- uses humor to lighten difficult family situations; feels fear; others see him/her as being immature; limited by bringing humor to all situations even if inappropriate
- this individual most popular in the family; brings fun and humour into the family
- learn to work hard at getting attention and making people laugh especially when the anger and tension of substance use are dangerously high
- often named a class clown in school; frequently demonstrates poor timing for the comic relief; most people don't take this child

seriously
- often hyperactive, charmers, or cute
- inside, they feel lonely knowing no one really knows the real person behind the clown's mask
- may grow up unable to express deep feelings of compassion
- may put themselves down often as well as cover up their pain with humor
- accepts laughter as approval, but the humor serves to hide inner painful feelings
- the laughter prevents healing rather than produces it

Mascot's purpose: to provide levity to the family; to relieve stress and tension by distracting everyone.

_____Lost Child

-Phlegmatic personality would be prone to this role.
- no connection to family; brings relief to family by not bringing attention to the family; feels lonely; does not learn communication and relationship skills
- has much in common with scrapegoat - neither feels very important
- disappears from the activity of the family
- sees much more than is vocalized
- reinforced for causing no problems
- build quiet lives on the edges of family life and are seldom considered in family decisions
- they hide their hurt and pain by losing themselves in the solitary world of short-term pleasure including excessive TV, computer, reading, listening to music, drugs, object love, eating and fantasy
- favorite places for the lost child are in front of the T.V. as well as in his/her room
- due to the sedentary lifestyle, a lost child tends to have issues with weight
- as adults they feel confused and inadequate in relationships
- may end up as quiet loners with a host of secondary issues such as: sexuality problems, weight problems, excessive materialism, or

heavy involvement in fantasy
Lost child's purpose: does not place added demands on the family system; he/she is low maintenance.

U.____ Undifferentiated Ego Mass--Members of dysfunctional families are enmeshed in each others boundaries. If mom is scared, all feel scared. Members feel for other members and don't have the ability to differentiate thoughts, desires and feelings. The boundaries are either enmeshed, which basically means there are no boundaries because they are all over run or 'walled' boundaries which are thick and there can be no interaction or intimacy. These families look good on the outside but on the inside there is no contact because each are playing their respective roles. So they play rigid roles in an enmeshed family and no one is in touch with their feelings, needs, or wants. Because they are all pretending, no one really knows anyone else.

Perhaps it is best described this way, if you have a spectrum of cohesions from low to high connectedness, low would be disconnected and "walled" and high would be overly connected which is enmeshment. Both being imbalanced, but the middle would be connected and balanced.

N.____ Needs Sacrificed to the System—Members don't get their needs met and as a result there is always low grade anger and depression in the family.

C._____ Conflicted Communication—The communication style is either open conflict which falls under the family rule of incompletion. Don't complete transactions. Keep the same fights and disagreements going for years. or the agreement never to disagree (confluence). There is rarely ever any real contact.

T._____ Together Polarity Dominates—Individual differences are sacrificed for the needs of the family system. The individual exists for the family. In discussing the stages of development I will highlight the polarity issues.

I._____ Irrevocable Rules—The rules are usually rigid and unchanging. Such rules are usually control, perfection, blame, no-talk rule, etc.

Control: One must be in control of all interactions, feelings and personal behavior at all times. Control is the major defensive strategy for shame. Control gives each member a sense of power, predictability and security.

Perfectionism: Always right in everything you do. There is a competitive aspect to this rule. There is a one-up, better-than-others aspect to this rule that covers the shame. The members live according to an image. They avoid what is bad wrong or inferior.

Blame: Whenever things don't turn out as planned, blame yourself or others. Since a shame-based person cannot feel vulnerable or needy without being ashamed, blame becomes an automatic way to avoid one's deepest feelings and true self. Blame is used to regain the illusion of control. Blaming is also a way to deflect shame away from yourself and onto others.

No-talk Rule: Don't talk openly about any feelings, thoughts or experiences that focus on the pain and loneliness of the dysfunctionality.

Myth-Making—Always look at the bright side. Reframe the hurt, pain and distress in such a way as to distract everyone from what is really happening.

Unreliability—Don't expect reliability in relationships. Don't trust anyone and you will never be disappointed. They live with the illusion of self-sufficiency. By acting either aloof and independent (walled boundaries) or needy and dependent (enmeshed boundaries), everyone feels emotionally cut off and incomplete. No one gets their needs met in a functional manner.

O._____ Open Secrets— The open secrets are part of the vital lie which keeps the family frozen. Everyone knows what everyone pretends not to know. It is the classic elephant in the room.

N._____ Non-changing Closed System—Everyone plays their role to control the controlling distress. The more each plays their role, the more the system stays the same.

A.____ Absolute and Grandiose Will—This is in reference to the disabled will that I wrote about earlier. The denial of conflict and frustration creates a situation in which one wills to will. This gives the illusion of doing something about the problem.

L.____ Lack of Boundaries—the equivalent of giving up one's identity – The loss of self comes as the result of being in dysfunctional families where stress often goes on for years. The degree of stress ranges in intensity from mild (chronic fear) to severe (traumatic events). Adult children of a dysfunctional family learns to survive by developing certain patterns of behavior. These behaviors are the survival behaviors which were the actual responses to the violence. As the child from that family grows up, these survival behaviors continue even though they are now disconnected from the original source of distress. These survival behaviors feel normal since they are the patterns one used every day of his early life in order to survive. As an adult they are not only unnecessary, they are actually unhealthy. While once they were protective now they are destructive.

> Robert Firestone has compared these defenses to the body's physical reaction in forming pneumonia. "In pneumonia, the body's defensive reaction is more destructive than the original assault. The presence of organisms in the lungs evokes cellular and humoral defenses that lead to congestion that can destroy the organism.
>
> Fire stone writes: "In a like manner, defenses that were erected by the vulnerable child to protect…against a toxic environment may become more detrimental than the original trauma. In this sense one's psychological defenses become the core of one's neurosis." (*Fantasy Bond*)

Survival behaviors are hard to give up. They are old friends who served us well. We did survive. But we survived by developing a kind of power that resulted from sacrificing ourselves. We learned to control people by playing our roles, i.e., Caretakers, Perfect Child, Scapegoat, etc. In the end it has left us powerless and spiritually bankrupt.

This loss of self is what we call co-dependence and is a symptom of abandonment, neglect, abuse and enmeshment. Co-dependence is a loss of one's inner reality and an addiction to outer reality. The denial and repression of self often results in sexual repression. This repression of sexuality is what sets up the wild and shameful sexual acting out in our addictions.

Co-dependence is a core addiction. It is a diseased form of life. Once a person believes that their identity lies outside themself in a substance, activity or another person, They have found a new god, sold his soul and became a slave. It is a "conflict of god's."

In growing up in a dysfunctional family the child will grow up to be an adult child. Again using an Acronym from Bradshaw ADULT CHILDREN OF DYSFUNCTIONAL FAMILIES, place an "X" beside the letters that indentify yourself. I have integrated certain exercise to work through as you identify characteristics of you. This is not meant to be exhaustive but to begin you on the journey of healing.

ADULT

A.____ Abandonment Issues—You were physically abandoned by one or both of your parents. Your parent(s) were there, but not emotionally available to you. You were physically, sexually or emotionally violated by someone in your family. Your developmental dependency needs were neglected. You were enmeshed in your parent's neediness or in the needs of your family system. You stay in relationships fare beyond what is healthy.

D.____ Delusion and Denial--- After reading this material you still think your family was perfect.

U.____ Undifferentiated Ego Mass—You carry feelings, desires and secrets of other people in your family system.

L.____ Loneliness and Isolation—You have felt lonely all or most of your life. You feel isolated and different.

T.____ Thought Disorders—You get involved in generalities or details. You worry, ruminate and obsess a lot. You stay in your head to avoid your feelings. You read about your problems, rather than taking action.

CHILDREN

C.___ Control Madness—You try to control yourself and everyone else. You feel extremely uncomfortable when you're out of control. You mask your efforts to control people and situations by "being helpful."

H.___ Hypervigilant and High Anxiety—You live on guard. You are easily startled. You panic easily.

I.___ Internalized Shame—You feel flawed as a human being. You feel inadequate and hide behind a role or an addiction or character trait, like control, blame, criticism, perfectionism, contempt, power and rage.

D.___ Disabled Will—You are willful. You try to control other people. You are grandiose. With you it is all or nothing.

R.___ Reactive and Reenacting—You react easily. You feel things that are not related to what is happening. You feel things more intensely than the event calls for. You find yourself repeating patterns over and over.

E.___ Equifinality—No matter where you begin, your life seems to end at the same place.

N.___ Numbed Out—You don't feel your feelings. You don't know what you feel. You don't know how to express what you feel.

OF

O.___ Offender with or without offender status—You are actually an offender, or you are not an offender, but you do in fact play that role sometimes.

F.___ Fixated Personality—You are an adult, but your emotional age is very young. You look like an adult, but feel very childlike and needy. You feel like the lifeguard on a crowded beach, but you don't know how to swim.

DYSFUNCTIONAL

D.____ Dissociated Responses—You have no memories of painful events of your childhood; you have a split personality; you depersonalize; can't remember people's names or even the people you were with two years ago. You are out of touch with your body and your feelings.

Y.____ Yearn for Parental Warmth and Approval, Seek it in other Relationships—You still try to gain your parent's approval. You yearn for the "perfect relationship". You have an exaggerated need for others' approval. You fear offending others. You find emotionally unavailable partners (just like your parents were), who you try to make love you. You will go to almost any length to care and help your partner. Almost nothing is too much trouble. Having had a little nurturing yourself, you find people who need nurturing and take care of them.

S.____ Secrets—You carry lots of secrets from your family of origin. You've never talked to anyone about how bad it was in your family, and you carry lots of secrets about your own life. You also carry lots of sexual secrets which you would not want to tell anyone.

F.____ Faulty Communication—You have had trouble communicating in every relationship you've been in. No one seems to understand what you say. You feel confused a lot in communicating with others. When talking to parents no matter how good your intentions are to be sane and clear, it winds up the same—conflict and confusion.

U.____ Underinvolved—You stand on the sidelines of life wishing you were a participant. You don't know how to initiate a relationship, a conversation, an activity. You are withdrawn and would rather bear the pangs of being alone than risking interaction. You are not spontaneous. You allow yourself very little excitement or fun.

N.____ Neglect of Developmental Dependency Needs—You have a hole in the cup of your psych (soul). You never seem to be satisfied. No matter how much you anticipate something, soon after it is over, you feel restless and unsatisfied. You are childish and feel like a child a lot of the time. You cry when someone says really beautiful things about you. You feel like you don't really belong a lot of the time.

C.___ Compulsive/Addictive—You have been or are now in an active compulsive addictive behavior(s), i.e., sexual addiction.

T.___ Trance—You still carry the family trance. You are fantasy bonded and still idealize your parents. You still play the role(s) you played in your family system. Nothing has really changed in your family of origin. Same dialogue—same fights—same gossip. Your marriage or your relationship is just like your parents.

I.___ Intimacy Problems—You have trouble in relationships; you've been married more than twice; you choose partners who embody the same emotional patterns of your primary caretakers. You are attracted to seductive psychopathic partners; you are not attracted to partners who are kind, stable, reliable and interested in you. You find "nice" men/women boring. When you start getting too close, you leave a relationship. You confuse closeness with compliance; intimacy with fusion.

O.___ Overinvolved—You are drawn to people who are needy. You confuse love with pity. You are drawn to people who have problems that you can get involved in fixing. You are drawn toward people and situations that are chaotic, uncertain and emotionally painful.

N.___ Narcissisitically Deprived—You feel empty and childishly helpless inside. You compensate with addiction as a way to feel important and worthwhile.

A.___ Abuse Victim—You were physically, emotionally, sexually abused as a child. You have become a victim in life and play that role in all areas of your life. You feel hopeless about changing anything. Or you were abused and have become an offender. You identified with the abusing parent or caretaker and act just like they did.

L.___ Lack of Coping Skills—You never learned how to do many things necessary for a fully functional life. Your methods of problem-solving do not work but you continue to use the same ones over and over. You learned ways of caring for your wounds that, in fact, perpetuated them. There are a whole set of models of what's normal that you have never seen. You have no real knowledge of what is normal. Your bottom line tolerance is quite abnormal.

FAMILIES

F.___ False Self—Confused Identity—Your self-worth depends on your partner's success or failure. When you're not in a relationship, you feel an inner void. You feel responsible for making your partner happy. You take care of people to give yourself an identity. You wear masks, calculate, manipulate, and play games. You act out rigid family roles and /or sex roles.

A.___ Avoid Depression Through Activity—You get involved in unstable relationships. The more your active and in your head, the more you can avoid your depression.

M.___ Measured, Judgmental and Perfectionistic—You have unrealistic expectations of yourself and others. You are rigid and inflexible. You are rigid and judgmental of yourself and others. You are stuck in your attitudes and behavior, even though it hurts to live the way you do.

I.___ Inhibited Trust—You really don't trust anyone, including your own feelings, perceptions and judgments.

L.___ Loss of Your Own Reality—Damaged and Weak Boundaries—You take more than 50% responsibility, guilt, and blame for whatever happens in a relationship. You know others feelings or need before you know your own feelings and needs. Rather than take any risk of abandonment, you have withdrawn and refuse to get involved. Any change in the status quo of a relationship is experienced as a threat by you. You feel embarrassed by what others do and take responsibility for their behavior.

I.___ Inveterate Dreamer—In your relationships you are in touch with your dreams of how it could be, rather than with the reality of your life and situations. You live according to an ideal image of yourself, rather than what your true reality is. You have a grandiose and exaggerated notion of yourself. You fantasize and catastrophize and exaggerate the seriousness of decisions and events.

E.___ Emotional Constraint (with or without dramatic outburst)—You believe that controlling your emotions is a way to control your life. You attempt to manage your life and your emotions. You have dramatic outbursts of emotions that have been repressed for long period of time. You have inappropriate outbursts of emotions. You compulsively expose your emotions. You do this so that you don't have to feel them for very long.

S.___ Spiritual Bankruptcy—You live totally oriented to the outside believing that your worth and happiness lies outside of you. You have no awareness of your "inner life" since you spend all of your energy avoiding your shame-based self.

By doing this exercise it was not my purpose to depress you but to consider how family has impact your own personality and soul. In addiction recovery it is about reconnecting with the true self, the person who God made you to be not what you thought everyone wanted you to be. One does not experience recovery without addressing the roots of shame in their life, and you don't deal with shame without looking at the dysfunctional family and all the false messages and rigid rules.

Erik Erikson in his work in Developmental Psychology states, adolescence is marked by what he calls the "Identity Crisis." To be honest I don't think it is limited to adolescence. I believe most of us don't know who we are given not only the number of dysfunction families in our nation, but our culture. If I went on the street today and asked people who they are in body, soul (personality) or spirit, they probably couldn't tell me. I am sure they would define themselves by what they do or where they live, most don't know there body type and its needs, their personalities and its needs and most definitely have no relationship with God in terms of positional truths.

Whether you've identified with co-dependency or not, everyone in recovery needs to consider their family of origin as you work through the Twelve steps. It is a process of surrender motivated by the acceptance of shame. For the addict surrender is the first step to freedom since beginning the addiction. The only way out of the compulsive/addictive shame cycle is to embrace the shame.

Using Bradshaws acronyms, the STAGES of RECOVERY is to UNCOVER so we can DISCOVER who we really are, the true self in regards to our soul.

STAGES:

S. - Surrender to Pain-

Surrender means I give up trying to control my compulsive /addictive behavior. I am willing to let others help me and do it their way. I am willing to go to any lengths to get well.

- Separation Process – Leaving Home- We leave home by giving up our scripts and rigid roles. We played the rigid roles out of loyalty to our dysfunctional family systems. We got power and control from these roles, but they have cost us dearly. Leaving home means giving up the idealizations and the fantasy of being bonded to our parents. Only by leaving and becoming separate can we have the choice of having a relationship with our parents. Relationships demands separation and detachment.

Separation demands that we forgive ourselves and we forgive our parents. It means that we give up the resentments and release the energy that has kept us in bondage. We can then love our parents as the real wounded people they are, not as a mythologized deity (gods). Only by breaking the spell with our family of origin can we have a life of our own choosing.

T. – Trust and Telling Your Secrets –

As you seek help, you are willing to trust enough and ask for help. You need to label your addiction, your disease, it is not your label, it is the disease that is being labeled. "The" addiction, not I am the addiction.

Practice asking for help by asking questions: Don't just take people's words without asking for clarification. As a child you lived in a trance and confusion and never asked questions for fear of the response, now we can seek clarification. If you're confused about someone's feelings or needs, ask them questions until you feel less confused. Tell your inner child that it is not easy to understand others or yourself so we need to ask lots of questions.

Practice active listening: You can become more conscious of other person's process. Listening also helps us check out what the other person is saying. Few of us grew up seeing this kind of communication modeled in our family systems.

A. - Affiliation Needs –
As you surrender to others, a group, sponsor, etc, you are coming out of isolation. We need a new mirroring, warmth and trust. This sometimes means that we have to change our friends and associates. Those who will encourage our recovery decisions, rather than thwart them at every turn. Eventually we can move into solitude where you enjoy your time alone and have more self-discovery.

G. - Group Support -
You now belong to a new family that models healthy messages and flexible rules and connectedness. You receive education on the nature of addiction and raise your awareness. It raises our God consciousness. We pray and /or meditate daily. You move from being lonely or frightened. This can happen in a recovery group or a therapeutic based church.

E. – Embracing Your Incomparable Inner Child:
The following idea is taken from the "index of suspicion" from the pioneering work of Hugh Missildine in his book *Your Inner Child of the Past* and the incorporation of Erik Erikson's Model of Developmental Stages. Answer yes or no to the following questions. There are degrees of woundedness if you answer yes to any of the questions it indicates that you may have had wounding, the more yes's means more wounding. Take your time, after you read each question take a moment and get in touch with what you feel.

<u>Infant Stage 0-9 months</u>

1. Do you have or have you had in the past an ingestive addiction (overeating, overdrinking, drugging, smoking)? Yes____ No____

2. Do you have trouble trusting your ability to get your needs met? Do you believe you must find someone to meet them for you? Yes____ No____

3. Do you find it hard to trust other people? Do you feel you must be in control at all times? Yes____ No____

4. Do you fail to recognize body signals of physical need? For example, do you eat when you're not hungry? Or are you often not aware how tired you are? Yes____ No____

5. Do you neglect your physical needs? Do you ignore good nutrition or fail to get enough exercise? Do you get to a doctor or dentist only in an emergency? Yes____ No____

6. Do you have deep fears of abandonment? Do you feel, or have you ever felt desperate because a love relationship ended? Yes____ No____

7. Have you considered suicide because a love relationship has ended (your lover has left you; your spouse filed for a divorce)? Yes____ No____

8. Do you often feel that you don't truly fit in or belong anywhere? Do you feel that people don't really welcome you or want your presence? Yes____ No____

9. In social situations, do you try to be invisible so that no one will notice you? Yes____ No____

10. Do you try to be so helpful (even indispensable) in your love relationships that the other person (friend, lover, spouse, child, parent) cannot leave you? Yes____ No____

11. Is oral sex what you most desire and fantasize about? Yes____ No____

12. Do you have great need to be touched and held? (This is often manifested by your needing to touch or hug others often without asking them.) Yes____ No____

13. Do you have a continual and obsessive need to be valued and esteemed? Yes____ No____

14. Are you often biting and sarcastic to others? Yes____ No____

15. Do you isolate yourself and stay alone a lot of the time? Do you often feel it's not worth trying to have a relationship? Yes____ No____

16. Are you often gullible? Do you accept others' opinions or "swallow things whole" without thinking them through? Yes____ No____

This stage is called the symbiotic stage because they are completely co-dependent on their mother. They are undifferentiated or enmeshed with the mother and their dependency needs are for thinking, imagining, feeling, competence, skills, decisions, doing, being and purpose. They need mirroring to discover their I AMness. If the mother is there an "interpersonal bridge" or bond is formed. If mom is not there they will come to believe that they have no right to depend on anyone and feel insecure that if something goes wrong there is no assurance that someone will be there for them, to help and protect them. The child will feel about themselves what the mom feels about them. The child needs to be touched when the child needs to be touched. The infant needs to hear welcoming, peaceful, warm voices around them. They need lots of echoing coos! And oohs! And ahs! They need to hear a safe, sure voice that signaled a high degree of safety. This forms the basis of trust and hope. If the world is basically trustworthy, then becoming who "I am" is possible. Pam Levin sees this first stage as one in which the power of being is developed.

Speaking from personal experience, being a parent can be a very difficult job under the best of circumstances. A very good parent has to be mentally and spiritually healthy and that is rare. Most of us have unresolved wounded shamed children living inside of us. As a result we parent with this fear, shame and self preservation. We either do a lot of what our parents did or we do just the opposite. Two wrongs don't make a right, I have often told individuals in my counseling that my parents loved me perfectly imperfectly, in other words they did the best they knew how as I did with my children. In either case if we as parents are seeking to meet our own needs, we will not be able to accurately assess and adequately supply our children's needs.

Children who do not develop a basic sense of trust, will often develop insatiable cravings and may act out with ingestive addictions, or they may need to be continually validated. Others may have an insatiable craving to be touched and hugged. Most of all when our infancy needs are not met, it sets you up to feel ashamed of yourself, to feel deep down that something is wrong with you. You feel emotional deprivation and abandonment, this deep sense of shame and hurt. To survive the self-defense mechanism kicks in and these feelings become locked, the limbic system shuts the door and they remain unresolved but ever longing to be met. So how do we resolve this thirst and craving to be loved and feel connected on the soul level. If you checked off several yes's in the Index of Suspicion then it would be helpful to do the following exercise.

Exercise: Reconnecting to your Infant self

Step 1 Debriefing – Get all the information you can about your family system. For example, what was going on when you were born? Where you wanted or deemed a "mistake?" What kind of families did your mother and father come from? Were they expecting the opposite sex and disappointed? Was your mom and/or dad an adult child.

Step 2 Share with a trusted friend/sponsor/ counselor – What you have written as much as you know about your infancy, it is important to talk about it and to read it out load to someone. What is important is to have someone hear you and validate your original pain as an infant. The listener should not question you, argue with you, or give advice. It is not advisable to share this with a parent or other family members.

Step 3 Feeling the Feelings – If you have a picture of yourself as an infant, take a long look at it. If you don't have a picture, spend some time looking at an infant and notice its innocents. The infant didn't ask to be born but all it wants is to be loved and nourished.

Step 4 Writing a Letter – imagine that you're a wise old adult and you want to adopt a child. Imagine that the infant you want to adopt is you as an infant. Further, imagine that you need to write this infant child a letter. It is okay that the infant child can't read. It doesn't need to belong, maybe just a paragraph or two. Tell your infant self that you want them and will give them the time they need to grow and develop. Assure them that you know what they need and will give it to them and that you will work hard to see them as the precious and wonderfully unique person they are. When you finished with the letter read it out load very slowly and notice your feelings. It's okay to be sad and cry if you want to.

Step 5 Letter from your Inner Infant – Now, although you might think it very strange, I want you to write yourself a letter from your inner infant. Write with your non-dominant hand. This helps you to not use the more controlling, logical side of your brain. Again we know an infant can't write but if they could what might they say, i.e., Dear (your name) I want you to come and get me I want to matter to someone. I don't want to be alone. Love, (little your name)

Step 6 Affirmations – If your infancy needs were not met, then it still needs nurturing and words of love and support. Saying new and empowering words can touch our original pain and trigger great healing.

Positive affirmations reinforce our beingness and can heal the spiritual wound. Repeated positive messages are emotional nutrients.

Here are some loving words you can say to your inner infant during the meditation. (Use whichever ones you like best).

Welcome to the world, I've been waiting for you.
I'm so glad you're here.
I will not leave you, no matter what.
Your needs are okay with me.
I'll give you all the time you need to get your needs met.
I'm so glad you're a boy/girl.
I want to take care of you and I'm prepared to do that.
I like feeding you, bathing you, changing you, and spending time with you.
God smiled when you were born.

<u>Toddler Stage: 9 months -3 years</u>

1. Do you have trouble knowing what you want? Yes___ No___

2. Are you afraid to explore when you go to a new place? Yes___ No___

3. Are you afraid to try out new experiences? If you do try them, do you always wait till someone else has tried first? Yes___ No___

4. Do you have great fears of abandonment? Yes___ No___

5. In difficult situations, do you long for someone to tell you what to do? Yes___ No___

6. If someone gives you a suggestion, do you feel you ought to follow it? Yes___ No___

7. Do you have trouble actually being in your experience? For example, when you're on vacation looking at an exciting sight, are you worrying about the tour bus leaving without you? Yes___ No___

8. Are you a big worrier? Yes___ No___

9. Do you have trouble being spontaneous? For example, would you be embarrassed to sing in front of a group of people just because you were happy? Yes___ No___

10. Do you find yourself in frequent conflicts with people in authority? Yes___ No___

11. Do you often use words that center on defecation or urination—like asshole, shit, or piss? Does your sense of humor focus on bathroom jokes? Yes____ No____

12. Are you obsesses with men's or women's buttocks? Yes____ No____

13. Are you often accused of being stingy with money, love, showing emotions, or affection? Yes____ No ____

14. Do you tend to be obsessive about neatness and cleanliness? Yes____ No____

15. Do you fear anger in other people or in yourself? Yes____ No____

16. Will you do almost anything to avoid conflict? Yes____ No____

17. Do you feel guilty when you say no to someone? Yes____ No____

18. Do you avoid saying no directly, but often refuse to do what you've said you would in a variety of indirectly manipulative and passive ways? Yes____ No____

19. Do you sometimes "go berserk" and inappropriately let go of all control? Yes____ No____

20. Are you often excessively critical of other people? Yes____ No____

21. Do you act nice to people when you're with them and then gossip about and criticize them when they go away? Yes____ No____

22. When you achieve success, do you have trouble enjoying or even believing in your accomplishments? Yes____ No____

Questions 1 through 9 cover ages 9 months to 18 months which is called the exploration stage because it involves crawling, touching, tasting, and in general being curious and eager to explore the world around them.

Questions 10 through 22 cover ages 18 months to 3 years. This period is called the separation stage. It is a counter dependence stage and is characterized by oppositional bonding. The child will say things like "No," and "I won't." The child is still bonded, but must oppose the parents in order to separate and be himself. It is seen as the second birth or psychological birth. It marks the true beginning of I AM Me.

If the child has established a basic level of trust in the first 9 months, the child will begin to naturally go exploring in their environment.

Erikson calls it the incorporation stage, because they take everything in and try to incorporate it into their lives.

Muscles develop in terms of holding on and letting go. They learn balance and willpower. It also requires a balance of emotions. Developmental polarity is between autonomy verses shame and doubt. The toddler learns that as mom and dad sets limits conflict occurs and they can be angry at mom and dad and they will still be there. Healthy shame is simply an emotion of limits and it safeguards our spirit by teaching us that it is okay not to be perfect and know we are not God. Healthy willpower is the goal of this stage because it is the power of doing.

Without healthy willpower we have no discipline. We don't know how to hold on or to let go appropriately. We either let go inappropriately (act with license) or hold on inappropriately (hoard, over control, become obsessive/compulsive). They also don't have a good sense of balance as adults they either don't know when to say no or they always say no. Sometimes they say yes and then say no in inconsistent and manipulative ways. Shame-based adults with no limits are set up for addiction. Without balance they either see themselves as good or bad, never both. They develop boundary problems because they don't know when to hold on or let go.

Exercise: Reconnecting to your toddler self

Step 1: Debriefing – Use the following questions as a guideline. Who was around when you were 2 or 3? Where was your dad? Did he play with you often? Spend time with you? Did Dad and Mom stay married? Where was your mom? Was she patient? Did she spend time with you? Were either or both parents addicts?

How did your mom and dad discipline you? If physical—What exactly was done to you—give details. If emotional, how were you terrorized? Were you told you would be spanked or punished when your father got home? Did you have any older brothers or sisters? How did they treat you?

Who was there for you? Who held you when you were scared or crying? Set firm but kind and gentle limits when you were angry? Who played, laughed, and had fun with you?

Pay attention to anything you now know about family secrets that you couldn't have known as a child. For example, was Dad a sex addict, having lots of affairs? Is either parent an untreated victim of physical, sexual, or emotional violence. Family secrets are always about the family's toxic shame. Focus on all the ways you were shamed—all the ways your feelings, needs, and desires were repressed. Consider lack of discipline or too much discipline. Write about any traumatic incidents and be detailed and concrete as possible. Details bring us back to the actual experience which comes closer to touching our actual feelings.

Step Two: Share the Toddler with a Friend – Telling your story of violation to your support person is a way of reducing your toxic shame. It pulls us out of isolation and we begin to learn that we can depend on others.

Step Three: Feeling your Feelings – If you have a photograph of yourself as a toddler, get it out. See how small and innocent you were. If you don't have a photo, spend some time with a toddler. Focus on the normalcy of this developmental stage. Toddlers get into things, they are curious and interested in things. They say no to begin a life of their own. Feel whatever feelings come up for you.

Step Four: Letter Writing – To the toddler self. For example you might say Dear little (your name), I know you are very lonely and scared to get angry. You can't be scared or afraid because that is for sissies. NO one really knows the wonderful person you are and what your really feel.

I am from your future and I know better than anyone what you've been through! I love you and want you to be with me always. I'll let you be exactly the way you are. I'll teach you some balance and let you be mad, sad, afraid, or glad. Please consider letting me be with you always. Love Big (your name)

Step Five: Letter from the Toddler – Write a letter from your wounded inner toddler. Write with your non-dominant hand, i.e., Dear Big (your name) Please come and get me, I've been in a closet for forty years, I'm terrified, I need you. Little (your name)

After you have written the letter, sit quietly and let whatever feelings you have come up. Read the letter out loud to one of your supports.

Step Six: Affirmations – Go back into the past and find your inner toddler and give them the affirmations they needed to hear.

Little (your name), it's okay to be curious, to want, to look, to touch and taste things. I'll make it safe for you to explore.
I love you just the way you are.
I'm here to take care of your needs. You don't have to take care of mine.
It's okay for you to be taken care of.
It's okay to say no. I'm glad you want to be you.
It's okay for both of us to be mad. We will work our problems out.
It's okay to feel scared when you do things your way.
It's okay to feel sad when things don't work out for you.
I'll never leave you no matter what!
You can be you and still count on my being there for you.
I love watching you learn to walk and talk. I love watching you separate and start to grow up.
I love and value you.
Read over these affirmations slowly and let their meaning sink in.

<u>Preschool Stage: 3 -6 years of age</u>

1. Do you have severe identity problems? Yes____ No____ To aid you in answering this , consider the following question. Who are you? Does an answer come easily? No matter what your sexual preference, do you feel like you're really a man? A women? Do you overdramatize your sex?

2. Even when you have sex in a legitimate context, do you feel guilty? Yes____ No____

3. Do you have trouble identifying what you are feeling at any given moment? Yes____ No____

4. Do you have communication problems with the people you are close to? Yes____ No____

5. Do you try to control your feelings most of the time? Yes____ No____

6. Do you try to control the feelings of those around you? Yes____ No____

7. Do you cry when you're angry? Yes____ No____

8. Do you rage when you're scared or hurt? Yes____ No____

9. Do you have trouble expressing your feelings? Yes____ No____

10. Do you believe that you are responsible for other people's behavior or feelings? (For example, do you feel that you can make someone sad or angry?) Yes____ No____ Also do you feel guilty for what has happened to your family members? Yes____ No____

11. Do you believe that if you just behave a certain way, you can change another person? Yes____ No____

12. Do you believe that wishing or feeling something can make it come true? Yes____ No____

13. Do you often accept confusing messages and inconsistent communication without asking for clarification? Yes____ No____

14. Do you act on guesses and unchecked assumptions, treating them as actual information? Yes____ No____

15. Do you feel responsible for your parents' marital problems or divorce? Yes____ No____

16. Do you strive for success so that your parents can feel good about themselves? Yes____ No____

At age three you start asking the question "why," amongst many other questions. Prior to age 6 children are truly unable to understand the world from another person's point of view. They are very independent and ask many questions forming their beliefs, envisioning the future, and trying to figure out how the world works and what makes things happen. As they develop a more sophisticated sense of cause and effect, is learned and how they can influence things. A little boy bonds with his dad, he wants to be like him. He begins to imitate his dad's behavior. They discover I am someone, male or female.

Erikson speaks of ego strength. He believes that strength of purpose arises out of a sense of identity. If healthy development has taken place up to the preschool age, a child can say: I can trust the world, I can trust myself, and I am special and unique. Power comes out of having an identity—the power to initiate and to make choices. They think, I can be me and all of life is ahead of me. The polarity of relationship is between initiative and guilt, in finding a sense of purpose.

Growth disorders at this age means that they cannot form intimate relationships when they are adults. Having lost their I AMness, authentic selves, they can't give themselves to their partners because they don't have themselves to give. When adult children marry they choose a person who is a projection of their parents—someone who is both positive and negative aspects of their parents and who compliments their family-system roles. For example a family Hero Caretaker will often marry a victim.

Exercise: Reconnecting to your Preschool self

Step 1: Debriefing – Use the following questions as a guideline. Who was around when you were 3-6 years of age? Where was your dad? Did he play with you often? Spend time with you? Did dad and mom stay married? Where was your mom? Was she patient? Did she spend time with you? Who was your role model that you most identified with?

How did your mom and dad discipline you? If physical—What exactly was done to you—give details. If emotional, how were you abused? Were you told you would be spanked or punished when your father got home? Did you have any older brothers or sisters? How did they treat you?

Who was there for you? Who held you when you were scared or crying? Set firm but kind and gentle limits when you were angry? Who played, laughed, and had fun with you?

Pay attention to anything you now know about family secrets that you couldn't have known as a child. For example, was dad a sex addict, having lots of affairs? Is either parent an untreated victim of physical, sexual, or emotional violence. Family secrets are always about the family's toxic shame. Focus on all the ways you were shamed—all the ways your feelings, needs, and desires were repressed. Consider lack of discipline or too much discipline. Write about any traumatic incidents and be detailed and concrete as possible. Details bring us back to the actual experience which comes closer to touching our actual feelings.

Step Two: Share the Preschool Child with a Friend – Telling your story of violation to your support person is a way of reducing your toxic shame. It pulls us out of isolation and we begin to learn that we can depend on others. Focus on any incidents of violation that you can remember.

Step Three: Feeling your Feelings – If you have a photograph of yourself at preschool age, get it out. See how small and innocent you were. If you don't have a photo, spend some time with a preschool child. Focus on the normalcy of this developmental stage. Feel whatever feelings come up for you. You may have an old doll, toy, or teddy bear from this age that may help you to remember and feel.

Step Four: Letter Writing – To the preschool self. For example you might say Dear little (your name), I know you are very lonely and scared to get angry. You can't be scared or afraid because that is for sissies. No one really knows the wonderful person you are and what your really feel.

I am from your future and I know better than anyone what you've been through! I love you and want you to be with me always. I'll let you be exactly the way you are. I'll teach you some balance and let you be mad, sad, afraid, or glad. Please consider letting me be with you always. Love Big (your name)

Write a letter to your mom and dad, a paragraph dedicated for each of them. You may say "I needed you to protect me. I was scared all the time. I needed you to play with me. I wish we could have gone fishing. I wish you would have taught me things. I wish you weren't drinking all the time. Mom I needed you to praise me. To tell me you loved me. I wish you hadn't made me take care of you. I needed to be taken care of...

After you have written the letter, sit quietly and let whatever feelings you have come up. Read the letter out loud to one of your supports.

Step Five: Dysfunctional Family-System Roles – Identify and write down the roles your wounded inner preschooler chose in order to matter in your family. What feelings did you have to repress in order to play your role. Close your eyes and imagine that you couldn't play your major role anymore! How does it feel to give up that role? Think of three new behaviors you could use to stop your role.

Write down all the ways your family-system enmeshment has had life-damaging consequences. Connect with your feelings of loss and share them with your trusted person.

Step Six: Affirmations – Go back into the past and find your inner pre-school child and give them the affirmations they needed to hear.

I will be here for you to test your boundaries and find out your limits.
It's okay for you to think for yourself. You can think about your feelings and have feelings about what you're thinking.
It's okay to find out the difference between boys and girls.
I'll set limits for you to help you find out who you are.
I love you just the way you are.
It's okay to be different; to have your own views on things.
It's okay to imagine things without being afraid they'll come true.
I'll help you separate fantasy from reality.
I like it that you're a boy/girl.
You can ask for what you want.
You can ask questions if something confuses you.
You are not responsible for your parent's marriage
You are not responsible for the family problems
It's okay to explore who you are.

<u>School Age Stage: 6 years of age to Puberty</u>

1. Do you often compare yourself to other people and find yourself inferior? Yes____ No____

2. Do you wish you had more good friends of both sexes? Yes____ No____

3. Do you frequently feel uncomfortable in social situations? Yes____ No____

4. Do you feel uncomfortable being part of a group? Yes____ No____ Do you feel most comfortable when your alone Yes____ No____

5. Are you sometimes told that you are excessively competitive? Do you feel like you must win? Yes____ No____

6. Do you have frequent conflicts with the people you work with? Yes____ No____

With the people in your family? Yes___ No___

7. In negotiations, do you either (a) give in completely or (b) insist on having things your own way? Yes___ No___

8. Do you pride yourself on being strict and literal, following the letter of the law? Yes___ No___

9. Do you procrastinate a lot? Yes___ No___

10. Do you have trouble finishing things? Yes___ No___

11. Do you believe you should know how to do things without instructions? Yes___ No___

12. Do you have intense fears about making a mistake? Yes___ No___ Do you experience severe humiliation if you are forced to look at your mistakes? Yes___ No___

13. Do you frequently feel angry and critical of others? Yes___ No___

14. Are you deficient in basic life skills (ability to read, speak or write with good grammar, ability to do necessary math calculations)? Yes___ No___

15. Do you spend lots of time obsessing on and /or analyzing what someone has said to you? Yes___ No___

16. Do you feel ugly and inferior? Yes___ No___ If yes, do you try to hide it with clothes, things, money, or make-up? Yes___ No___

17. Do you lie to yourself and others a lot of the time? Yes___ No___

18. Do you believe that no matter what you do, it is not good enough? Yes___ No___

The school age child learns that I am capable. The developing polarity is industry verses inferiority. The child is to learn competence. The child enters a new stage of socializing and skill building. School age should be a time of play and work. School should verify our sense of self. If we are competent, then we can be industrious and competent. "Because I am capable, I can be what I choose to be."

By age 7 or 8 children are able to think logically, but theirs is still a concrete kind of thinking. Not until puberty will they be able to abstract and entertain contrary-to-fact propositions. Only then will a child begin to idealize and idolize. I stated in an earlier section that children are egocentric and believe adults to be benevolent.

This brings me to another environmental impact on our belief system and I AMness. I don't want to come across as totally negative, but I believe the school system had a tremendously negative impact on my false belief system. Our schools, like our homes can be very dysfunctional. It may not provide an environment that affirms who we are. It may not treat us as unique people that we truly are.

Milton Erickson said," There is no people who understand the same sentence the same way." In my case I can actually recall when my inner child was crushed by the burden of conforming to the perfectionistic school system. You either become hopeless about your chance of success and drop out, or you got taken up into the conformity trance were your soul is murdered in the process. Over the last 25 years there have been some strides for improvement but for the most part schools continue to reward conformity and memorization rather than creativity and uniqueness. Given that I was poor at memorization and had difficulty concentrating, my conclusion as a child—"I am stupid, and a failure." Parents can unknowingly feed into this shame-based system when the report cards come home and the child is chastised for not measuring up to this rigid empirical system of conformity and performance. Parker Palmer challenged this system by stating that as educators we should know the landscape of our students.

While there are many courageous, creative, and nurturing teachers, there are also lots of very angry, abusive teachers. I know I was taught by some of them. In some cases classmates themselves were also the offenders, further wounding the soul and reinforcing the false beliefs.

Exercise School age

Step one: Debriefing - Who was around when you were 6 years of age to puberty? Where was your dad? Did he play with you often? Spend time with you? Did dad and mom stay married? Where was your mom? Was she patient? Did she spend time with you? Who was your role model that you most identified with?

How did your mom and dad discipline you? If physical— What exactly was done to you—give details. If emotional, how were you terrorized? Were you told you would be spanked or punished when your father got home? Did you have any older brothers or sisters? How did they treat you?

Who was there for you? Who held you when you were scared or crying? Set firm but kind and gentle limits when you were angry? Who played, laughed, and had fun with you?

Pay attention to anything you now know about family secrets that you couldn't have known as a child. For example, was dad a sex addict, having lots of affairs? Is either parent an untreated victim of physical, sexual, or emotional violence. Family secrets are always about the family's toxic shame. Focus on all the ways you were shamed—all the ways your feelings, needs, and desires were repressed. Consider lack of discipline or too much discipline. Write about any traumatic incidents and be detailed and concrete as possible. Details bring us back to the actual experience which comes closer to touching our actual feelings. When considering teachers, clergyman, older kids etc, write out each person's name and comment on whether they were nurturing or spiritually wounding.

Write about the three most important events of each year.

6 years old:

1. Started first grade
2. Peed in my pants one day and was humiliated in front of my class.

7 years old:

1. Passed to second grade.
2. Got a record player for Christmas
3. Was in a car accident

Continue the list until age 13. Remember pleasant and unpleasant memories.

Step Two: Share your school-age child's history with a support person – Read your story to a friend, spouse, sponsor or therapist.

Step Three: Feeling the Feelings - If you have a photograph of yourself at school age, get it out. See how small and innocent you were. If you don't have a photo, spend some time with a school child. Focus on the normalcy of this developmental stage. Feel whatever feelings come up for you.

Step Four: Letter Writing – To the preschool self. For example you might say Dear little (your name), I know you are very lonely and scared to get angry. You can't be scared or afraid because that is for sissies. No one really knows the wonderful person you are and what your really feel.

I am from your future and I know better than anyone what you've been through! I love you and want you to be with me always. I'll let you be exactly the way you are. I'll teach you some balance and let you be mad, sad, afraid, or glad. Please consider letting me be with you always. Love Big (your name)

Write a letter to your mom and dad, a paragraph dedicated for each of them. You may say "I needed you to protect me. I was scared all the time. I needed you to play with me. I wish we could have gone fishing. I wish you would have taught me things. I wish you weren't drinking all the time. Mom I needed you to praise me. To tell me you loved me. I wish you hadn't made me take care of you. I needed to be taken care of...

Another very powerful writing exercise at this age is to write a fairy tale about your childhood. Your story should have two parts. Part one should begin with "Once upon a time," and describe the events you have chosen, focusing on how they created the wound. Part two should begin with "And when she/he grew up," and should focus on the later life-damaging effects of the spiritual wounds.

After you have written the letter, sit quietly and let whatever feelings you have come up. Read the letter out loud to one of your supports.

Step Five: Dysfunctional Family-System Roles – Get in touch with any new roles that you took on during the school age years and work with them as you did earlier. Focus on life damaging consequences of those roles.

Step Six: Affirmations –

It's okay to learn to do things your own way.

It's okay to think about things and try them out before your make them your own.

You can trust your own judgments; you need only take the consequences of your choices.

You can do things your own way and it is okay to disagree.
I love you just the way you are.
You can choose your own friends
You can dress the way the other kids dress, or you can dress your own way.
I'm willing to be with you no matter what.
I love you

Adolescence Stage: 13-26

1. Are you frequently in conflict with authority figures (bosses, police, and other officials)? Yes____ No____

2. Do you feel enraged by "senseless rules and regulations" that others seem to accept? Yes____ No____

3. When you visit your parents, do you quickly fall into the role of the obedient (or rebellious) child? Yes____ No____

4. Are you confused about who you really are? Yes____ No____

5. Do you feel superior to others because your life-style is offbeat and nonconformist? Yes____ No____

6. Do you still follow unquestioningly the religion of your youth? Yes____ No____

7. Are you able to form close relationships only with people of the opposite sex? Yes____ No____

8. Are all your non-work relationships with the opposite sex sexual or romantic? Yes____ No____

9. Are you a dreamer, preferring to read romance novels or science fiction, rather than taking action in your life? Yes____ No____

10. Do people sometimes tell you to "grow up"? Yes____ No____

11. Do you find it almost impossible to speak your opinion when it goes against an accepted norm? Yes____ No____

12. Do you rigidly follow a guru or hero, or are you deeply attracted to cults secret groups? Yes____ No____

13. Do you talk a lot about the great things you are going to do, but never do them? Yes____ No____

14. Do you believe that no one has ever been through the things you've had to go through, or that no one could really understand your unique pain? Yes____ No____

Adolescence is the leaving home stage. There is a sense of regeneration, and the discovery of the unique self. Some developmental theorist state that is the stage of counter-dependence where they develop a new identity, new competence, new skills, new purpose, new choices and trust. The developmental polarity is identity verses role confusion.

I would tend to agree with Erikson who calls it "reformed identity." In order to achieve this, one must integrate our genetic abilities and personality strengths and skills cultivated earlier with the opportunities offered by our culture's social roles and family systems. It is an accrued confidence that our inner sameness and continuity prepared in the past are matched by the sameness and continuity of one's meaning for others, as evidenced in the tangible promise of a "career." When our body (physically and biologically), soul(personality) and spirit(identity in Christ) are aligned with who God created us to be, our unique I AMness, foundation is well laid for ongoing transformation and maturity.

I have stated throughout the book that when we know our spiritual identity in Christ then our two primary spiritual drives for significance and security are met and we know longer strive in the soul to have these needs met for self-worth. When we are secure in our spiritual I AMness then our personalities can have their full expression and be affirmed with its two primary needs. To quote Freud's famous two marks of maturity: love and work. That our personality is then able to love and accept others (giving "security") without the hidden agenda of trying to get love and security. Secondly work, (being "significant" to others) fulfilling our sense of purpose as we serve others, not to get significance but to extend volitionally what we have positionally.

A wounded inner child can be a devastating force of contamination during one's adolescence. Even a person with a healthy inner child will still have to "refight many of the battles of earlier years." For normal adolescence is one of the stormiest times in the life cycle. Bradshaw's acronym in his book *Home Coming* best describes normal

ADOLESCENCE and captures the developmental needs of an adolescent.

A – Ambivalence:

Refers to the emotional upheavals and mood swings. For example abhor parents' presence one day and desire heart-to-heart talks with them the next day.

D – Distancing from parents:

In order to leave home, they need to make their parents unattractive. Peer group is the vehicle by which adolescents achieve distancing, a kind of peer group parent.

O – Occupation:

Several studies have shown that the number-one worry on teenagers' minds is career: What kind of work will I do? What am I going to do when I grow up?

L – Loneliness:

No matter how many peer group buddies a person has, they feel an emptiness inside. They are still discovering their I AMness, body, soul and spirit. Because of a newly emerged ability to think abstractedly, the future becomes a problem for the first time in a person's life. They have a wounded inner child, this experience is intensified by the degree they have been wounded.

E – Ego Identity:

The question of "who am I" and "where am I going?"

S –Sexual Exploration:

With a sex drive, genital masturbation opens up the throttle. Other forms of exploration often follow. Sex is who we are rather than something we have. The first thing we notice about another person is there sex. When sex is shame-based and determined to be bad, we conclude we are bad and become ashamed of our sexuality. This at any stage of development becomes a strong predisposing factor for sexual addiction.

C – Conceptualization:

The ability to think in abstract, logical terms, moving beyond the concrete literal thinking. Another manifestation of this new cognitive structure is idealization. They become dreamers and dreaming and idealizing create models that motivate. They will attach themselves to idols like rock stars and movie stars, it also suggests that it is a time when they are most religiously ready.

E – Egocentric Thinking:
Unlike the egocentrism of earlier stages, adolescents are fully capable of grasping another person's point of view. This is more about an acute self-consciousness which believes "everyone is looking at me."

N – Narcissism:
They are obsessed with their own reflection in the mirror, they spend hours looking at themselves. This flows from their intense self-consciousness.

C – Communication Frenzy:
Talking endlessly to one's friends is a way to feel wanted and connected.

E – Experimentation:
They experiment a great deal with ideas, styles, roles, and behaviors. They are often in opposition to their parents' style and values. Experimentation is a way to expand one's horizons, to try on other ways of behaving before finalizing one's identity. All and all, adolescence is an integration and reformation of all the previous childhood stages. Out of this reformation a new identity begins to emerge.

It is in adolescence that we begin to act out our original pain and unmet needs. Criminality is a way to steal back what was lost in childhood. Drug use dulls the pain of the dysfunctional-family loneliness. They often act out their families' unexpressed secrets. Sexual acting out is natural during this time of emerging sexual energy. Mom's rigid repression of her shamed sexuality may come out in daughter's early promiscuity. Adolescents are often the scapegoats for the family. The most significant role one has played in the family system up to this point becomes the most available way to have an identity. For me it was the "Lost Child" seeking to be invisible and not cause any negative impact on the family system. Isolated, lonely, withdrawn and no voice in any family decisions, I simply existed with no emotional connection.

Underneath this false identity remained a lonely, confused and terrified little boy. After coming to know Christ my role changed to "Caretaker" in the family of God, but my false identity remained the same, driven out of the fear of failure and rejection.

Exercise Adolescent Stage

Step One: Debriefing - Who was around when you were 13-26? Where was your dad? Spend time with you? Did dad and mom stay married? Where was your mom? Was she patient? Did she spend time with you? Who was your role model that you most identified with?

How did your mom and dad discipline you? If physical—What exactly was done to you—give details. If emotional, how were you impacted? Were you punished when you deviated from the family rules, morals, when you experimented? Did you have any older brothers or sisters? How did they treat you?

Where you able to talk about your sexuality? Who and How were you taught about sex? Who was there for you? Who played, laughed, and had fun with you? How did your wounded inner child contaminate your adolescent life? Who was your peer group? What did you feel was peer pressure?

Pay attention to anything you now know about family secrets that you couldn't have known as a child. For example, was dad a sex addict, having lots of affairs? Is either parent an untreated victim of physical, sexual, or emotional violence. Family secrets are always about the family's toxic shame. Focus on all the ways you were shamed—all the ways your feelings, needs, and desires were repressed. Consider lack of discipline or too much discipline. Write about any traumatic incidents and be detailed and concrete as possible. Details bring us back to the actual experience which comes closer to touching our actual feelings. When considering teachers, clergyman, older kids etc, write out each person's name and comment on whether they were nurturing or spiritually wounding.

Write about the three most important events of each year.

13 years old:

1. Started grade first grade
2. Peed in my pants one day and was humiliated in front of my class.

14 years old:

1. Passed to second grade.
2. Got a record player for Christmas
3. Was in a car accident

Continue the list until age 26. Remember pleasant and unpleasant memories.

Step Two: Share your adolescent history with a support person – Read your story to a friend, spouse, sponsor or therapist.

Step Three: Feeling the Feelings - If you have a photograph of yourself at school age, get it out. See how small and innocent you were. If you don't have a photo, spend some time with a school child. Focus on the normalcy of this developmental stage. Feel whatever feelings come up for you.

Step Four: Dysfunctional Family-System Roles – Get in touch with any new roles that you took on during the school age years and work with them as you did earlier. Focus on life damaging consequences of those roles.

Step Five: Letter Writing – Home coming meditation

Step Six: Affirmations –

It's okay to learn to do things your own way.
It's okay to think about things and try them out before your make them your own.
You can trust your own judgments; you need only take the consequences of your choices.
You can do things your own way and it's okay to disagree.
I love you just the way you are.
You can choose your own friends
You can dress the way the other kids dress, or you can dress your own way.
I'm willing to be with you no matter what.
I love you

Step Seven: Forgiveness – Real harm was done to us and it needs to be legitimatized and validated. When we acknowledge the real harm that was done, we demythologize our parents. We free them for the real wounded human beings they actually are (were). We see that they were adult children acting out their own contaminations.

Only by demythologizing our parents can we grasp the real harm that was done to us and allow us to own our feelings about being violated. Once we have connected with and expressed those feelings, we are free to move on. Forgiveness allows us to leave our parents. Our frozen grief formed the deep resentments that kept us attached to them. Resentments cause us to recycle the same feelings over and over again. Forgiveness is the way we leave home.

Once we reclaim who we really are, we must make a decision about our real parents. What kind of relationship will we have with them? If they are still offenders stay away from them and keep healthy boundaries. As Jesus, perhaps we need to say, "forgive them for they know not what they do." In the Greek, it suggests that he repeated that phrase over and over again, there are times we need to do the same.

As we reconnect to our true identity, our I AMness in soul, it opens the way for our soul to reconnect with our spirit. We can tell our inner child about our personal relationship with our Higher Power Jesus Christ. You can let the child know that he makes you feel safe and protected and in times of trouble you call on him. Tell the child that Jesus came into the world as a child and grew up to be a man and his name was Jesus. Jesus tells me that God is both my mother and father. Jesus tells me I can have a friendship with him. He tells me that he made me the way that I am and wants me to grow and expand in my I AMness. He tells us not to judge others and to forgive. Jesus modeled His own I AMness. That is why He said "I am the truth." I can talk to Him. He loves me just the way that I am. In fact, my I AMness is like God's I AMness. When I truly am, I am most like God. We need to let our inner child know that God loves us and will always protect us and be with us. There is a power we can call on that is greater than both of us.

When we reconnect with the I AMness of our soul, our personality, strengths, gifts and abilities, we feel a renewed hope, purpose, initiative, and competence, we will feel a reconnection with our spirit and our I AMness in Christ.

It also reconnects us to family. It is imperative to let the inner child know that we have been adopted into a new family, the family of God.

A new family is necessary in order to give our child protection while we form new boundaries and do corrective learning. We also need to keep a safe distance and work on finding a new, non-shaming, supportive extended family. This could be a support group of friends, your 12 Step Group or your local church.

This will mean that as family we need to live by a new set of rules that are not shaming. Scott Peck states good discipline involves rules that allow a person to be who he is. Such rules enhance our being and protect our I AMness. The following is a set of rules to teach our inner child.

1. It's okay to feel what you feel. Feelings are not right or wrong. They just are. There is no one who can tell you what you should feel. It's good and it's necessary to talk about feelings.

2. It's okay to want what you want. There's nothing you should or should not want. If you're in touch with your spirit, you will want to expand and grow. It's okay and it's necessary to get your needs met. It's good to ask for what you want.

3. It's okay to see and hear what you see and hear. Whatever you saw and heard is what you saw and heard.

4. It's okay and it's necessary to have lots of fun and play.

5. It's essential to tell the truth at all times. This will reduce life's pain. Lying distorts reality. All forms of distorted thinking must be corrected.

6. It's important to know your limits and to delay gratification some of the time. This will reduce life's pain.

7. It's crucial to develop a balanced sense of responsibility. This means accepting the consequences for what you do and refusing to accept the consequences for what someone else does.

8. It's okay to make mistakes. Mistakes are our teachers—they help us to learn.

9. Other people's feelings, needs and wants are to be respected and valued. Violating other people leads to guilt and to accepting the consequences.

10. It's okay to have problems. They need to be resolved. It's okay to have conflict. It needs to be restored.

RECOVERY:

R. – Relativize the Absolutist Will – Live by the Serenity Prayer, one day at a time, learn to delay gratification. Accept your limitations and what you can't change.

E. – Experience Emotions – You are no longer psychically numb. You start to experience your emotions. You grieve, feel the shame, anger, embarrassment. You can't heal what you don't feel. Remember that feelings are our primary biological motivators. What you feel at any given moment is the core of your authentic reality at that moment. Growing up in a dysfunctional home means that your shame is so enmeshed with shame that to feel anything is to feel shame. So we need to tell ourselves that it is safe to express our feelings.

Practice for twenty-one days, spending thirty minutes a day just noticing you're feeling. Listen to music or watch a movie or TV show because it may trigger feelings. Instead of pushing down the feelings, take a deep breath and really let yourself have it. Exaggerate it physically as fully as you can. Try to name the emotions your feelings because wounded children get confused between thoughts and feelings.

Practice expressing current anger: Take assertive training courses. Follow the STEPS:

S-Situation: Describe what has occurred
T-Thoughts: Describe what you are thinking
E-Emotions: Describe what your feeling and stick to feeling words.
P-Plans: Describe what you have done, are doing, or plan to do, to deal with the situation.
S-Statement of valuing: I care more about our relationship than being right.

Some people find it easier to write these out first before verbally expressing. Practice what you want to say out loud and when ready contact the person. Sooner is better than later. You might want to preface what you say by saying something like, "When I was growing up my dad would always say we were going to do something and then he wouldn't show up and I would be devastated, so when you…" Remember we choose to be angry, no one is powerful enough to make us angry.

C. – Collapse Grandiosity – You have given up your denials about being able to control your addiction. You are more realistic and have more realistic expectations of yourself and others. You can laugh at more things. They are not so dramatic or serious.

O. – Oneness with Self – You are starting to accept yourself. You are accepting the responsibility for your life and know your happiness will depend on you. Your starting to trust your feelings, perceptions and wants. Toxic guilt denies you the right to be your unique self. It enhances your spiritual wound. Toxic guilt is twofold. One form of it results from living in a dysfunctional family system. With the rigid roles if someone tries to change they are often quilted. The second form of guilt results from anger turned against oneself. As a child you were angry at your parents but you were not allowed to express that anger. To work on this guilt you need to express the underlying anger directly.

> Practice by making a list of childhood events about which you were made to feel guilty. Redo these events in your imagination and assert your rights. You may say something like, "Hey, I'm just a normal 5 year old who loves to play. I'm trying to set my boundaries. I'm angry at you for spoiling my fun."

V. – Values Restored – Feel good about living according to your values. You have a sense of cleanness about yourself.

E. – Externalizing Shame – You have come out of hiding. You are asking for help to be vulnerable. As you embrace the shame, you discover that you're not that bad. Shame is now a feeling not a state of being.

R. – Rigorous Honesty – Working on Step 4 and 5 about your character defects such as perfectionism, judgment, manipulation, personality weakness, defense mechanism, you are becoming aware when you are being dishonest.

Y. – Yin/Yang Balance – Your life is becoming balanced. It's not all or nothing. The peaks and valleys are not as dramatic.

UNCOVER:

U. – Uncovering Your Interpersonally Transferred "carried shame." It is a long process by which we transform the shame back into a feeling then reduce the shame by giving back to those "shameless" significant others who transferred it to us. Realizing how we were abandoned and expressing our feelings about it is the beginning.

N. – Normalcy and Averageness – Normalcy is being within certain limits that define the range of normal functioning and averageness is the state of being that is average; indicates normality but with connotations of mediocrity.

C. – Corrective Experiences Concerning Basic Needs- This involves uncovering the lost child that hides within us. As adults, many opportunities arise for us to embrace the child within us and do the work of reparenting ourselves. Allowing God's voice as our heavenly father, speak into our souls by His authority. This is TRUTH telling and cognitive restructuring. We can also learn, as adults, to let the nurturing we get from others be parenting.

O. – Original Pain-Greif Work for Abandonment – It begins with shock and denial. It proceeds to a kind of bargaining, then to anger, guilt, remorse, sadness, hurt and finally acceptance. Give up the illusion of a happy childhood, can free us. See your childhood as a sacrifice to come to a place of discovering what true unconditional love is in God.

V. – Values Formation – One internet writer best summarizes the formation of values, at www.significanceofvalues.com/formayinon/index.html, by stating forming values starts in our childhood.

> First we learn to appreciate things that fulfill our basic needs, but we value especially those people that provide them to us. Their behavior towards us becomes the main reference of what is valuable.

Thus, our character and personality are molded through the attitudes and behavior of the people who raise us, whether they're our parents or other relatives. Their behaviors determine in large part what will subsequently become our most important beliefs and principles.

We learn to value the substance and the form of everything they say and do, and what they don't say and don't do. Each gesture or comment affects how we learn to make choices. We also learn to differentiate between the theory and practice of values. The latter is what marks us the most.

So the consistency and coherence of our parents' behavior is what strengthens our formation. If they practice what they preach, our personality will be stronger than if they don't.

Later, when we are students, we start feeling social pressures and the pressure of values that are different from ours, as we relate to other people. The strength of the values formed through our parents is put to the test.

Values are often confused with habits, and many parents hope that school will form the values that were not instilled at home. This is not possible, because school does not fulfill the basic needs of life... that is the responsibility of those who raise us.

Teachers, leaders, and value models at school can reinforce what was formed at home, but they cannot replace them. If the convictions formed at home are not solid, they will soon be exposed to an intense social competition against other beliefs.

Why is it so difficult to form values? Because, unlike norms, values are convictions; they are behaviors we gladly decide to follow and produce satisfaction. We can follow norms against our will, but values have the support of our will. We have learned their importance due to the benefits they produce, individually and collectively.

Those who play a leadership role in our lives are most powerful at conveying to us their values. They are our parents, elder siblings, grandparents, some relatives, teachers, peers we admire, professors, and bosses.

However, to convey something, we must first possess it. Values are only conveyed through the example of our daily attitudes and behaviors. They can seldom be formed by explaining them or through a list of what is considered correct or incorrect. Memorizing their theoretical meaning does not guarantee their implementation.

E. – Ego Repair and Boundary Work – No one in a dysfunctional family has a right to any autonomy and separateness. This lack of differentiation means that no one had the right to be different. Therefore, to be autonomous and different is to feel guilty. Guilt is the symptom of family enmeshment and no personal boundaries.

Establish your own separate domain: A useful practice in changing enmeshed or co-dependent relationship is to make a list of what belongs to you. You may also want to make a time chart which indicates which times belong to you for privacy and solitude, and what times you are willing to share.

Practice Confrontation: A good model to use is the "awareness model." I modify it to include the five powers each of us possesses in order to interact with the world. These are our senses, our minds, our emotions, and our wills and love. You use "I" messages to convey the truth of my awareness. I statements are self-responsible statements. It looks like this:

I see, hear, etc..(senses-body)
I interpret… ….(mind, thinking-Soul)
I feel… … … … ..(emotions-Soul)
I want… … … ..(desire-soul)
I need… … … … (love: accurate assessment and adequate supply-spirit)

Confronting is honest and creates trust; therefore, it is an act of love. When I confront, I value myself and set a boundary. I trust and value enough to tell you what's going on in me.

Practice "Fight-Fair Rules:" The ones I like are:

-Stay in the now, fight about what just happened, not about something in the distant past.
-Avoid scorekeeping. The child in us wants to save things up and later dump them on people.
-Stay with the concrete, specific behavioral detail. Remember a child does better with things it hears, sees and touches verses statements like "you make me sick."
-Be honest
-Avoid blame and judgment. These are cover-ups for your shame. Stay with the "I" statements and use the awareness model.
-Use the listening rule, which has you repeat to the other person what you heard him/her say before you go the answer. The child rarely listens if they are shame-based and defensive.
-Avoid arguing about details.
-Avoid withdrawing, stay in there until you find resolution, unless it is abusive, for your personal boundaries sake, leave.

Practice saying "no," this is usually pretty scary if you were punished and/or abandoned for saying "no" as a child. Practice on your own, repeating it 20 times in the mirror, then move on to practice with another person. Lastly say "no' to someone and mean it. You can say something like, "thanks for asking me! But no..." Remember you're not responsible for the other persons' feelings. Some "no's" are much harder than others. It is hard when you want something or when it touches a vulnerable area of unfulfilled need. A person who is starving to be touched and held may experience great difficulty in turning down a sexual come-on.

Practice physical boundaries: Develop a statement like, "I have the right to determine who can touch me. I will tell others when and how they may touch me. I can withdraw from physical contact anytime it feels unsafe to me. I can do so without explanation. I will never let anyone violate my body."

Practice setting emotional boundaries: A statement may sound something like this," Emotions are not right or wrong. They simply are. What you feel about me is about your emotional history; what I feel about you is about my emotional history. I will respect and value your emotions and I ask you to do the same for me. I will not be manipulated by your anger, sadness, fear, or joy."

R. – Recycling Childhood Needs as an Adult - Offers adults the opportunity to make choices about what, how and whom they want to be. This approach enables the adult to initiate and direct their life with the support of interested and responsive others. They construct their own knowledge from their experiences and interactions with the world around and fosters growth and development of their inner child's interests, needs and strengths within a safe and caring environment.

DISCOVER:

D. – Differentation – Individuation – You are realizing your true self. You love and affirm yourself for your uniqueness. This exercise is from Corrina and Steve Andrea and their book *Heart of the Mind*. It is recommended that you record the process or have a friend or therapist walk through these steps with you. Find a quite space where you will not be distracted.

Step One: The Enmeshed Parent - Close your eyes and focus your attention on memories of the parent you feel the most enmeshed with. Really see, feel, or hear that person in your internal experience. Let them be present to you in their most attractive behavior. Your unconscious will know exactly what that behavior is…
Trust the first thing that comes to your mind. If you cannot visualize your parent, just sense or pretend that he or she is there.

Step Two: Feeling the Enmeshment – Now see your wounded school age inner child standing next to that parent… Notice what the child is wearing… Hear your child talking to the parent… Now float into your inner child's body and look out of his/her eyes at your parent… Look at your parent from different angles… Notice how your parent sounds… How your parent smells… Now walk over and embrace your parent… What does it feel like to be in physical contact with that parent?...In what ways do you feel over-connected? How do you experience that parent as attached to you? Is it a physical attachment? Is it an attachment to some part of your body? Is there a cord or some other means of attachment between you? Get a full experience of the quality of this connection.

Step Three: Temporarily Breaking the Enmeshment – Now sever this connection for a moment… Just allow yourself to notice what it would be like. If you are attached by a cord, imagine cutting it with scissors… If you are attached to your parents' body, imagine a laser beam severing you and heals the wound simultaneously… You will feel discomfort separating at this point… This is a signal that this connection serves an important purpose in your life. Remember that you are not disconnecting. You are only experiencing what it feels like to separate temporarily.

Step Four: Discovering the Positive Purpose of the Enmeshment – Now ask yourself, "What do I really get from this parent that satisfies my basic needs?"..."What do I really want from that parent?"... Wait until you get an answer that touches you to the core—such as safety, security, protection from death, feeling that you matter, that your are lovable and worthwhile... Now reconnect the attachment to your parent.

Step Five; Using Your Adult Potency – Now turn to the right or left and see yourself as wise. Become aware that this older you is capable of giving you what you want and believe you are getting from your enmeshed parental relationship. Really look at your resourceful adult self... Notice how this part of you looks, moves, and sounds. Go over and embrace your grown-up self... Feel the power and potency of your adult... Realize that the worst thing you've always feared has already happened to you... You were violated and abandoned by being enmeshed,... and your adult part has made it,...your adult has survived and functioned in spite of it.

Step Six; Transforming the Connection with Your Parent into a Connection with Yourself – Turn again to your enmeshed parent... See and feel the connection... Sever the connection and immediately reconnect with your adult self in the same way you were connected to your parent... Enjoy feeling interdependent with someone you can completely count on: yourself. Thank your adult for being there for you. Enjoy receiving from your adult what you wanted from your parent. Your adult is the person that you can never lose.

Step Seven; Rejecting Your Enmeshed Parent – Now look at your enmeshed parent and notice that he has choice...He can reconnect the cord to his adult self. Remember that your parent has the same options for reclaiming and wholeness if he/she stays attached to you... You are loving them by giving them a chance for wholeness. Also notice that you now have an opportunity for a true relationship with them for the very first time.

Step Eight; Relationship with Self – Now float back into your adult self... Feel the interconnection with your wounded inner school-age child. Realize that you can now love and cherish this child and give him what he needed from his parent.

Final Step; Finish with a Fairy Tale. Here's how my story ends…

I. – Intuitive Vision- You are having powerful insights. At times you experience an immediate knowledge of God's presence.

S. – Spiritual Disciplines – You are practicing meditation. You put time aside each day to make conscious contact with God.

C. – Creativity – Creative Love – You trust your sensations, feelings and thoughts. You are committed to service. You are creative in your love.

O. – Oneness –Unification of Polarity – You do not see the world as black and white. You see there is no joy without pain, no light without darkness. Thinking in extremes is devastating to relationships. No one can love unconditionally including you.
Practice polarity thinking: Look at peoples' assets and liabilities. Tell yourself everyone has plus and minuses. We all have an "as is" tag, some defects are just more obvious in some than others, and others are just really good at hiding it. Don't set people up to be god, so they can fail you.

V. – Values Concerned with Being – You are most concerned about truth and honesty. You are less possessive and attached. Your life is less complex and more attached

E. – Energized and Empowered – You feel one with yourself and are in less internal conflict.

R. – Reverence for Life - Peacemaking – You want to leave the world a better place.

Appendix XI
Soul Design: Personality Profile

Who am I? If we stay true to the Trinitarian nature of who we are then we do need to ask the question three different ways, body, soul and spirit. I have explored the question as it has related to our spirit and secondly to whom we are physically and biologically as it relates to our body?

Now I ask the question in relationship to your personality, the psychology of our soul as we have come to know it. Our aim in completing the profile and studying the temperaments is to assess our basic strengths and realize that we are people of value and worth; to become aware of our weaknesses and set out to overcome them; to learn that just because other people are different doesn't make them wrong or that there is something wrong with us; and to accept the fact that since we can't change them we might as well love them as they are.

What pressure it takes off of us when we realize that we are not responsible for the behavior of those other people. How liberating it is when we realize God created us as unique individuals and we don't have to conform to someone else's image. The philosophical Socrates said, "To know thyself is the beginning of wisdom."

God created each one of us to be unique creations, special blendings of the four humors—Sanguine, Choleric, Melancholy, and Phlegmatic.

As we use these terms from Hippocrates as tools in following God's command that we examine ourselves and understand how people have tampered with God's original plan for our life, we should gain a better understanding not only of our personality and traits but also of those other members of our family.

Christian people are longing for some sense of identity and self-worth. They study the Word; they know they are created in God's image and made slightly lower than the angels; they've been crucified in Christ and have taken off the old clothes and put on the new. They have gone to church, knelt at the alter, and taught Bible studies. And yet still remain stifled and confused in their soul identity, trying to be someone they were never meant to be.

As sex addicts we have underlying needs that we don't always communicate clearly to others. We think if they really loved us, they would know what we needed. To prevent this type of problem in your life or to heal underlying wounds you need to first identify what your personality or soul needs are.

Personality Needs

The Sanguine needs attention and approval. While they want to have fun in life and appear to have no serious requirements for happiness, underneath they have a craving for approval. They need to know that they are accepted. They feed on compliments and criticism wounds them deeply. Given praise and encouragement the Sanguine will go to extremes to please you, for they want to be loved. They are sexually tempted when their significant other doesn't give compliments or laugh at their humor. Because they get desperate for love and excitement they may find it in the wrong place. They are most prone to depression when life's no fun and there is too much criticism. There is fear in being alone and unpopular. Getting old and lonely and running out of money. There stress relief is shopping, partying with friends or eat to cheer up. Spiritually their barrier to becoming a Christian is it doesn't sound like fun and those people are too serious. They get hung up with the idea of holiness and purity. They see that there are too many strict rules and commandments.

The Choleric has the emotional need for achievement and appreciation. They are born leaders and have a need to see things accomplished and have a mental progress list in their brain. They have an insatiable need to get things done now. If there is a block to their accomplishment they will suggest, list, demand and threat, or storm off in anger. They are sexually tempted when their significant other doesn't get things done and doesn't appreciate his/her achievements. They like the chase and conquest more than commitment. They feel the need to be in control of relationships. They are prone to depression when life's out of control and there's no appreciation. They fear losing control, being sick or weak. When they are stressed they work harder, exercise more and stay away from unyielding situations. They have a problem becoming a Christian because they don't want to give up control especially someone they can't see. They have trouble with the authority of God and too little control of their own destiny.

The Melancholy needs order and sensitivity. They are perfectionist who must have their life in order and hopefully everyone else's as well. They have a deep need to be understood and long for others to respond with sensitivity to their inner struggles and to commiserate with them over a flippant comment made by shallow people attempting to be funny. Because they are unwilling to express their needs, they throw others into a constant guessing game. "If you really loved me, you would be sensitive enough to my needs to figure them out. They are sexually tempted when their significant other lacks sensitivity to their needs and life is no longer in order. They long for deep meaningful relationships and likes romance, candles and music. They are prone to depression when life's a mess and there's no hope. They fear making mistakes, failing or having to compromise standards. When they are stressed they tend to withdraw from people, read, meditate or go to bed early. Melancholics have a barrier to believing in Christ because they don't believe they will be perfect enough. They have trouble with forgiveness for those who don't deserve it and feel that there's too much unconditional love.

Phlegmatic's need respect and a feeling of worth. Their goal in life is to keep the peace, and when this is not possible they will sometimes withdraw and shut down until some facsimile of peace is restored. They will often feel useless and of no value because they are not crying out for attention. They are sexually tempted when their mate takes them for granted and they feel worthless. They want someone who makes them feel worthwhile and won't ridicule or demand too much action. They are prone to depression when life's full of problems and there's no peace. They fear being pressured, facing conflict or being left to hold the bag. When they are stressed they tend to tune out on life, turn on the TV, eat and sleep. The barrier to them becoming a Christian is that they would have to change. They also have trouble with truth and responsibility before God. They believe there is too much emphasis on good works.

Directions: In each of the following rows of four words across, place an X in front to the word that most often applies to you. Continue through all forty lines. Be sure each number is marked. If you are not sure of which word "most applies," ask spouse or a friend, and think of what your answer would have been when you were a child.

Personality Profile
Strengths

1.____Adventurous ____Adaptable ____Animated ____Analytical
2.____Persistent ____Playful ____Persuasive ____Peaceful
3.____Submissive ____Self-sacrificing ____Sociable ____Strong-willed
4.____Considerate ____Controlled ____Competitive ____Convincing
5.____Refreshing ____Respectful ____Reserved ____Resourceful
6.____Satisfied ____Sensitive ____Self-reliant ____Spirited
7.____Planner ____Patient ____Positive ____Promoter
8.____Sure ____Spontaneous ____Scheduled ____Shy
9.____Orderly ____Obligingly ____Outspoken ____Optimistic
10.____Friendly ____Faithful ____Funny ____Forceful

11.___Daring ___Delightful ___Diplomatic ___Detailed

12.___Cheerful ___Consistent ___Cultured ___Confident

13.___Idealistic ___Independent ___Inoffensive ___Inspiring

14.___Demonstrative ___Decisive ___Dry Humor ___Deep

15.___Mediator ___Musical ___Mover ___Mixes easily

16.___Thoughtful ___Tenacious ___Talker ___Tolerant

17.___Listener ___Loyal ___Leader ___Lively

18.___Contented ___Chief ___Chart maker ___Cute

19.___Perfectionist ___Pleasant ___Productive ___Popular

20.___Bouncy ___Bold ___Behaved ___Balanced

Personality Profile Weaknesses

21.___Blank ___Bashful ___Brassy ___Bossy

22.___Undisciplined___Unsympathetic___Unenthusiastic ___Unforgiving

23.___Reticent ___Resentful ___Resistant ___Repetitious

24.___Fussy ___Fearful ___Forgetful ___Frank

25.___Impatient ___Insecure ___Indecisive ___Interrupts

26.___Unpopular___Uninvolved__Unpredictable___Unaffectionate

27.___Headstrong ___Haphazard ___Hard to Please ___Hesitant

28.___Plain ___Pessimistic ___Proud ___Permissive

29.___Anger easily ___Aimless ___Argumentative___Alienated

30.___Naive ___Negative attitude ___Nervy ___Nonchalant

31.___Worrier ___Withdrawn ___Workaholic ___Wants Credit

32.___Too sensitive ___Tactless ___Timid ___Talkative

33.___Doubtful ___Disorganized ___Domineering___Depressed

34.___Inconsistent ___Introverted ___Intolerant ___Indifferent

35.___Messy ___Moody ___Mumbles ___Manipulative

36.___Slow ___Stubborn ___Show-off ___Skeptical

37.___Loner ___Lord over ___Lazy ___Loud

38.___Sluggish___Suspicious___Short-tempered___Scatterbrained

39.___Revengeful ___Restless ___Reluctant ___Rash

40.___Compromising___Critical___Crafty___Changeable

Now transfer all your "X's" to the corresponding words on the personality scoring sheet and add up your total.

Created by Fred Lettauer

Personality Scoring Sheet not to be reproduced—Copies may be ordered from 1814 Commercenter West Suite E, San Bernadino, CA 92408 or (714) 888-8665 or at the back of the Florence Littauer's book Your Personality Tree

Personality Strengths and Weaknesses

Exercise: Go through your previous answers and circle the corresponding words below under the personaliy strenghts and weaknesses. Also circle the "Emotions, Work, and Friends" characteristics that are best describe you under all the Personality Profile strengths and weaknesses.

Sanguine:(Talker)

Sanguine Personality strengths

Character: Animated, playful, Sociable, Convincing, Refreshing, Spirited, Promoter, Spontaneous, Optimistic, Funny, Delightful, Cheerful, Inspiring, Demonstrative,, Mixes easily, Talkier, Lively, Cute, Popular, Bouncy.

Emotions: Appealing personality, talkative, storyteller, life-of-the-party, good sense of humor, memory of color, physically holds onto listener, emotional and demonstrative, enthusiastic and expressive, cheerful and bubbling over, curious, good on stage, wide-eyed and innocent, lives in the present, changeable disposition, sincere at heart, always a child.

Work: Volunteers for jobs, thinks up new activities, looks great on the surface, creative and colorful, has an energy and enthusiasm, start in a flashy way, inspires others to join, charms others at work.

Friends: Makes friends easily, loves people, thrives on compliments, seems exciting, envied by others, doesn't hold grudges, apologizes quickly, prevents dull moments, likes spontaneous activities.

Sanguine Personality Weaknesses:

Character: Brassy, Undisciplined, Repetitious, Forgetful, Interrupts, Unpredictable, Haphazard, Permissive, Angered easily, Naive, Wants credit, Talkative, Disorganized, Inconsistent, Messy, Show-off, Loud Scatterbrained, Restless, Changeable.

Emotions: Compulsive talker, exaggerates and elaborates; dwells on trivia, can't remember names; scares others off, too happy for some, has restless energy, egotistical, blusters and complains, naive, gets taken in, has loud voice and laugh, controlled by circumstances, gets angry easily, seems phony to some, never grows up.

Work: Would rather talk, forgets obligations, doesn't follow through, confidence fades fast, undisciplined, priorities out of order, decides by feelings, easily distracted, wastes time talking.

Friends: Hates to be alone, needs to be center stage, wants to be popular, looks for credit, dominates conversations, interrupts and doesn't listen, answers for others, fickle and forgetful, makes excuses, repeats stories.

Choleric (The Worker)

Choleric Personality Strengths:

Character: Adventurous, Persuasive, Strong-willed, Competitive, Resourceful, Self-reliant, Positive, Sure, Outspoken, Forceful, Daring, Confident, Independent, Decisive, Mover, Tenacious, Leader, Chief, Productive, Bold.

Emotions: Born leader, dynamic and active, compulsive need for change, must correct wrongs, strong-willed and decisive, unemotional, not easily discouraged, independent and self-sufficient, excludes confidence, can run anything.

Work: Goal-oriented, sees the whole picture, organizes well, seeks practical solutions, moves quickly to action, delegates work, insists on production, makes the goal, stimulates activity, thrives on opposition.

Friends: Has little need for friends, will work for group activity, will lead and organize, is usually right, and excels in emergencies.

Choleric Personality Weaknesses:

Character: Bossy, Unsympathetic, Resistant, Frank, Impatient, Unaffectionate, Headstrong, Proud, Argumentative, Nervy, Workaholic, Tactless, Domineering, Intolerant, Manipulative, Stubborn, Lord over others, Short-tempered, Rash, Crafty.

Emotions: Bossy, impatient, quick-tempered, can't relax, too impetuous, enjoys controversy & arguments, won't give up when losing, comes on too strong, inflexible, in not complimentary, dislikes tears and emotions, is unsympathetic.

Work: Little tolerance for mistakes, doesn't analyze details, bored by trivia, may make rash decisions, may be rude or tactless, manipulates people, demanding of others, end justifies the means, work may become his god, demands loyalty in the ranks.

Friends: Tends to use people, dominates others, decides for others, knows everything, can do everything better, is too independent, possessive of friends and mate, can't say, "I'm sorry," may be right, but unpopular.

Melancholy (The Thinker)

Melancholy Personality Strengths:

Character: Analytical, Persistent, Self-sacrificing, Considerate, Respectful, Sensitive, Planner, Scheduled, Orderly, Faithful, Detailed, Cultured, Idealistic, Deep, Musical, Thoughtful, Loyal, Chart maker, Perfectionist, Behaved.

Emotions: Deep and thoughtful, analytical, serious and purposeful, talented and creative, artistic and musical, philosophical and poetic, appreciative of beauty, sensitive to others, self-sacrificing, conscientious, idealistic.

Work: Schedule-oriented, perfectionist, high standards, detail-conscious, persistent and thorough, orderly and organized, neat and tidy, economical, sees the problems, finds creative solutions, needs to finish what he starts, likes chart, graph, figures, lists.

Friends: Makes friends cautiously, content to stay in background, avoids causing attention, faithful and devoted, will listen to complaints, can solve others problems, deep concern for other people, moved to tears with compassion, seeks ideal mate.

Melancholy Personality Weaknesses:

Character: Bashful, Unforgiving, Resentful, Fussy, Insecure, Unpopular, Hard to please, Pessimistic, Alienated, Negative attitude, Withdrawn, Too sensitive, Depressed, Introvert, Moody, Skeptical, Loner, Suspicious, Revengeful, Critical.

Emotions: Remembers the negatives, moody and depressed, enjoys being hurt, has false humility, off in another world, low self-image, has selective hearing, self-centered, too introspective, guilt feelings, persecution complex, tends to hypochondria.

Work: Not people-oriented, depressed over imperfections, chooses difficult work, hesitant to start projects, spends too much time planning, prefers analysis to work, self-depreciating, hard to please standards often too high, deep need for approval.

Friendships: Lives through others, insecure socially, withdrawn and remote, critical of others, holds back affection, dislikes those in opposition, suspicious of people, antagonistic and vengeful, unforgiving, full of contradictions, skeptical of compliments.

Phlegmatic (The Watcher)

Phlegmatic Personality Strengths:

Character: Adaptable, Peaceful, Submissive, Controlled, Reserved, Satisfied, Patient, Shy, Obliging, Friendly, Diplomatic, Consistent, Inoffensive, Dry humor,

Mediator, Tolerant, Listener, Contented, Pleasant, Balanced.

Emotions: Low-key personality, easygoing and relaxed, calm, cool, and collected, patient, well-balanced, consistent life, quiet, but witty, sympathetic and kind, keeps emotions hidden, happily reconciled to life, all-purpose person.

Work: Competent and steady, peaceful and agreeable, has administrative ability, mediates problems, avoids conflicts, good under pressure, finds the easy way.

Friends: Easy to get along with, pleasant and enjoyable, inoffensive, good listener, dry sense of humor, enjoys watching people, has many friends, has compassion and concern.

Phlegmatic Personality Weaknesses:

Character: Blank, Unenthusiastic, Reticent, Fearful, Indecisive, Uninvolved, Hesitant, Plain, Aimless, Nonchalant, Worrier, Timid, Doubtful, Indifferent, Mumbles, Slow, Lazy, Sluggish, Reluctant, Compromising.

Emotions: Unenthusiastic, fearful and wounded, indecisive, avoids responsibility, quiet will of iron, selfish, too shy and reticent, too compromising, self-righteous.

Work: Not goal-oriented, lacks self-motivation, hard to get moving, resents being pushed, lazy and careless discourages others, would rather watch.

Friends: Dampens enthusiasm, stays uninvolved, is not exciting, indifferent to plans, judges others, sarcastic and teasing, resists change.

Are You Wearing A Mask?

	Yes	No
1. Personality Profile comes out with relatively even splits between Sanguine and Melancholy or when you are half Choleric with half Phlegmatic.		
2. Did you have trouble taking the Personality Profile Test?		
3. Were you uncertain on many of the words and not sure which one to choose?		
4. Did you feel you needed someone else's opinion to help you decide?		
5. Do you lack assurance that the way your scores came out is the real you?		
6. Do you come out differently each time you do the profile test?		
7. Do you feel confused as to who you really are?		
8. Have you been insecure about you self worth for as long as you can remember?		
9. Do you think you were one person as a child and someone different as an adult?		
10. Do you sometimes wonder if people can see through you?		
11. Do you often wish you were someone else?		

Causes of Masking

(Put a check mark beside the one's that relate to you)

1.____A Domineering Parent: A parent who constantly requires the child to conform to the personality he or she wants the child to have forces the child to wear a mask.

2.____ A Domineering and Controlling Spouse: A spouse can have the same effect as a domineering parent, when trying to conform a personality.

3.____ An Alcoholic Parent: A child who has an alcoholic parent feels unnatural pressures to perform or contribute to the household, often assuming parental roles not natural for the child or his or her God-given birth personality. They will often feel responsible for the chaos around them. Even when they don't understand what is happening.

4.____ A Legalistic Religious Household: Everyone is expected to be a spiritual giant, living up to the letter of the law.

5.____Strong Feelings of Rejection in Childhood: Often parents are so busy earning money that they have little eye-to-eye contact with their children. They perceive that the giving of money and gifts satisfies the children's need for love. Sometimes the other parent overprotects the child or depends on that child for his or her happiness. All children who are abused in any form also have feelings of rejection.

6.____Feeling of Rejection as an Adult: Due to loss of job, friends, mate, or children. Other causes include put-downs, feelings of exclusion, and inferences of stupidity. No one seems to like them, and they are often ignored.

7.____A Single-Parent Home: A first-born, may often be required to fulfill some of the roles of the absent parent. If they move back and forth between parents in a divorce situation their feelings of rejection are renewed each week. The confusion will be even greater if one parent has one set of standards that is drastically different from the others.

8.____Any form of Verbal, Emotional, or Physical Abuse: It will imply worthlessness, shame and give them the message that they are a bad person. Many parents consider themselves to be loving parents but in fact they are taking out their insecurities and anger on their children.

9.____Childhood Sexual Interference: Any form of touching the child in a sexual way or having the child touch the adult in an inappropriate manner. The child subconsciously rationalizes, maybe if I would just be good enough, he would leave me alone.

10.____Abuse Received as an Adult: This may be any type of abuse--verbal, emotional, physical, or sexual—received after the age of eighteen. If you felt hurt and ashamed when it happened, it was abuse. Emotionally stable people will not allow themselves to be victimized more than one or two times before taking action. The person who was abused as a child usually will not go for help until the seventh major attack, according to reports from spouse abuse centre.

If you have checked off any of the above, I would suggest using Fred & Florence Littauer's book, "*Get a Life Without the Strife.*"

Exercise:

What personality traits have become character defects and contribute to your addiction?

____

____

____

What are three personality weaknesses that you would like to see changed?

1.______________________________________

____

____

2.______________________________________

____

____

3.______________________________________

____

____

What are three emotional needs that you like to have met by a significant other in your life?

1.______________________________________

____

____

2.______________________________________

____

____

3.____

What personality mask have you been wearing? Why? And When?

Give three examples when you experienced rejection in your life and replace them with a truth statement.

1.____

2.____

3.____

List those who abused you emotionally, physically, sexually or otherwise, explain.

List those you need to forgive.

Pull up the weeds: Read Exodus 20:6, Deuteronomy 4:40, 7:9; Isaiah 48:18; Matthew 15:13; Hebrews 12:1, 15 Having thought about families and their personalities, you will have seen some distorted roots, what roots do you need to take an axe too. ____________________

Burn the dead branches: Read John 15:6; Jeremiah 11:16 What dead branches have you been saving from the fire? ____________________

____

____

Repair the wastelands: Read Isaiah. 61:4; Joel 2:25; I Peter 2:9 remember that God often gets our attention by sending us to the desert. What did you learn from your wilderness experience? Write down the periods of waste. ____________________

____

____

Produce Fruit: Read Isaiah 61:9, Deuteronomy 5:29; Psalm 51:3 How has God showed you mercy? ____________________

____

____

Tips:

Popular Sanguine: Learn to listen, don't interrupt, don't laugh everything off. Accept the fact that life is full of strife. Face reality, and don't expect others to protect you forever.

Perfect Melancholy: Don't take everything personally. Realize life may not be quite as bad as it seems at the moment.

Powerful Choleric: Don't expect everyone to want to do it your way. Don't assume you know everything. Let people offer opinions without cutting them off or putting them down. Don't get angry if others disagree. They might be right.

Peaceful Phlegmatic: Speak up, make decisions, move into action, and say what you mean. Don't procrastinate and expect others to do your work. Be willing to take a risk. You probably have the best idea of all.

Appendix XII
Body Work: Stress Management

In the 12 Step program you will hear the acronym HALT used which stands for Hungry, Angry, Lonely and Tired. If you haven't figured it out already, I like acronyms, primarily because it helps me to remember things. So in the case of HALT when we feel any of these feelings, both physically (body) and emotionally (soul), they are indicators of potential relapse, hence the need to "halt" or stop and address one or more of those needs. One or all of these symptoms in and of themselves have the potential to cause stress and anxiety on our overall body system.

So when we consider our recovery we need to consider nutrition and exercise as a vital part to our recovery. I spoke at length about the physical, biological and psychological effects of our sexual addiction. It only makes sense that we consider exercise and nutrition and how they benefit and help to rebalance what has become very imbalanced over time. As I stated early in the book, I have a Diploma in fitness and nutrition and was certified years ago as a Fitness Instructor. That does not make me an expert but indicates that I strongly believe in the benefits of exercise and nutrition. I do however have a niece who is currently finishing up her degree to be a homeopathic doctor. If given the chance she would stand on a mountain top and proclaim the importance of regular exercise and the medicinal benefits of good nutrition. I have found the book *Prescription for Nutritional Healing* by James and Phyllis Balch" to be an excellent source of self-help information. I have listed the book in the bibliography as a source.

Exercise

A reliable body of scientific evidence supports the immeasurable value of exercise and relaxation, and affirms both as critical to total health and well being. For doctors and researchers, debate about physical and mental exercise is a nonissue. It is widely recognized among health professionals that cardiovascular improvement through exercise is a life and brain extender. An effective exercise program can reduce your brain stress and body stress, improve health, firm muscles, and help you lose weight. The study defined "exercise" as planned workout time rather than normal, everyday-life-related activities.

If you recall I stated in the book that one of the areas that addicts have difficulty with is managing stress in both the body and soul. It has long since been proven that one of the most effective ways to manage stress is through developing a balanced life style with regular exercise and a healthy nutritional diet. So it is important to your recovery program to design one that is most helpful for your personal needs. A good way to get started is to have a few sessions with a fitness trainer to assess your fitness level, body type and determined what exercise program will work best for you. It may also be helpful, especially if you are currently on lots of pharmaceuticals for depression, anxiety, etc, to see a homeopathic doctor to re-evaluate your prescriptions (and no my niece did not tell me to say that).

If you want to try to go it alone there are lots of very good books out there for both men and women to help you get started and determine what is going to work best for your body type. I do suggest, however, that you at least get a medical assessment. Set reasonable goals and ease into it slowly and pace yourself. Remember as addicts we tend to be all or nothing and jump in with both feet with unrealistic expectations. So schedule your exercise time when you are not extremely tired but alert, are you an A.M. person or a P.M. person? Listen to your body so not to be counter-productive and cause chronic fatigue or injuries. Remember the goal is to reduce stress and anxiety not to cause more.

Give yourself some rewards and it is helpful for some people to have a partner. Perhaps most of all find something that is fun, you deserve it.

If one of the goals of exercise is to improve overall fitness, then we need to know what that means. Body and brain fitness means a well-conditioned, well-nourished muscular and brain system. Your brain, heart, muscles, and other vital organs need regular exercise to stay fit. Your body fitness is important for a healthy brain. You are fit if you can carry out daily mental tasks and challenges without feeling fatigue or being irritable, impatient, or upset. Secondly, that you can climb one or two flights of stairs without gasping for air or feeling fatigue in your legs. Thirdly carry out daily tasks with little or no struggle and have energy to spare.

Stretching, aerobic exercise and some kind of muscle resistant training is vital to overall body wellness. The benefits of regular exercise reduce overall risk of death from all causes, including cardiovascular disease and cancer, by about seventy percent. Some studies show that exercise promotes development of new coronary arteries if existing arteries are blocked due to blood fats. Regular exercisers are also less likely to suffer from stroke, high blood pressure, and other circulatory disorders. Exercise can also increase blood flow to the brain, improving mental ability. Lest I forget to mention that exercise is also key to reducing anxiety both physically and psychologically which is key to the addiction recovery. The addict has learned to self medicate when stressed and anxious; exercise is the healthy alternative.

Exercise is also a healthy way for the body to process the chemicals that are secreted during a stressful event. During the fight-or-flight process, your brain and body is made to believe that you are in danger and hormones electrify your system for action, and blood rushes to the vital organs to help you face the challenge. When this happens, you vasoconstrict in other parts of your body which means that the blood vessels tighten up in the extremities of your body, causing the heart to pump harder to push blood to the feet and the fingers. This state of alertness causes the hormones and nervous system to ignore other important bodily functions. The sympathetic nervous system not only triggers the negative effects, it also suppresses the activities in the parasympathetic nervous system, the other half of the autonomic nervous system that I discussed earlier in the book.

The parasympathetic nervous system controls many crucial mind-brain-body functions such as sleep, relaxation, and internal calmness—and is involved in quiet meditation and prayer. It is active in bodily recovery and healing process. It also promotes growth, energy, storage, blood pressure control, correct heart rhythms, maintenance of essential materials, and positive cognitions. Parasympathetic activity is also associated with controlling many of our emotions, including anger, rage, and irrational fears. But this half of our autonomic nervous system is generally inactive during a stress response.

Without having gone into great detail, it is clear that stress is hazardous to our health and our recovery. But just as exercise aids us in dealing with the stress hormones—corticotropin (CRF) and glucocorticoid along with epinephrine and norepinephrine in a healthy way so are there ways to prepare your body nutritionally for the onslaught of stress. Proper food will boost your immune system and help your bodily systems get back to normal after a sudden stressor.

Nutrition

The kind of food you eat affects measurably your mind, brain, body, emotions, and consequently your Christian walk and recovery. So you need to eat foods that help you view stressors positively.

Epidemiological research, have given us the knowledge to confirm that foods do have specific medicine—like properties to be used as immune protectors, cancer fighters, antihypertensives, antidepressants, sedatives, tranquilizers, analgesics, antibiotics and anti-inflammatory agents, to name a few uses. A term that has become quite vogue in this generation is "antioxidants." I don't know how many people really know what it means, but I like what Dr.Thomas Whiteman, Dr. Sam Verghese and Randy Petersen in their book *The Complete Stress Management Workbook* call it, "The Oxygen War." They tell us to imagine two opposing forces in our bodies, engaged in battle. The valiant defenders of health and vitality are the antioxidants, and the deficient defectors are the oxidants.

"In this war oxygen is the bad guy. It's actually a two-edged sword. Though it sustains life, oxygen can also damage our cells the same way it can rust iron. A combination of environmental pollutants, poor nutrition, smoking, and a normal cellular metabolic processes (such as breathing and immune functions) can rob normal oxygen atoms of crucial electrons. This produces unstable oxygen molecules with an insufficient number of electrons (free radicals). These are simply waste products, but they possess fierce destructive potency.

When our bodies are exposed to chronic stress, free radicals gain strength and attack our immune system. Antioxidants strive to protect our bodies by fending off these destructive oxidants.

The free radicals take various forms. Since the molecules of the free radical atoms lack one of the electrons that is required to keep them stable, they furiously travel throughout the body in search of the missing electron. In the process, they steal electrons from good but weak cells and create more free radical renegades. Then they continue their savage journey. This robbing and pairing of electrons creates a damaging free radical chain reaction in our bodies that erodes our cell membranes and can alter the many cells that encode genetic information in the DNA, these cells mutate. This is the first step on the path to cancer and other illnesses.

Only the free radical scavengers that occur naturally in our body can neutralize the radicals. This neutralization process is accomplished chiefly by antioxidant substances such as vitamin A and beta-carotene, vitamins C and E, glutathione, coenzyme Q10, selenium, lycopene, and other nutrients. You can get a sufficient supply of antioxidants by eating lots of fruits and

> vegetables. This will help maintain tissue concentration of these vital nutrients and although your B-complex vitamins are not an antioxidant, I just want to state they do play a key role in helping our nervous system battle against stress."

The following is a simple checklist of common complaints that might be remedied through better nutrition or vitamin supplements. Indicate which of the following most clearly corresponds to you in the past three to six months.

____Under chronic stress

____Tense and anxious

____Irritable

____Tire easily

____Restless sleep

____Trouble falling asleep

____Frequent headaches

____Can't relax

____Smoker

____Negative feelings

____Heavy smoker

____Constant stomach problems

____Can't make decisions

____Depressed

____Poor eating habits

____Teeth grinding

____Family history of cancer

____Feel like a social outcast

____Need coffee, alcohol, etc. to function

____Suffer premenstrual symptoms

____Prone to colds and infections

____Recovery from surgery

___Suffer "sugar blues"

___Cravings for sweets

___Family history of high blood pressure

___Family history of heart disease

___Family history of diabetes

___Sweaty palms

___Hostile

___Constant conflicts at work

___Frequently late to work or appointments

___Worry

___Chest tightness

___Moody

___Lack of concentration

___Exposed to toxic substances

___Elderly

___Feel helpless

___Chronic fatigue

___Family problems interfering with work

___Tempted to use drugs or alcohol as an escape

___Poor attention and concentration skills

___Non assertive

___Low self-esteem

Taken from the Complete Stress Management Workbook

With this list it is not difficult to see connectedness of the body and soul. It is for this reason, you need to adopt an eating style that will pave the way for you to reduce health risks and meet the stresses of your life and promote recovery.

Here are a few examples of positive messages. Look them over and decide whether you can claim any of them as your own. But don't look only at the present or past, look at the future too. In the space at the left, write "now" (if it is something that is true already) or "soon" or "someday" (depending on when you think this will be true of you).

______I love the feeling of being in good shape and being attractive and thin.

____I find it easy to lose weight gradually and safely.

____I deserve to be healthy.

____My body is healthier, attractive, and stronger.

____I am confident in myself and about losing weight.

____I am in control of my attitude and behavior toward eating.

____I don't eat because I am angry and /or frustrated and upset.

____I keep a food diary until I get used to eating nutritiously.

____I drink a glass of water or diluted juice twenty minutes before eating.

____My desire for salt, sugar, fat, and junk food decreases.

____I munch on veggies for snacks.

____I am satisfied with smaller portions and stop eating before feeling stuffed.

____I like staying on a low-fat diet.

____I visualize myself as a disciplined eater and shopper.

____I read labels on food and buy only healthy food.

____My investment in my well-being is profitable.

____I eat about four hours before going to sleep.

____I brush my teeth after every meal.

____I like the feeling of being in control of my body and my eating habits.

____I am very happy that I am losing weight permanently.

____Other ____

According to nutrition scientists, the human body requires over forty nutrients to maintain food health. These are classified as vitamins, minerals, amino acids, essential fatty acids, carbohydrates, enzymes, and water. What you want to strive for is a balanced diet based on your needs. Like exercise I am not going to suggest a specific diet, there are many books and nutritionists out there that can help with that, but I am going to suggest the basic building blocks to a healthy diet and its portions.

Protein: 15 to 20 percent of total calories
Carbohydrates: 55 to 60 percent of total calories
Fat: 20-30 percent of total calories (mostly monounsaturated fat)
Fiber: 40-50 grams per day
Water: 6-8 eight-ounce glasses per day
Such a plan includes the six basic food groups:
Vegetables: all types, especially dark green and leafy.
Fruits: all kinds, including berries, melons, and citrus fruits.
Whole grains: rice, cereals, legumes (peas and beans), nuts, seeds and added fiber.
Dairy products: non fat or low-fat milk, including natural cheese and non fat yogurt. Soy milk is a good substitute for some.
Meats: fish, lean meats, poultry (skin and fat removed), and vegetable protein.
Liquids: clear water, unsweetened and diluted juices (pulped), and drinks that are caffeine free, and artificial-sugar free.

Be sure to eat every meal, and breakfast is the most important meal of the day, because calories consumed early in the day are given more opportunity to be converted into energy. It goes without saying, watch out for sweets and hidden sweets and reduce salt.

As you look back over the material on exercise and relaxation, list three to five changes you would like to make in this area. Include exercise habits you'd like to begin as well as other factors, such as cutting back on alcohol or tobacco, or getting more sleep. ______________

____
____
____
____
____
____
____
____

As you look back over the material on diet and nutrition, list three to five changes you would like to make in your diet to become healthier.

____
____
____
____
____
____
____
____
____

____Each week chart your progress:

How successful was I this week in adopting this change?__________
____
____

Were there factors that made it more difficult than I expected? How will I overcome these?______________________________________
____
____

Do I need to revise my goals?______________________________
____
____

What strategies will help me do better in the next week?________
____
____

Bibliography

Alcoholics Anonymous, New York, NY: Alcoholics Anonymous World Services Inc. 1976.

Anderson, Neil T. A Way of Escape, Eugene Oregon: Harvest House Publishers, 1994

Anderson, Neil T. & Quarles, Mike and Julia, Freedom from Addiction, Ventura, California:

Anderson, Neil T. The Bondage Breaker, Eugene Oregon: Harvest House Publishishing, 1990, 1993

Arterburn, Stephen Healing is a Choice, Nashville Tenn.: Thomas Nelson 2005

Arterburn, Stephen Every Man's Battle, Colorado Springs, Col.: WaterBrook Press, 2000

Arterburn, Stephen& Stoop, David The Book of Life Recovery, Tyndale House Publishers, 2012

Backus, William and Chapian, Marie Telling Yourself the Truth, Minneapolis Minn.: Bethany Press International 1980, 1981, 2000

Balch, James & Phyllis Prescription for Nutritional Healing, Garden City Park, NY: Avery Publishing Group1997

Bourne, Edmund J. The Anxiety & Phobia Workbook, Oakland, CA: New Harbinger Publications, Inc., 1995

Bradshaw, John Home Coming: Reclaiming and Championing Your Inner Child, New York, NY: Bantam Books 1990, 1992

Bradshaw, John The Family: A Revolutionary Way of Self-Discovery, Pompano Beach, Florida: Health Communications, Inc. 1988

Carnes, Patrick A Gentle Path through the Twelve Steps, Center City: Minn.: Hazelden 1993

Carnes, Patrick Contrary to Love, Minneapolis, Minn.: CompCare Publishers 1989

Carnes, Patrick Don't Call it Love, New York, NY: Bantam Books 1992

Carnes, Patrick Out of the Shadows, Center City, Minn.: Hazelden 2001

Carnes, Patrick Sexual Anorexia, Center City, Minn.: Hazelden 1997

Cooper, Al Sex and the Internet, New York, NY: Brunner-Routledge, 2002

Crabb, Lawrence, Jr. Connecting: healing ourselves and our relationships, Nashville, Tenn.: W. Publishing Group 1997

Crabb, Lawrence, Jr. Effective Biblical Counseling, Grand Rapids, Mich.: Zondervan 1977

Crabb, Lawrence, Jr. Understanding People, Grand Rapids, Mich.: Zondervan 1987

Crabb, Lawrence, Jr. Shattered Dreams, Colorado Springs, Col.: WaterBrook Press 2001

Dayton, Tian Emotional Sobriety, Deerfield Beach, FL, Health Communications 2007

Horrobin, Peter J. Healing Through Deliverance, Grand Rapids, Mich.: Chosen Books 1991, 2003

Laaser, Mark R. Healing the Wounds of Sexual Addiction, Grand Rapids, Mich.: Zondervan 1992, 1996, 2004

Leman, Kevin Dr. The Birth Order Book, Grand Rapids, MI, Baker Book House Co. 1998

Littauer, Florence. Your Personality Tree, Dallas TX, Word Publishing 1986

Littauer, Fred & Florence. Get A Life Without the Strife, Nashville, TN, Thomas Nelson Publishing 1993

Littauer, Fred. The Promise of Healing Your Hurts & Your Feelings, Nashville, TN, Thomas Nelson Publishing 1994

Kruger, C. Baxter Across All Worlds, Jackson MS.: Perichoresis Press 2007

Maltz, Larry & Wendy The Porn Trap, New York, NY: HarperCollins Publishers 2008

Pearce, Josheph Chilton, The Biology of Transcendence A Blueprint of the Human Spirit, Rochester, Vermont, Park Street Press, 2002

Penner, Joyce Counseling for Sexual Disorders, Dallas Texas: Word Publishing 1990

P.D.N.E.C. Hope and Recovery, Minneapolis, Minn.: CompCare Publishers 1987

Sexaholics Anonymous, Washington, DC: Library of Congress, 1989

Sex Addict Anonymous, Houston, TX: International Service Organization of SAA, 2005

Southern, Jill Sex God's Truth, Landcaster, Eng.: Sovereign World Ltd 2006

Stedman, Ray C. Spiritual Warefare: How to Stand Firm in the Faith, Grand Rapids, Mich.: Discovery House 1999

Schwarzenegger, Arnold Total Recall My Unbelievably True Life Story, New York, New York, Simon & Schuster 2012

The Comparative Study Bible, Grand Rapids, Mich.: Zondervan Publishing 1984

Therman, Chris The Lies We Believe, Nashville, Tenn.: Thomas Nelson Publishers 1989

Virkler, Henry A. Broken Promises, Dallas Texas, Word Publishing, 1992

Warkentin, Henrey Answers and Hope for the Struggling Christian, Belleville, ON: Guardian Books 2001

White John EROS Defiled, Downers Grove, Ill.: InterVarsity Press 1977

White, Tom Breaking Strongholds, Ann Arbor, Mich.: Servant Publications 1993

White, Tom The Believers Guide to Spiritual Warfare Ann Arbor, Mich.: Servant Publications 1990

Wommack, Andrew Spirit, Soul & Body Colorado Springs, CO.: Andrew Wommack Ministries 2005

Work Books

A Spiritual Journey: The Twelve Steps, San Diego, CA. Recovery Publications 1988

Cairnes, Patrick Facing the Shadow Carefree, Arazona: Gentle Path Press 2001-2008

Backus, William Learning to Tell Myself the Truth, Minneapolis, Minn.: Bethany House Publishers 1994

McGee, Robert S. The Search for Significance, Nashville Tenn.: W Publishing 1998

Schiraldi, Glenn R. The Self-Esteem Workbook, Oakland, CA.: New Harbinger Publications, Inc. 2001

Thurman, Chris The Lies We Believe, Nashville Tenn.: Thomas Nelson Publishers 1995

Whiteman, Thomas; Verghese, Sam; Petersen, Randy The Complete Stress Management Workbook, Grand Rapids, MI: Zondervan Publishing House 1996

CPSIA information can be obtained at www.ICGtesting.com
Printed in the USA
LVOW07*0724060915

452988LV00002B/2/P

9 781460 241776